AMERICAN JOURNAL of PUBLIC HEALTH
MARCH 2025
Issue 3

AJPH

A PUBLICATION OF THE
AMERICAN PUBLIC HEALTH ASSOCIATION

115 YEARS OF ADVANCING PUBLIC HEALTH

What Comes Next?, p. 245

Public Health in a New Political Era
by Georges Benjamin, Mary Bassett, Daniel Dawes, Jerome Adams, David Michaels, Sherry Glied, Laura Magaña, & Nancy Krieger, pp. 304 to 325

Also in this issue:

LOCAL PUBLIC HEALTH WORKFORCE
Racial/Ethnic Representation, pp. 271 and 333

ABORTION FOR OLDER MINORS
Parental Consent Requirements, pp. 262 and 397

CONTRACEPTIVE ACCESS
Utah's Family Planning, pp. 259 and 387

Standard Methods for the Examination of Dairy Products, 18th edition

Edited by Jeffrey L. Kornacki, PhD, Elliot T. Ryser, PhD, and Cynthia M. Mangione; Managing Editor: H. Michael Wehr, PhD

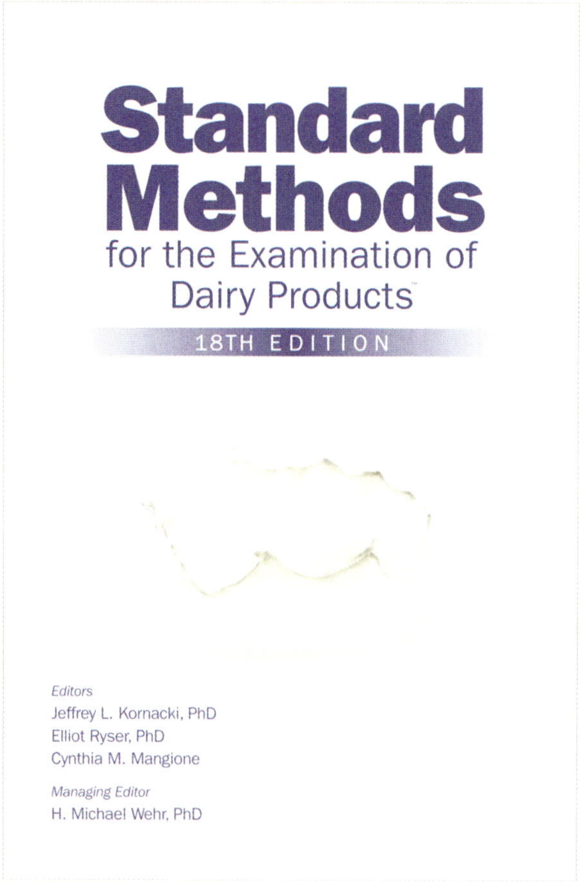

9780-887553-3421, SOFTCOVER, 1144 PP, 2024

Standard Methods for the Examination of Dairy Products is a widely-recognized source of methods to assess the safety and quality of dairy products. It is an overview of microbiological, chemical and physical methods for analyzing milk and dairy products, designed for use by regulatory, industry and commercial laboratories. As with earlier editions, the 18th edition of Standard Methods for the Examination of Dairy Products:

- Highlights test methods that are a critical component of both government and industry analytical programs.
- Provides methods that foster uniformity in the testing of milk and milk programs.

This new 18th Edition of SMEDP updates and expands upon earlier editions of this authoritative reference, including:

- Comprehensive revision to chapters on antibiotic drug residues, pathogens, chemical and physical methods, and methods for heat process verification.
- Updates on both automated, and molecular-based methods.

APHABOOKSTORE.ORG

APHA PRESS

AN IMPRINT OF AMERICAN PUBLIC HEALTH ASSOCIATION

APHA
AMERICAN PUBLIC HEALTH ASSOCIATION
For science. For action. For health.

AJPH®, published monthly, is the official Journal of the American Public Health Association®, 800 I St NW, Washington, DC 20001-3710; (202) 777- APHA; TDD (202) 777-2500. APHA is a nongovernmental professional society founded in 1872, representing all disciplines and specialties in public health.

The *American Journal of Public Health*® (*AJPH*) (print ISSN: 0090-0036; electronic ISSN: 1541- 0048), first published in 1911, is the official journal of the American Public Health Association® (APHA). The oldest and largest organization of public health professionals in the world, APHA represents approximately 30 000 members from more than 50 occupations of public health.

Submissions: Visit www.editorialmanager.com/ajph or ajph.edmgr.com for online manuscript preparation and submission guidelines. Contributions of original unpublished research, social science analyses, scholarly essays, critical commentaries, departments, and letters to the editor are welcome. Questions? Write ajph.submissions@apha.org or call APHA at (202) 777-2469.

Print plus online subscriptions: Institutional price (print copy with online access for a single institution and all authorized users, regardless of geographic location) varies by size of organization and ranges from $993–$1445 for US organizations, and $1073–$1526 for international organizations (air delivery); multiple campuses not permitted without special arrangement. Details of the tiered pricing system at https://subscriptionoffice.com/pages/apha-landing-page. To order, write apha.subscriptions@apha.org.

Online-only subscriptions: Institutional price for one institution and its authorized users (regardless of geographic location) is $878–$1307. To order, write apha.subscriptions@apha.org. For academic consortia or multisite corporate subscriptions, contact apha.subscriptions@apha.org.

Print-only subscriptions: Institutional price is US $701, $782 international.

Back print issues: A limited number of print issues are for sale. Single copies are US $65, $75 international (air delivery). Shipping included; prepay only. To order, write apha.subscriptions@apha.org.

Reprints: For prices and ordering information on 50 or more reprints, check the Reprints section at www.ajph.org. To order smaller quantities of reprints (rush delivery), use the "Purchase Article" link on the article site itself.

Electronic access: Online articles more than 10 years old are available free for personal use at www.ajph.org. Recent articles are available through pay-per-view: single PDF article for $24, single issue access for 24 hours for $33, or entire site access for 24 hours for $38.

Postal information: Periodicals postage paid at Washington, DC, and additional mailing offices. Postmaster: Send address changes to American Journal of Public Health, 800 I St NW, Washington, DC 20001-3710.

Address changes: Send to AJPH, Membership Department (members) or AJPH Subscriptions (subscribers), APHA, 800 I St NW, Washington, DC 20001-3710. Or write to membership.mail@apha.org (members) or apha.subscriptions@apha.org (subscribers).

Advertising: For pricing and other information, see www.ajph.org. Please write to brian.selzer@apha.org or call (202) 777-2470 for other advertising opportunities. Ask about special exhibit packages and sponsorships. Acceptance of advertising by the *Journal* does not imply endorsement of products.

Indexes: Publications that index or abstract articles from *AJPH* include the following: Ageline, Assia (Applied Social Science Index and Abstracts), Biological Abstracts, Chemical Abstracts, CINAHL, Criminal Justice Abstracts, EMBASE, EMCare, Environmental Abstracts, e-psyche, ERIC, ETOH (Alcohol and Alcohol Problems Science Database), Excerpta Medica, Food Science and Technology, General Science Index, Grateful Med, Hospital Literature Index, Human Resources Abstracts, International Pharmaceutical Abstracts (IPA), Medline, Physical Education Index, Pollution Abstracts, Psychological Abstracts, PsychINFO, Safety Science Abstracts, Sage Family Studies Abstracts, Sage Human Resources Abstracts, Science Citation Index, SCOPUS, SIIC Data Bases, Social Work Research and Abstracts, and Statistical Reference Index (SRI)/LexisNexis.

Medscape Publishers' Circle

AJPH
A PUBLICATION OF THE
AMERICAN PUBLIC HEALTH ASSOCIATION

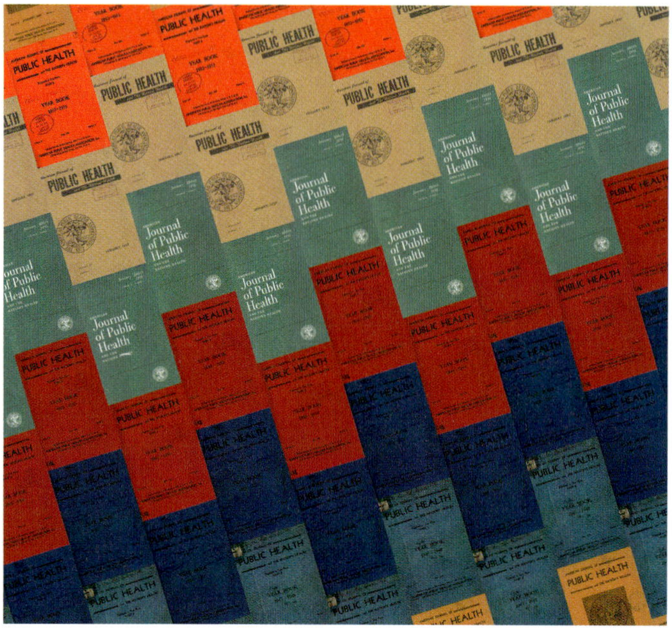

COVER: In 1911, when the *American Journal of Public Health* launched, the APHA understood the need for an independent place to publish the science that underpins public health policy. Nearly 115 years later, that mandate remains and *AJPH* continues to be a beacon of knowledge in the field. But what of the future when the threats to democracy are threats to public health? The future cannot be predicted. But we are ready and will continue to play our role as an independent source of knowledge—a place where all science-based opinions can dialogue.

Cover concept and design by Aleisha Kropf.

APHA
AMERICAN PUBLIC HEALTH ASSOCIATION
For science. For action. For health.

Promoting public health research, policy, practice, and education is the *AJPH* mission. As we widen our scope to embrace global issues, we also sharpen our focus to support the needs of public health practitioners. We invite contributions of original unpublished research, opinion and commentary, and letters to the editor.

The *Journal* is printed on acid-free recycled paper.

AJPH March 2025, Vol. 115, No. 3

OPEN ACCESS ONLINE ONLY PODCAST DATA SUPPLEMENT AVAILABLE

EDITOR'S CHOICE

245 115 Years of Advancing Public Health: What Comes Next?
A. Morabia

OPINIONS, IDEAS, & PRACTICE

EDITORIALS

247 Vaccinating During Pregnancy: Are We Failing to Protect Our Mothers and Infants?
A. B. Berenson

250 The Continuing Need for HIV Telehealth Services Following the COVID-19 Pandemic
T. G. Heckman, B. D. Heckman, and J. C. Markowitz

253 Amplifying the Voices of Low-Wage Workers in Health and Well-Being Research to Promote Health Equity
B. W. Sherman

255 Paradox of Progress: NIH-Funded Research on Sexual and Gender Minority Populations, 2012–2022
M. R. Friedman, T. Taggart, and R. W. S. Coulter

259 Expanding Access, Elevating Equity: Lessons From Utah's Family Planning Elevated Contraceptive Access Program
H. E. M. Riley

262 Parental Involvement Laws and the Best Interests of Minors: A Need for Reform
J. D. Rosen

265 Health Care Stereotype Threat: The Danger and Damage of Stigma and Discrimination in Health Care
R. E. Turpin

268 Measurement Matters for Transgender Veterans' Visibility in the Electronic Health Record
J. G. Patterson

271 Building a Representative Local Public Health Workforce: Progress, Promise, and Looming Challenges
L. E. Masselink

PERSPECTIVES

274 The Effects of Racial Exclusion and Racial Othering on South Asian American Identity and Population Health
R. Rastogi, V. V. Raval, T. Yip, J. A. Chen, and C. H. Liu

279 Public Health Data to Action: Reframing Surveillance to Build Trust in Public Health
T. J. Stopka, J. Cordes, D. Bernson, R. Bayly, and C. Bauer

NOTES FROM THE FIELD

282 Real-Time Linkage of Public-Facing Jail Registers and Syphilis Testing and Treatment Monitoring Data, Washington State, 2023–2024
S. J. Erly, L. O. Hill, K. B. Gavigan, K. L. Haecker, and R. M. Amiya

287 Improving Participation in HIV Preexposure Prophylaxis via an Informatics Approach—a Process-Improvement Project
J. J. Mandia, C. H. Keltner, R. C. Haynes III, L. Cruz, K. Solveson, and L. E. Mease

292 Medical Care or Deportation: Examining Interior Border Checkpoints and Access to Higher-Level Medical Care for Undocumented Immigrants in South Texas
C. C. Blackburn, M. Rico, J. Hernandez, and M. Lee

296 Increasing Access Through Integration: Behavioral Health Services and Beyond
D. H. Carter, M. C. Meimers, and E. F. Bemben

AJPH 115TH ANNIVERSARY

301 Celebrating 115 Years of *AJPH*: Perspectives on Public Health in a New Political Era
A. Morabia, B. E. Coston, P. Erwin, L. Ferguson, B. Ojikutu, W. E. Parmet, and J. S. Tenorio

304 Speaking Truth to Power: Making Optimal Health a Top National Priority
G. C. Benjamin

307 Threats to Democracy and the Right to Health
M. T. Bassett

310 Wide Awake: The Movement for Health Equity Continues
D. E. Dawes

313 The Imperative Link Between Civic Engagement and Public Health: Insights From a Former US Surgeon General
J. Adams

316 Bearing Witness and Spurring Action for Worker Safety and Health
D. Michaels and G. R. Wagner

319 Four Distinct Dimensions Through Which Government Actions May Affect Health Insurance Coverage
S. Glied

321 *AJPH*'s Coverage of Education in Public Health in the Age of Democracy's Crisis
L. Magaña

324 Buyer's Remorse, Betrayal, and Blame: Who Will Be Held Responsible for the Adverse Health Impacts of the US Elections?
N. Krieger

RESEARCH & ANALYSIS

HISTORY

326 Trusted Messengers: Public Health Education and Advocacy in 20th Century Black American Newspapers
W. Muigai

OPEN-THEMED RESEARCH

333 Racial and Ethnic Representation of the Local Public Health Workforce
C. P. Balio, H. Leslie, and M. B. Meit

344 Impacts of State COVID-19 Vaccine Mandates for Health Care Workers on Health Sector Employment in the United States
Y. Wang, K. Callison, J. H. Hernandez, and C. Stoecker

349 Health Care Facility Characteristics Associated With Providing Telehealth HIV Care Services During the COVID-19 Pandemic
E. E. Valverde, L. Beer, D. Pepin, S. Crim, and J. Weiser

354 Uptake of Recommended Vaccines During Pregnancy Among Publicly and Privately Insured People in the United States, December 2020–September 2022
S. L. Rowe, S. G. Sullivan, F. M. Munoz, M. M. Coates, O. A. Arah, and A. K. Regan

364 Direct Estimation of Alcohol-Attributable Fractions for Suicide in the United States, 2021
J. Robitaille, Jürgen Rehm, M. S. Kaplan, C. Kilian, L. Llamosas-Falcón, and S. Lange

369 Parental Factors Associated With Measles–Mumps–Rubella Vaccination in US Children Younger Than 5 Years
E. G. Zhou, J. Cantor, A. Gertz, B. Elbel, J. S. Brownstein, and B. Rader

374 Research Funded by National Institutes of Health Concerning Sexual and Gender Minoritized Populations: A Tracking Update for 2012 to 2022
B. C. D. Weideman, A. M. Ecklund, R. Alley, B. R. S. Rosser, and G. N. Rider

387 Changes in Contraceptive Services During Utah's Family Planning Elevated Contraceptive Access Initiative: A Prospective Assessment of Intervention and Control Sites
R. G. Simmons, A. Gero, G. Carter, J. N. Sanders, C. Quade, J. Baayd, M. Mullholand, S. Elliott, K. Myers, E. Torres, J. D. Smith, and D. K. Turok

397 Changes to Parental Consent Requirements for Abortion in Massachusetts and Impact on Timeliness of Care for Adolescents Aged 16 to 17 Years
I. Fulcher, K. Kimball, Z. Rosen, J. Fortin, N. Arunkumar, D. Gelfand, E. Janiak, and L. Ireland

403 Impact of Gender Identity Field in the Veterans Health Administration Electronic Health Record, 2016–2023
S. M. Leder, A. A. McConnell, S. Lamba, C. Sonnier, A. R. Matza, W. E. Meriwether, G. R. Brown, J. C. Shipherd, M. R. Kauth, and K. T. Jones

414 Predictors of Persistent COVID-19 Vaccine Refusal Among Previously Infected Patients in Nebraska
H. (Julia) Bai, D. Brett-Major, Y. Du, S. Paritala, E. S. Peters, K. L. Ratnapradipa, and P. Maloney

425 Health Care Stereotype Threat During the COVID-19 Pandemic Among Sexual and Gender Minority Individuals
W. D. Manning, C. K. Dush, and K. Gustafson

BACKMATTER

OTHER DEPARTMENTS

440 Subscription Form

115 Years of Advancing Public Health: What Comes Next?

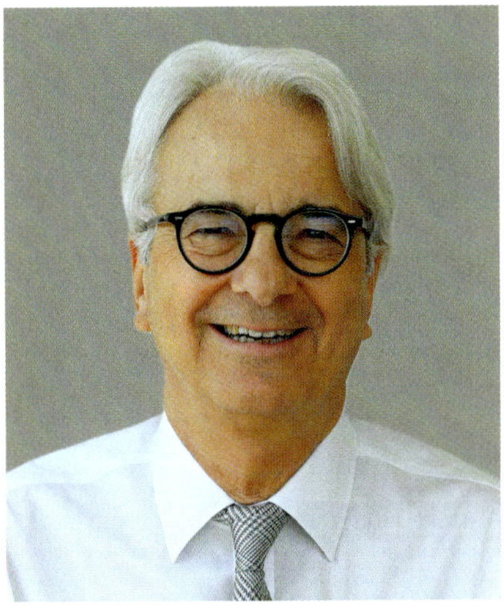

Alfredo Morabia, MD, PhD
Editor in Chief, *AJPH*

In 1911, the American Public Health Association (APHA) inaugurated its own journal, which became the *American Journal of Public Health* (*AJPH*) in 1912. The APHA understood the need to provide an independent place for the science it hoped would underpin public health policy, a place independent from corporate or partisan interests. For more than a century, *AJPH* has played exactly that role, and sometimes has been supported at great cost by the APHA through difficult economic times.

The history of *AJPH* has been told several times (https://bit.ly/408SI2r; https://bit.ly/4frDXMo; https://bit.ly/3BxIlpZ).

The version of the *Journal* I have been the Editor-in-Chief of appeared with its first new format in January 2016. We published since then so many groundbreaking works that it is not easy to single out just one topic covered by year among them. The covers of those I have selected are printed here: the drinking water disaster in Flint, Michigan (2016); the estimated prevalence of transgender persons in the United States (2017); the 100-year anniversary of the great 1918 flu, which was prescient of the coming COVID-19 pandemic (2018); 350 years of slavery in North America after 1619 Jamestown (2019); "We are not all in this pandemic together" (2020); the evolving theory and practice of intersectionality (2021); the harassment of the public health workforce (2022); population-based public health monitoring (2023); and excess mortality because of COVID-19 in US states (2024).

AJPH is a beacon of knowledge in the field of public health. What is its future? We have decided to place this yearlong celebration under the theme of "Threats to democracy are threats to public health" and invite our editors, authors, reviewers, and other involved parties to reflect on this new political and institutional context in the United States and in many other parts of the world, in which people having a declared antiscience stand are accessing the handle of public health institutions and threatening to wipe out decades of progress.

We are confident that most of our populations support public health.

Continued on page 246...

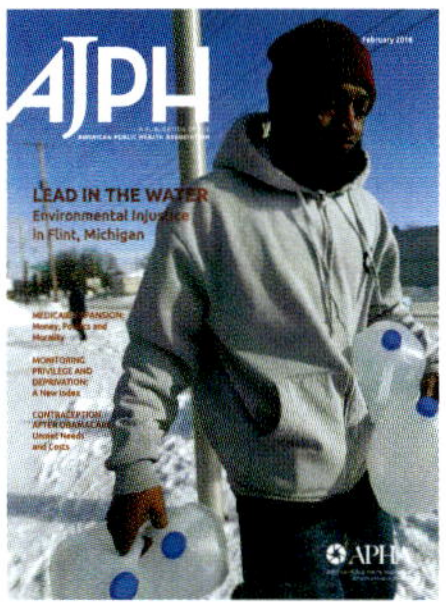

February 2016

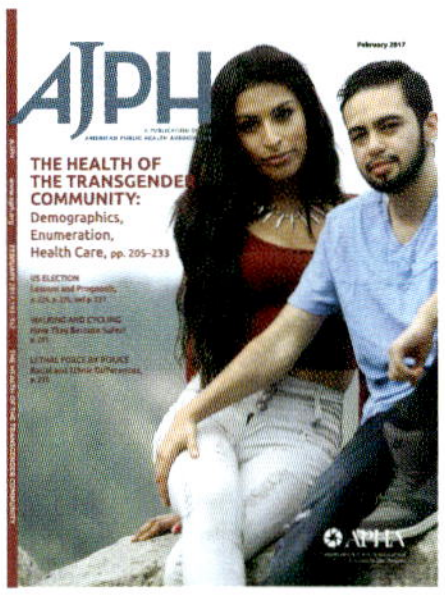

February 2017

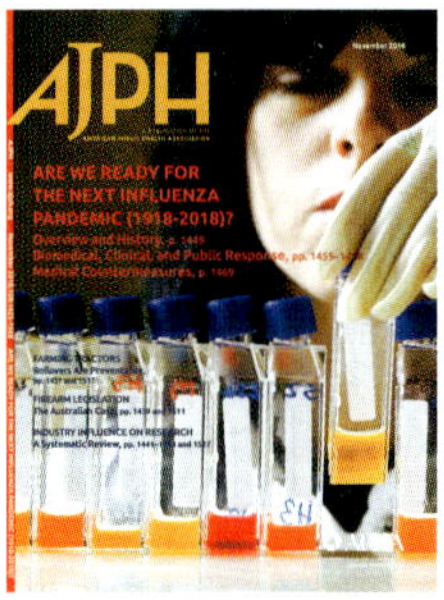

November 2018

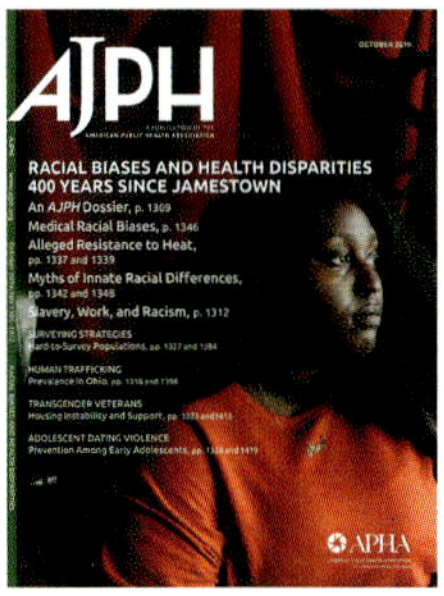

October 2019

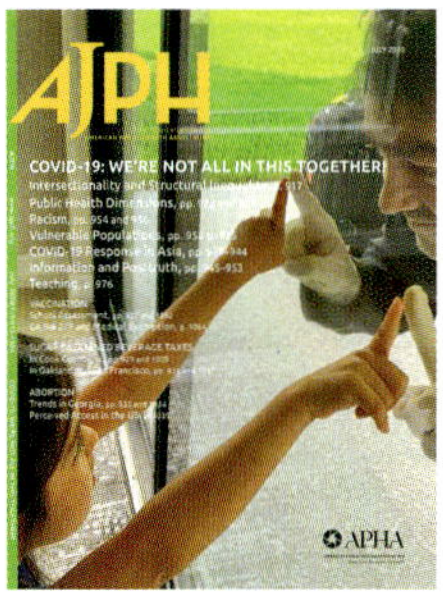

July 2020

AJPH March 2025, Vol. 115, No. 3

They showed it in getting vaccinated in unexpectedly high proportions in all states during COVID-19 and in complying with public health mandates. The paradox is that the noisy minority that does not trust public health may find itself at the head of the Department of Health and Human Services, Centers for Disease Control and Prevention, the Food and Drug Administration, the Environmental Protection Agency, and the Office of the Surgeon General.

We still need to see what they will do in practice, but we will keep playing our role as an independent source of scientific knowledge and a place where all opinions that are science-based can dialogue. AJPH

DOI: https://doi.org/10.2105/AJPH.2024.307976

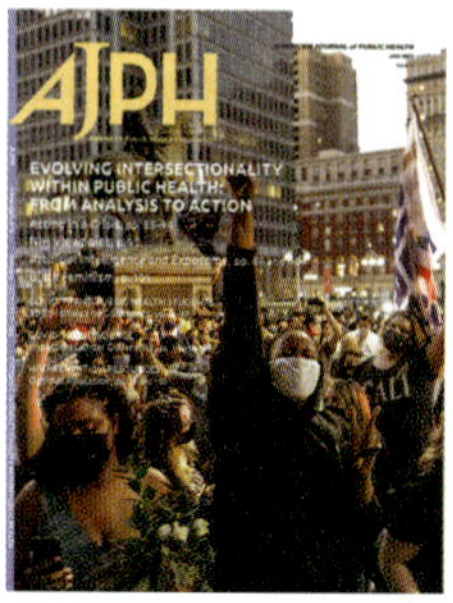

January 2021

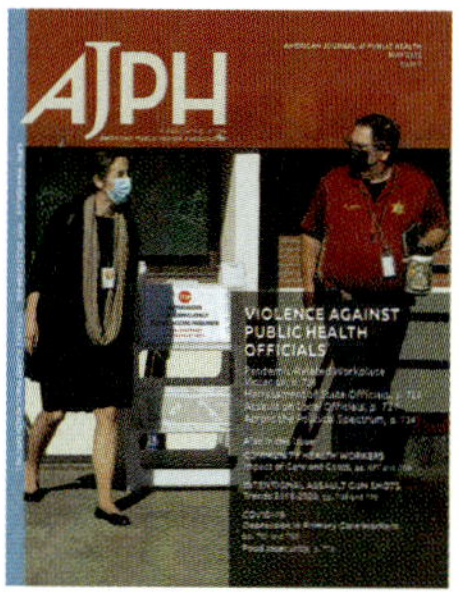

May 2022

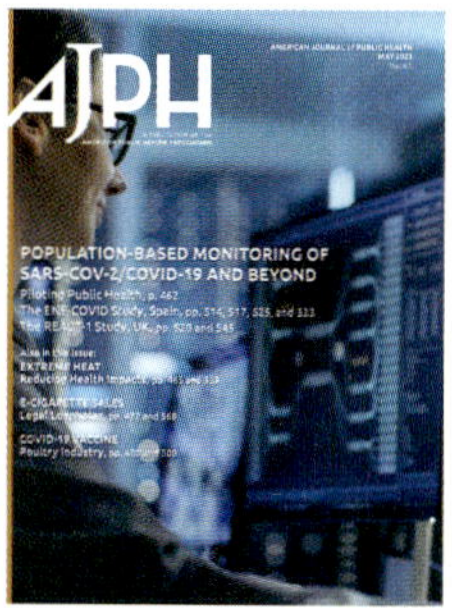

May 2023

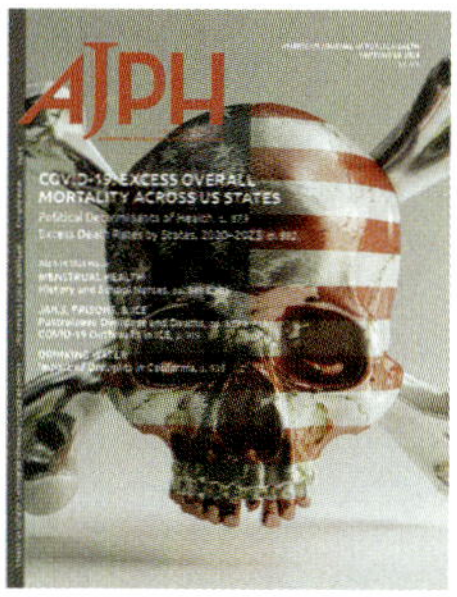

September 2024

Vaccinating During Pregnancy: Are We Failing to Protect Our Mothers and Infants?

Abbey B. Berenson, MD, PhD

ABOUT THE AUTHOR

Abbey B. Berenson is with the Department of Obstetrics and Gynecology and director of the Center for Interdisciplinary Research in Women's Health, The University of Texas Medical Branch, Galveston.

See also Rowe et al., p. 354.

Vaccines indisputably save lives and reduce the cost burden of disease on the US health care system. For example, the Centers for Disease Control and Prevention estimates that between 2010 and 2023, influenza infections resulted in as many as 51 000 deaths in a single year,[1] and as recently as 2022, COVID-19 was estimated to be the underlying cause of death for more than 186 000 individuals.[2] The economic burden of these vaccine-preventable diseases is equally striking. One previous study of several vaccine-preventable diseases (hepatitis A; hepatitis B; herpes zoster; human papillomavirus; influenza; measles, mumps, and rubella; meningococcal disease; pneumococcal disease; tetanus, diphtheria, and pertussis; and varicella) estimated that the cost is around $9 billion, with unvaccinated individuals accounting for roughly 80% ($7.1 billion) of this.[3] A more recent estimate of the annual cost of four major vaccine-preventable diseases (influenza, pneumococcal, herpes zoster, and pertussis) among individuals aged 50 years and older was $26.5 billion in 2013.[4]

Vaccines are especially critical for pregnant women, as they are more susceptible to morbidities associated with infectious diseases. For example, SARS-CoV-2 infection (the causative agent of COVID-19) places pregnant women at higher risk for maternal mortality, as well as for preeclampsia, eclampsia, preterm labor, and thromboembolic disease.[5] In addition, neonates born to mothers infected with SARS-CoV-2 are more likely to be admitted to the neonatal intensive care unit after birth. Infection of pregnant women with influenza has also been linked to an increased risk of stillbirths.[6] Moreover, vaccinations during pregnancy protect the infant through the transplacental transfer of antibodies.[7]

Although many factors influence a person's decision to vaccinate, having any type of health insurance is one of the greatest predictors of vaccination. Among the general US population, for example, the vaccination rates of individuals with any type of insurance between 2015 and 2018 were 43.6% for influenza and 62.6% for tetanus.[8] Among the uninsured, the numbers dropped to 16.3% for influenza and 50.1% for tetanus. The situation among pregnant women is analogous. In one study of pregnant women from 2012 to 2018, only 15% of uninsured pregnant women self-reported having received the influenza vaccine, compared with 41% of pregnant women with any type of insurance.[9] However, vaccination rates differ by type of insurance.

In this issue of *AJPH*, Rowe et al. (p. 354) highlight that 4.9%, 12.4%, and 40.9% of pregnant women with public insurance were vaccinated against COVID-19, influenza, and pertussis, respectively. By comparison, for those with private insurance, the respective vaccination rates were 21.4%, 24.8%, and 68.1%. A closer look at these numbers reveals an even darker truth. Astonishingly, pregnant women with public insurance are sometimes vaccinating at an even lower rate than the uninsured.

The reasons for discrepancies in vaccination rates between the publicly and privately insured are complex. Contributing factors include differences in insurance coverage and benefits. During the 2020–2022 period examined by Rowe et al., Medicaid coverage for the three vaccines was not consistent across state programs. In fact, vaccines recommended by the Advisory Committee on Immunization Practices (ACIP) were not required to be covered by all state Medicaid programs. This was true even with the expansion of Medicaid established through the Patient Protection and Affordable Care Act of 2010. Although the legislation mandated that adults falling under the new expansion group receive all ACIP-recommended vaccines at no cost, merely 37.6% of adults enrolled in Medicaid qualified for this benefit as recently as fiscal year 2019. An equal share of adults enrolled in Medicaid (38.2%) during fiscal year 2019 were not a part of the expansion group and remained subject to state-specific variations in vaccine coverage.[8] Even for

AJPH March 2025, Vol. 115, No. 3

those who were covered, some were still required to share the costs. This presents yet another barrier to vaccination, as one study on the flu vaccine previously found that for every dollar of copayment, the vaccination rate decreases between 1% and 6%.[10] Confounding matters further, Medicaid frequently does not reimburse providers adequately for vaccinations. The scientific literature has shown that physicians report losing money when vaccinating Medicaid beneficiaries. Not only are the median Medicaid payments for vaccines below that reported for private sector prices, they are also below the average estimated cost of vaccination for the providers.[8] Another study found that the median cost of vaccination was substantially higher for obstetrics and gynecology practices, further compounding the issue for pregnant women. Fortunately, a remedy was passed into law via the Inflation Reduction Act of 2022. Under this legislation, Medicaid programs are required to cover in full, without cost sharing, all Food and Drug Administration–approved vaccines recommended by the ACIP as of October 1, 2023. The coverage also applies to nearly all full-benefit Medicaid beneficiaries aged 19 years and older.[11] Still, more must be done.

As Rowe et al. also point out, provider hesitancy to recommend vaccines during pregnancy has been implicated in low vaccine coverage for COVID-19 and influenza. This reality must change, as provider recommendations are the most important predictors of vaccination during pregnancy. This is true even for patients that previously refused vaccination. One underlying cause may be a gap in communication training for obstetricians, who sometimes have little to no training on how to address vaccine hesitancy among their patients. Fine-tuning how we recommend vaccines to pregnant women is also key, as multiple studies have found that mothers prefer information that focuses on the benefits and safety of vaccines for their infants, more so than for themselves. Even the mode of delivery can influence the success of a provider recommendation, as educational pamphlets appear superior to educational text messaging and video-based education.[7]

If we ask ourselves as a medical community, are we adequately protecting our mothers and infants from vaccine-preventable diseases, the current answer is no. Despite the heightened need to protect this vulnerable population, maternal vaccination rates are currently lagging by every standard, especially among those with public insurance. However, the means to change this exist. We must ensure that Medicaid continues to cover the costs of vaccines for its beneficiaries, at rates that preclude health care providers from losing money. We must ensure that our Medicare recipients are receiving strong recommendations to vaccinate from their providers. We must ensure that our obstetricians are receiving the necessary training to address vaccine hesitancy. We must ensure that obstetricians continue to recommend vaccinations at each prenatal visit, even if a patient refuses at first. Finally, we must ensure that our messaging on vaccinations during pregnancy are both framed effectively and delivered through the appropriate forms of media. As a medical community and society, we must do better to ensure that we are adequately protecting both our mothers and infants from vaccine-preventable diseases. AJPH

CORRESPONDENCE

Correspondence should be sent to Abbey B. Berenson, MD, PhD, Center for Interdisciplinary Research in Women's Health, The University of Texas Medical Branch, 301 University Blvd, Galveston, TX 77555-0587 (e-mail: abberens@utmb.edu). Reprints can be ordered at https://www.ajph.org by clicking the "Reprints" link.

PUBLICATION INFORMATION

Full Citation: Berenson AB. Vaccinating during pregnancy: are we failing to protect our mothers and infants? *Am J Public Health*. 2025;115(3):247–249.

Acceptance Date: November 17, 2024.

DOI: https://doi.org/10.2105/AJPH.2024.307946

ORCID iD:

Abbey B. Berenson https://orcid.org/0000-0002-5007-1080

ACKNOWLEDGMENTS

Nathaniel Girer, PhD, provided editorial assistance as paid staff within the Center for Interdisciplinary Research in Women's Health at the University of Texas Medical Branch.

CONFLICTS OF INTEREST

The author declares no perceived or actual conflicts of interest.

REFERENCES

1. Centers for Disease Control and Prevention. About estimated flu burden. October 7, 2024. Available at: https://www.cdc.gov/flu-burden/php/about/index.html. Accessed November 7, 2024.
2. Kochanek KD, Murphy SL, Xu J, Arias E. *Mortality in the United States, 2022*. Hyattsville, MD: National Center for Health Statistics; 2024. NCHS Data Brief no. 492.
3. Ozawa S, Portnoy A, Getaneh H, et al. Modeling the economic burden of adult vaccine-preventable diseases in the United States. *Health Aff (Millwood)*. 2016;35(11):2124–2132. https://doi.org/10.1377/hlthaff.2016.0462
4. McLaughlin JM, McGinnis JJ, Tan L, Mercatante A, Fortuna J. Estimated human and economic burden of four major adult vaccine-preventable diseases in the United States, 2013. *J Prim Prev*. 2015;36(4):259–273. https://doi.org/10.1007/s10935-015-0394-3
5. Smith ER, Oakley E, Grandner GW, et al. Adverse maternal, fetal, and newborn outcomes among pregnant women with SARS-CoV-2 infection: an individual participant data meta-analysis. *BMJ Glob Health*. 2023;8(1):e009495. https://doi.org/10.1136/bmjgh-2022-009495
6. Wang R, Yan W, Du M, Tao L, Liu J. The effect of influenza virus infection on pregnancy outcomes: a systematic review and meta-analysis of cohort studies. *Int J Infect Dis*. 2021;105:567–578. https://doi.org/10.1016/j.ijid.2021.02.095
7. Rand CM, Olson-Chen C. Maternal vaccination and vaccine hesitancy. *Pediatr Clin North Am*.

2023;70(2):259–269. https://doi.org/10.1016/j.pcl.2022.11.004

8. Medicaid and CHIP Payment and Access Commission. Chapter 2: vaccine access for adults enrolled in Medicaid. In: Report to Congress on Medicaid and CHIP. March 2022. Available at: https://www.macpac.gov/wp-content/uploads/2022/03/Chapter-2-Vaccine-Access-for-Adults-Enrolled-in-Medicaid.pdf. Accessed November 14, 2024.
9. Cambou MC, Copeland TP, Nielsen-Saines K, Macinko JA. Insurance status predicts self-reported influenza vaccine coverage among pregnant women in the United States: a cross-sectional analysis of the National Health Interview Study data from 2012 to 2018. *Vaccine.* 2021;39(15):2068–2073. https://doi.org/10.1016/j.vaccine.2021.03.026
10. Stoecker C, Stewart AM, Lindley MC. The cost of cost-sharing: the impact of Medicaid benefit design on influenza vaccination uptake. *Vaccines (Basel).* 2017;5(1):8. https://doi.org/10.3390/vaccines5010008
11. US Dept of Health and Human Services. Fact Sheet: Inflation Reduction Act changes to Medicaid & Children's Health Insurance Program (CHIP) adult vaccine coverage. June 2023. Available at: https://www.medicaid.gov/medicaid/quality-of-care/downloads/vaccinations-fact-sheet-06272023.pdf. Accessed November 14, 2024.

The Continuing Need for HIV Telehealth Services Following the COVID-19 Pandemic

Timothy G. Heckman, PhD, Bernadette D. Heckman, PhD, and John C. Markowitz, MD

ABOUT THE AUTHORS

Timothy G. Heckman is with the Department of Health Promotion and Behavior, College of Public Health, University of Georgia, Athens. Bernadette D. Heckman is with the Department of Counseling and Human Development Services, College of Education, University of Georgia, Athens. John C. Markowitz is with the Department of Clinical Psychiatry, Vagelos College of Physicians and Surgeons, Columbia University, and the New York State Psychiatric Institute, New York, NY.

See also Valverde et al., p. 349.

The Centers for Disease Control and Prevention (CDC) describes telehealth as an important part of Ending the HIV Epidemic in the United States, an initiative seeking to achieve a reduction of at least 90% in new HIV infections by 2030.[1] Telehealth is the use of electronic information and telecommunication technologies to support long-distance clinical health care, patient and professional health-related education, health administration, and public health.[2] HIV telehealth can promote early HIV diagnosis and treatment, sustained viral suppression, prevention of new HIV transmissions, and rapid responses to isolated HIV outbreaks.[1]

Remotely administered HIV services can circumvent barriers related to a shortage of health care professionals (particularly specialists) in the geographic vicinity, a lack of personal and public transportation, scheduling difficulties, the need to arrange child care, avoidance of long waits for appointments, and confidentiality concerns about being seen in or near HIV-related organizations.[3] A growing compendium of research, sufficiently large for the conduct of meta-analyses, shows that HIV telehealth interventions can improve rates of HIV counseling and testing, treatment initiation, retention in care, and treatment adherence and decrease depressive symptoms and improve quality of life in people living with HIV (PLHIV).[4] A US Veterans Affairs health system study found that veterans living with HIV with access to telehealth services had more treatment visits and slightly higher rates of viral suppression than patients who received only traditional in-person HIV care.[5]

TELEHEALTH DURING THE COVID-19 PANDEMIC

Remotely delivered HIV prevention and treatment services were critical during the COVID-19 pandemic, when PLHIV, some of whom were immunocompromised, sheltered in place while trying to remain in care. In this issue of *AJPH*, Valverde et al. (p. 349) present their survey findings from 1023 HIV care facilities that provided care to a large nationally representative sample of US adults diagnosed with HIV during the COVID-19 pandemic. Using data from the CDC's facility survey of the Medical Monitoring Project, they compared characteristics of organizations that provided HIV telehealth care to those that did not.

Encouragingly, more than 80% of facilities provided HIV telehealth services during the COVID-19 pandemic. Characteristics differentiating facilities that provided remote HIV care from those that did not were largely foreseeable. Facilities not providing remote HIV care during the pandemic were located in Primary Care Health Professional Shortage Areas and rural areas, had 50 or fewer HIV patients, received no Ryan White HIV/AIDS Program funding, did not accept Medicaid, and did not offer HIV pre-exposure prophylaxis.

Valverde et al. posited that these smaller rural facilities were less likely to offer HIV telehealth services because of limited finances (lack of Medicaid or Ryan White HIV/AIDS Program funding), staffing, and telehealth infrastructure (e.g., lack of high-speed Internet access). Because their article's brevity precluded in-depth discussion of potential solutions, this editorial takes the opportunity to expand upon potential solutions to the problem of some HIV care facilities' inability to offer HIV telehealth care.

TELEHEALTH FOLLOWING THE COVID-19 PANDEMIC

Interest in HIV telehealth services has not waned in the post–COVID-19 era. Prior to the pandemic, 57% of PLHIV expressed willingness to use telehealth services. After the pandemic, that percentage increased to 80%.[6] Considering the demonstrated effectiveness of

HIV telehealth in HIV prevention and treatment,[4] and high interest levels in its continuation, it is important to identify strategies that enable all HIV care facilities to deliver telehealth services to PLHIV.

Some ways of assisting facilities in providing HIV telehealth care, such as increasing financial resources (e.g., Ryan White HIV/AIDS Program) and reducing staffing shortages, though worth attempting, may not always prove feasible; even if enacted, they may prove difficult to sustain. HIV care facilities need more innovative and affordable strategies to provide care to PLHIV and those at elevated risk for HIV infection, particularly in rural and underserved areas.

EXTENSION FOR COMMUNITY HEALTHCARE OUTCOMES

Valverde et al. astutely recommend one potential solution: the Extension for Community Healthcare Outcomes (ECHO) Model.[7] The Georgia Telehealth Network offers one example of how a remote network of providers can enhance HIV care management. On an annual budget slightly exceeding $2 million, the Georgia Department of Public Health established a statewide comprehensive HIV telehealth system in all 159 counties. Dedicated circuits installed throughout the state ensure that all participating clinics have sufficient bandwidth to provide remote care through patients' local medical homes.[8] An Infectious Disease ECHO Program that leveraged the Georgia Department of Public Health Telehealth platform at no cost was established in 2019 to strengthen HIV provider capacity. The Infectious Disease ECHO Program, consisting solely of volunteers, helps providers (e.g., physicians, nurses, pharmacists, mental and behavioral health specialists, dieticians), particularly those in rural areas and with low HIV patient caseloads, learn from specialists across the state to manage care for their patients living with HIV.[9] ECHO team members volunteered all of their time in support of the ECHO Program, and these additional approved duties were not compensated. All speakers who provided their expertise through virtual ECHO presentations gave their time freely without honoraria or compensation.

This network not only improves HIV care capacity but likely reduces health care costs through fewer new HIV infections, improved treatment adherence, and fewer hospitalizations for PLHIV. Smaller and more rural HIV care facilities that connect with Project ECHO networks in their states could receive mentoring on establishing telehealth infrastructures as well as practical issues that might hinder efforts to offer telehealth services, such as reimbursement uncertainties, satisfying Health Insurance Portability and Accountability Act (HIPAA) requirements, and conducting telehealth training to ensure competence.

Evidence of the efficacy of HIV telehealth is increasing; however, barriers continue to preclude the equitable distribution of HIV telehealth services. These barriers must be mitigated before telehealth can become the boon that researchers, practitioners, patients, and family members hope it can be. Black and Hispanic PLHIV are less likely to engage in telehealth,[3,6] although some evidence to the contrary is emerging.[8] Older adults uncomfortable with or suspicious of telehealth technology and individuals with low telehealth literacy are also less likely to use remote technologies.[3,6] Moreover, integrating electronic health records into telehealth platforms can be difficult, concerns about privacy and data security linger, and disparities in access to digital devices and the Internet persist, especially in rural areas. Only 5% of houses with annual incomes above $75 000 lack broadband access, compared with 38% of houses with incomes below $20 000.[10] These factors further complicate efforts by HIV care facilities to provide telehealth services.

Valverde et al. found that 17% of HIV care facilities did not offer telehealth services during the COVID-19 pandemic. Additional research is needed to determine *why* these facilities did not offer remote services. Perhaps HIV telehealth was not standard of care at these facilities, and it was impractical to establish and offer remote services when COVID-19 emerged. In light of the growing consensus that remote HIV prevention and treatment services are just as efficacious as in-person services,[11] future dissemination and implementation science research is needed to transition efficacious HIV telehealth services from the research arena into community settings, perhaps with a particular focus on HIV facilities in rural and underserved areas.

HIV telehealth services can be delivered during periods of normalcy and crisis, as the COVID-19 epidemic showed. Optimal delivery of HIV telehealth services, however, will not be achieved until disparities affecting access to and delivery of HIV telehealth services are addressed. Valverde et al. showed that many HIV care clinics (one out of six) and even more rural HIV care clinics (one out of three) provided no telehealth services during the COVID-19 pandemic and identified characteristics of facilities unable to offer such services. In so doing, they provide a roadmap for future research to remove these barriers so that all HIV care facilities can offer telehealth care to people affected by HIV. AJPH

CORRESPONDENCE

Correspondence should be sent to Timothy G. Heckman, PhD, Department of Health Promotion and Behavior, College of Public Health, 327 Wright Hall, Health Sciences Campus, University of Georgia, Athens, GA 30602 (e-mail: heckman@uga.edu). Reprints can be ordered at https://www.ajph.org by clicking the "Reprints" link.

PUBLICATION INFORMATION

Full Citation: Heckman TG, Heckman BD, Markowitz JC. The continuing need for HIV telehealth services following the COVID-19 pandemic. *Am J Public Health*. 2025;115(3):250–252.

Acceptance Date: November 30, 2024.

DOI: https://doi.org/10.2105/AJPH.2024.307967

ORCID iD:

John C. Markowitz https://orcid.org/0000-0003-2364-8363

CONTRIBUTORS

All authors contributed equally to the preparation and revision of this editorial.

ACKNOWLEDGMENTS

We acknowledge Gregory S. Felzien, MD, AAHIVS, for reviewing several versions of this editorial.

CONFLICTS OF INTEREST

The authors report no conflicts of interest.

REFERENCES

1. Centers for Disease Control and Prevention. Telehealth for HIV prevention and care services. Available at: https://www.cdc.gov/hiv/effective-interventions/treat/telehealth/index.html. Accessed November 8, 2024.
2. Health Resources Services Administration. What is telehealth? Available at: https://www.hrsa.gov/telehealth/what-is-telehealth. Accessed November 9, 2024.
3. Smith E, Badowski ME. Telemedicine for HIV care: current status and future prospects. *HIV AIDS (Auckl)*. 2021:13;651–656.
4. Saragih ID, Tonapa SI, Osingada CP, Porta CM, Lee B-O. Effects of telehealth-assisted interventions among people living with HIV/AIDS: a systematic review and meta-analysis of randomized controlled studies. *J Telemed Telecare*. 2024;30(3):438–450. https://doi.org/10.1177/1357633X211070726
5. Ohl ME, Richardson K, Rodriguez-Barradas MC, et al. Impact of availability of telehealth programs on documented HIV viral suppression: a cluster-randomized program evaluation in the Veterans Health Administration. *Open Forum Infect Dis*. 2019;6(6):ofz206. https://doi.org/10.1093/ofid/ofz206
6. Labisi T, Regan N, Davis P, et al. HIV care meets telehealth: a review of successes, disparities, and unresolved challenges. *Curr HIV/AIDS Rep*. 2022;19:446–453. https://doi.org/10.1007/s11904-022-00623-z
7. Arora S, Kalishman S, Thornton K, et al. Project ECHO (Project Extension for Community Healthcare Outcomes): a national and global model for continuing professional development. *J Contin Educ Health Prof*. 2016;36(suppl 1):S48–S49. https://doi.org/10.1097/CEH.0000000000000097
8. Salgado S, Felzien G, Brumbeloe J. Georgia leverages telehealth to expand HIV care management in underserved areas. *Am J Prev Med*. 2021;61(5 suppl 1):S55–S59. https://doi.org/10.1016/j.amepre.2021.07.001
9. Felzien GS, Salgado S. Georgia utilizes telehealth & Project ECHO. Available at: https://targethiv.org/sites/default/files/RWNC2020/15698_Felzien.pdf. Accessed November 11, 2024.
10. Community Tech Network. Broadband equity and the digital divide. Available at: https://www.communitytechnetwork.org/blog/broadband-equity-and-the-digital-divide/#:~:text=Another%20helpful%20definition%20to%20know,their%20long%2Dterm%20needs.%E2%80%9D. Accessed November 17, 2024.
11. Fadul N, Regan N, Kaddoura L, Swindells S. A midwestern academic HIV clinic operation during the COVID-19 pandemic: implementation strategy and preliminary outcomes. *J Int Assoc Provid AIDS Care*. 2021;20:23259582211041423. https://doi.org/10.1177/23259582211041423

Amplifying the Voices of Low-Wage Workers in Health and Well-Being Research to Promote Health Equity

Bruce W. Sherman, MD

ABOUT THE AUTHOR

Bruce W. Sherman is with the Department of Medicine, Case Western Reserve University School of Medicine, Cleveland, OH, and the Department of Public Health Education, University of North Carolina, Greensboro.

Despite long-standing awareness of health inequities among different demographic subpopulations,[1] inequitable utilization of and outcomes from employer-sponsored health benefits among US employees have only recently been described. In order for employers and researchers to mitigate existing health inequities in commercially insured populations, two important considerations warrant attention. The first involves achieving a broader understanding of the drivers of health among low-wage employees. The second relates to ensuring that employer-sponsored health initiatives address the unique needs and preferences of low-wage workers. These are distinct but related and important concerns.

Many factors affect the health of employees who are low-wage earners. This subpopulation is disproportionately represented by racial and ethnic minorities, who have a greater prevalence of chronic conditions and associated health care cost liability than their higher-earning counterparts.[2,3] Employers inadvertently worsen low-wage worker health inequities through their use of "one-size-fits-all" benefit plan cost structures, which do not vary on the basis of employee wage. In fact, only 7% of employers report offering low-wage workers any type of financial subsidy for health benefits.[4] As a result, low-wage workers may need to spend a disproportionately greater percentage of their income on health care[5] to achieve equitable health outcomes.

In addition to affordability concerns, a myriad of other factors confound workforce health inequities. In the health care services setting, low-wage workers may also be challenged by unmet health-related social needs, health benefits access concerns, health and health benefits literacy limitations, implicit bias exhibited by clinicians, and medical mistrust.[6] Chronic stress[7] and weathering[8] experienced by many low-wage workers may also exacerbate health issues, particularly among minority populations. In the workplace, adverse environmental conditions, occupational exposure risks, and physical job demands represent additional potential contributors to employee health and well-being inequities. Employee mental health may also be adversely affected by a psychologically stressful workplace culture. Additionally, inequitable organizational policies that, for example, provide paid leave to salaried workers, but not to hourly workers, may also be discriminatory in relation to low-wage workers, further exacerbating health inequities.

An understanding of the lived experience of low-wage workers is essential to developing approaches to improve their health and well-being,[9] as claims-based analyses do not provide insight into the root causes of disparities or inequities in health care utilization.[10] In the absence of objective input from these individuals, assumptions about low-wage workers' likely participation in health and well-being programs, and how they perceive the value of these programs may not reflect the needs and priorities of the low-wage worker population. Targeted surveys and focus groups engaging low-wage workers represent two distinct approaches to gaining a better understanding of their unique health and well-being issues, and the potential steps necessary to meaningfully address them. Whereas focus groups may be more practical in smaller, single-site studies, for larger and geographically dispersed populations, surveys likely provide the most efficient and scalable means for data collection from low-wage workers.

In their analytic essay published in *AJPH*, Sabbath et al. provide pragmatic and useful insights into approaches to engage low-wage workers in survey-based research.[11] The authors use a series of five case studies from their published research experience, each including low-wage worker populations of different sizes and geographical distribution to characterize their approach to enhancing participation in survey research. In each scenario, the authors discuss a number of often contemplated yet frequently overlooked factors regarding low-wage worker participation, in addition to effective as well as ineffective approaches to enhancing survey participation rates. Four principal recommendations are provided: building trust with eligible employees, encouraging managers to permit workers to take surveys during work time, high-touch recruitment and support for interested employees, and in-person data collection.

Of these suggestions, building trust is likely the most consequential. Trust by employees in employers and employer-sponsored or supported initiatives is a foundational element upon which much successful participatory research relies. In the absence of trust, as Sabbath et al. have described, employee participation and engagement are less likely to occur. Participation bias among those low-wage workers who do elect to engage in survey research may further confound the interpretation of survey data. Acknowledging researchers as a distinct third-party entity separate from the employer can help to ensure employee confidentiality and willingness to participate, as can addressing employee concerns in an understandable, thoughtful, and direct manner. In that setting, it may also be helpful for a trusted individual, such as a respected supervisor, to endorse and attest to the trustworthiness and credibility of the researchers. Additionally, although not explicitly mentioned in the Analytic Essay, building trust by sharing the findings with survey participants as circumstances allow may also be helpful for encouraging participation in future survey research.

With the authors' recommendations, reported survey participation rates in their case studies ranged from 23% to 92% for various subpopulations, with mean rates above 50%. These results suggest that additional opportunities may exist to achieve still greater response rates, although the effort to do so may outweigh the incremental value of the additional responses. Although not explicitly mentioned by Sabbath et al., the growing prevalence of employee resource groups in many businesses represents an additional setting for survey research. Endorsement of research activities by peer leaders of employee resource groups may also increase employee participation. Further research and insights into best practices to improve low-wage worker participation rates in survey research are needed to enhance our understanding of their unique issues and concerns.

Low-wage workers represent a demographic subgroup whose health and well-being status warrants more attention from researchers, employers, and other stakeholders, including policymakers. Sabbath et al. provide practical, evidence-based recommendations to enhance survey-based research participation rates among this socioeconomic subgroup. Results can be used to gain a better understanding of workplace challenges, including physical hazards, psychological safety, well-being concerns, and perceived inequities. Insights from survey responses represent an important step for identifying factors that contribute to inequities and providing useful insights to resolve them. Every employee should have an equitable opportunity to thrive in all dimensions of health. AJPH

CORRESPONDENCE

Correspondence should be sent to Bruce W. Sherman, MD, 117 Kemp Rd East, Greensboro, NC 27410 (e-mail: bws@case.edu). Reprints can be ordered at https://www.ajph.org by clicking the "Reprints" link.

PUBLICATION INFORMATION

Full Citation: Sherman BW. Amplifying the voices of low-wage workers in health and well-being research to promote health equity. *Am J Public Health*. 2025;115(3):253–254.

Acceptance Date: November 30, 2024.

DOI: https://doi.org/10.2105/AJPH.2024.307966

ORCID iD:

Bruce W. Sherman https://orcid.org/0000-0002-0659-2129

CONFLICTS OF INTEREST

B. W. Sherman reports receiving honoraria or consulting fees from Merck, Amgen, Lilly, Compass Pathways, Pittsburgh Business Group on Health, National Alliance of Healthcare Purchaser Coalitions, American Heart Association, and the National Pharmaceutical Council.

REFERENCES

1. Institute of Medicine. *Unequal Treatment: Confronting Racial and Ethnic Disparities in Healthcare.* Washington, DC: National Academies Press; 2003.
2. Harris J, Huang Y, Hannon P, Williams B. Low-socioeconomic status workers: their health risks and how to reach them. *J Occup Environ Med.* 2011;53(2):132–138. https://doi.org/10.1097/JOM.0b013e3182045f2c
3. Adler N, Boyce T, Chesney M, et al. Socioeconomic status and health. *Am Psychol.* 1994;49(1):15–24. https://doi.org/10.1037/0003-066X.49.1.15
4. *Employer Health Benefits Survey.* San Francisco, CA: Kaiser Family Foundation; 2022.
5. Hager K, Emanuel E, Mozaffarian D. Employer-sponsored health insurance premium cost growth and its association with earnings inequality among US families. *JAMA Netw Open.* 2024;7(1):e2351644. https://doi.org/10.1001/jamanetworkopen.2023.51644
6. National Academies of Sciences, Engineering, and Medicine. *Ending Unequal Treatment: Strategies to Achieve Equitable Health Care and Optimal Health for All.* Washington, DC: National Academies Press; 2024.
7. Yaribeygi H, Panahi Y, Sahraei H, Johnston T, Sahebkar A. The impact of stress on body function: a review. *EXCLI J.* 2017;16:1057–1072.
8. Forde A, Crookes D, Suglia S, Demmer R. The weathering hypothesis as an explanation for racial disparities in health: a systematic review. *Ann Epidemiol.* 2019;33:1–18.e3. https://doi.org/10.1016/j.annepidem.2019.02.011
9. Sherman B, Stiehl E, Gupta R, Pratap P. The importance of human-centered design in equitable health promotion initiatives. *Am J Health Promot.* 2024;38(3):443–447. https://doi.org/10.1177/08901171241232057f
10. Sherman B, Gibson T, Lynch W, Addy C. Healthcare utilization and cost patterns vary by wage level in employer-sponsored plans. *Health Aff (Millwood).* 2017;36(2):250–257. https://doi.org/10.1377/hlthaff.2016.1147
11. Sabbath EL, Lovejoy M, Schneider DK, Diaz-Linhart Y, DeHorn G, Peters SE. Engaging low-wage workers in health and well-being survey research: strategies from 5 occupational studies. *Am J Public Health.* 2025;115(2):201–208. https://doi.org/10.2105/AJPH.2024.307875

Paradox of Progress: NIH-Funded Research on Sexual and Gender Minority Populations, 2012–2022

M. Reuel Friedman, PhD, MPH, Tamara Taggart, PhD, MPH, and Robert W. S. Coulter, PhD, MPH

ABOUT THE AUTHORS

M. Reuel Friedman is with the School of Public Health, Rutgers University, Newark, NJ. Tamara Taggart is with the Milken Institute School of Public Health, George Washington University, Washington, DC. Robert W. S. Coulter is with the School of Public Health, University of Pittsburgh, Pittsburgh, PA.

See also Weideman et al., p. 374.

In 2009, Randy Sell published an editorial in *AJPH* concluding that only a small fraction of US national surveys incorporated measures characterizing sexual and gender minority (SGM) populations.[1] This lack of national population-level data created impediments for researchers attempting to estimate the level of health disparities that SGM populations experience, thus making it difficult to effectively promote and target interventions to remediate these disparities and achieve health equity. Basic questions were empirically unanswerable given the available data: How many SGM people are there? What health inequities do SGM individuals experience, and at what magnitude? What social–structural factors drive these inequities? Are they spread evenly across SGM communities, or do particular communities experience them more?

HISTORICAL GAPS IN HEALTH DATA AND RESEARCH

Fifteen years ago, it was evident that gay men and transgender women had been devastated by the HIV epidemic, but our knowledge of the extent to which SGM populations experienced other health inequities was minimal. Efforts from National Institutes of Health (NIH)-funded investigators to address these gaps had been repeatedly challenged and, in the mid-2000s, researchers were subjected to defunding of SGM-related grants, tantamount to blacklisting, during politicized proceedings.

In 2011, the Institute of Medicine published an NIH-commissioned report detailing compelling potential indicators of profound health disparities experienced by SGM populations.[2] The Institute of Medicine report highlighted social–structural deficits (i.e., employment and housing discrimination, lower educational attainment and income, poorer health care access and insurance), stigma, and HIV/AIDS as key domains of inequity faced by SGM individuals. It recommended the harmonization of measures characterizing SGM populations across national surveys as well as increased NIH funding to more closely investigate the depth and breadth of health inequities in SGM populations.

In 2014, Coulter et al. developed a methodology to track SGM-related research using public NIH RePORTER (Research Portfolio Online Reporting Tools Expenditures and Results) data and showed that only 0.5% of funded projects centered on SGM populations from 1989 through 2011 (0.1% of projects, excluding HIV/AIDS funding).[3] The 2015 establishment of the NIH Sexual and Gender Minority Research Office acknowledged the historical elision of SGM research from NIH portfolios and formally created a conduit for intramural and extramural SGM health research advocacy, collaborations, NIH-wide strategic planning and tracking, and identification of barriers to conducting SGM-related health research.[4]

PROGRESS AND INEQUITIES IN HEALTH RESEARCH

Meanwhile, the research base has expanded. We now have a better idea of what the SGM population looks like and how it is growing: 3.2% of the US

AJPH March 2025, Vol. 115, No. 3

population identifies as gay or lesbian, 4.6% as bisexual, and 0.8% as transgender.[5] We also now have a better idea of what health inequities SGM populations face. In study after study, compared with the general population, SGM people experience a significantly higher prevalence of social–structural deficits, poor psychosocial health (e.g., depression, anxiety), alcohol and substance use disorders, violence victimization, and stigma and discrimination. We have begun to demonstrate empirically that these inequities are produced by minority identity–related adversities that can begin in childhood and persist across the life course, predisposing older SGM individuals to greater risk of social isolation and loneliness and precipitating earlier mortality.[6–9]

We now also are beginning to understand that in SGM populations, those who are made more vulnerable and historically and contemporaneously marginalized are most at risk for poor health outcomes. SGM communities of color, particularly Black and Latinx individuals, experience higher rates of health inequities than do White SGM individuals. Bisexual people experience higher odds of health inequities than do gay or lesbian people, likely as a result of higher rates of stigma and discrimination from both sexual majority and minority communities. Transgender people experience profoundly higher odds of health inequities than do cisgender people, including those who are lesbian, gay, or bisexual.

The timely article by Weideman et al. in this issue of *AJPH* (p. 374) shows that the proportion of SGM-related NIH-funded projects more than doubled from 2012 to 2022 and provides valuable data about the context of awarded projects. However, this doubling masks persistent underrepresentation. To pinpoint gaps in NIH funding of SGM research, we can compare the percentage of the US population identifying as in a sexual or gender minority with the percentage of SGM-related NIH-funded projects and funding.

We paired data from the US Census,[5] Weideman et al., the General Social Survey,[10] NIH's RePORTER, and the Sexual and Gender Minority Research Office[11] to quantify disproportionality in NIH support of SGM health research. Table 1 shows that from 2012 through 2022, NIH SGM-related research projects consistently constituted less than 1.0% of the NIH portfolio, even as SGM individuals constituted 4.5% to 8.2% of the US population.

We estimated that NIH-funded SGM research projects would have had to increase by an overall factor of 6.9 times (with funding increasing 9 times) to achieve population-based proportionality. Moreover, although bisexual people experience profound health inequities and constituted 2.7% to 4.6% of the US population, research on bisexual populations constituted merely 0.02% to 0.14% of NIH projects (0.16% of NIH funding). Projects related to bisexual health would have had to increase by 50 times (with funding increasing 28.3 times) to achieve allocative proportionality. In 2018 to 2022, although proportions of SGM-related research projects increased from 2012, they remained misaligned with US SGM population proportions. Overall, NIH funding for projects related to bisexual men, bisexual women, and lesbian women was disproportionate to their respective populations by factors of more than 10. We argue that these misallocation estimates are conservative, given that the health inequities SGM people experience likely require research efforts above and beyond allocations simply balanced across populations.[12]

INTERVENTION RESEARCH TRENDS AND FUTURE DIRECTIONS

A promising finding from Weideman et al. is that the NIH funded 436 projects from 2012 to 2022 dedicated to improving SGM health via interventions. Substantially fewer, however, were for non-HIV health outcomes: only 74 projects. These numbers are increases from the previous 23-year period during which the NIH funded 202 projects on SGM health–related interventions and only 26 on non-HIV health outcomes. This shift indicates the NIH's investment in advancing SGM health equity research in recent years. Although future NIH funding for SGM health is unknown, the need for SGM health equity research will persist, particularly because anti-SGM legislation is being enacted across the United States, the bulk of which, for now, has targeted transgender people. These forms of structural anti-SGM discrimination are hypothesized to yield negative impacts across numerous preventable health outcomes, presenting opportunities for research by using natural experiments to study contraindicated policies.

Although the specific mechanisms of NIH-funded SGM health interventions remain unclear, future research must prioritize community partnerships—both to codesign interventions and to develop strategies for studying how anti-SGM policies affect violence and discrimination against SGM populations. Developing and testing interventions to decrease violence and discrimination against SGM people by targeting non-SGM individuals, including in schools, health care systems, and families, are hypothesized to promote SGM health and mitigate the negative health impacts of anti-SGM legislation.

TABLE 1— Estimated Percentages of Sexual and Gender Minority (SGM) Populations and National Institutes of Health (NIH)–Funded Research Projects and Funding Related to SGM Health: United States, 2012–2022

SGM Population	No. Total NIH Research Projects[a] or Funding in $ Millions[b]	% of US Population Identifying[5,10,b,c]	NIH Awards Centered on SGM Health Subpopulation, No. Projects[11] (%) or Funding in $ Millions[c] (%)	No. Projects or Funding in $ Millions Necessary to Achieve Proportionality: Total Required	Additional Required	Factor of Disproportionality
2012 projects	57 682					
All SGM		4.5	279 (0.48)	2596	2317	8.3
Transgender		0.8	21 (0.04)	462	441	21.0
Bisexual		2.7	11 (0.02)	1557	1546	140.5
2018 projects	61 799					
All SGM		4.5	384 (0.62)	2781	2397	6.2
Transgender		0.8	76 (0.12)	494	418	5.5
Bisexual		2.7	55 (0.09)	1669	1614	29.3
2019 projects	63 731					
All SGM		4.5	408 (0.64)	2868	2460	6.0
Transgender		0.8	92 (0.14)	510	418	4.5
Bisexual		2.7	70 (0.11)	1721	1651	23.6
2020 projects	64 464					
All SGM		4.5	500 (0.78)	2901	2401	4.8
Transgender		0.8	116 (0.18)	516	400	3.4
Bisexual		2.7	91 (0.14)	1741	1650	18.1
2021 projects	67 693					
All SGM		8.2	546 (0.81)	5551	5005	9.2
Transgender		0.8	165 (0.24)	542	377	2.3
Bisexual		4.6	81 (0.12)	3114	3033	37.4
2012–2021 projects, mean						
All SGM						6.9
Transgender						7.3
Bisexual						49.8
2012–2022 funding, total	60 100.0					
All SGM		8.2	491.7 (0.82)	4928.2	4436.5	9.0
Transgender		0.8	115.2 (0.19)	480.8	365.6	3.2
Bisexual		4.6	94.2 (0.16)	2764.6	2670.4	28.3
Lesbian/WSW		1.0	36.6 (0.06)	601.0	564.4	15.4
Gay men/MSM		1.9	368.0 (0.61)	1141.9	773.9	2.1
Bisexual men		1.2	62.3 (0.10)	721.2	658.9	10.6
Bisexual women		2.9	31.9 (0.05)	1742.9	1711.0	53.6

Note. MSM = men who have sex with men; WSW = women who have sex with women.
[a]Project-related data from NIH RePORTER (Research Portfolio Online Reporting Tools Expenditures and Results) per fiscal year, aggregating funded projects from all NIH institutes except the Center for Scientific Review.
[b]Weideman et al., in this issue of *AJPH*, p. 374
[c]From 2012 to 2018, we used data extracted from the General Social Survey for "all SGM" and "bisexual" categories. For all others (including funding table), we used data extracted from the 2021–2022 US Census Household Pulse Survey, in which we included data of transgender people who do not identify as gay, lesbian, or bisexual, resulting in the addition of 0.4% of total population to the SGM category. Because transgender people also have sexual orientations, subcategories of SGM should not be considered mutually exclusive.

Fifteen years after Sell's editorial, SGM population research has inched forward but remains disproportionately underrepresented in the NIH portfolio, wherein it is consistently dominated by HIV-related research among gay male communities. Bisexual health remains severely underfunded. Although unlikely, it is possible that non-SGM–focused NIH projects proportionately enroll SGM individuals in research, but legislation has still not mandated SGM categories in NIH inclusion enrollment and clinical trials reports[1]; consequently, sexual orientation and gender identity information remains neither systematically recorded nor reported in resulting publications, as age and ethnoracial data are. The US Census only recently began to collect SGM-related information from respondents. These small, important steps demonstrated progress in the face of historical headwinds. In the short period between this editorial's acceptance and production, SGM Research Office and Census data related to SGM are no longer publicly available. The renewed adversities that SGM populations face spur us to action and remind us that NIH support for SGM health research will be more important than ever in the years to come. AJPH

CORRESPONDENCE

Correspondence should be sent to M. R. Friedman, One Riverfront Plaza, Suite 1000, Newark, NJ 07102-0301 (e-mail: mf1061@sph.rutgers.edu). Reprints can be ordered at https://www.ajph.org by clicking the "Reprints" link.

PUBLICATION INFORMATION

Full Citation: Reuel Friedman M, Taggart T, Coulter RWS. Paradox of progress: NIH-funded research on sexual and gender minority populations, 2012–2022. *Am J Public Health*. 2025;115(3): 255–258.

Acceptance Date: December 13, 2024.

DOI: https://doi.org/10.2105/AJPH.2024.307986

ORCID iD:

Tamara Taggart https://orcid.org/0000-0001-9240-1212

ACKNOWLEDGMENTS

In memory of Anthony J. Silvestre.

CONFLICTS OF INTEREST

The authors have no conflicts of interest to disclose.

REFERENCES

1. Sell RL. LGBTQ health surveillance: data = power. *Am J Public Health*. 2017;107(6):843–844. https://doi.org/10.2105/AJPH.2017.303798
2. Institute of Medicine Committee on Lesbian, Gay, Bisexual, and Transgender Health Issues and Research Gaps and Opportunities. *The Health of Lesbian, Gay, Bisexual, and Transgender People: Building a Foundation for Better Understanding*. Washington, DC: National Academies Press; 2011.
3. Coulter RWS, Kenst KS, Bowen DJ, Scout. Research funded by the National Institutes of Health on the health of lesbian, gay, bisexual, and transgender populations. *Am J Public Health*. 2014;104(2):e105–e112. https://doi.org/10.2105/AJPH.2013.301501
4. Alexander R, Parker K, Schwetz T. Sexual and gender minority health research at the National Institutes of Health. *LGBT Health*. 2016;3(1):7–10. https://doi.org/10.1089/lgbt.2015.0107
5. Glassman B. Financial insecurity and hardship in the Pulse: an in-depth look at gender identity and sexual orientation. April 20, 2023. Available at: https://www.census.gov/content/dam/Census/library/working-papers/2023/demo/SEHSD-wp2023-16.pdf. Accessed January 5, 2025.
6. Cochran SD, Björkenstam C, Mays VM. Sexual orientation and all-cause mortality among US adults aged 18 to 59 years, 2001–2011. *Am J Public Health*. 2016;106(5):918–920. https://doi.org/10.2105/AJPH.2016.303052
7. Stall R, Matthews DD, Friedman MR, et al. The continuing development of health disparities research on lesbian, gay, bisexual, and transgender individuals. *Am J Public Health*. 2016;106(5):787–789. https://doi.org/10.2105/AJPH.2016.303183
8. Hatzenbuehler ML, Lattanner MR, McKetta S, Pachankis JE. Structural stigma and LGBTQ+ health: a narrative review of quantitative studies. *Lancet Public Health*. 2024;9(2):e109–e127. [Erratum in: *Lancet Public Health*. 2024;9(4):e217. https://doi.org/10.1016/S2468-2667(24)00045-8]. https://doi.org/10.1016/S2468-2667(23)00312-2
9. Zachry CE, O'Brien RP, Clark KA, Ding ML, Blosnich JR. Mortality among sexual and gender minority populations: a systematic review. *PLoS ONE*. 2025;20(2):e0307688. https://doi.org/10.1371/journal.pone.0307688
10. Monto MA, Neuweiler S. The rise of bisexuality: US representative data show an increase over time in bisexual identity and persons reporting sex with both women and men. *J Sex Res*. 2024;61(6):974–987. https://doi.org/10.1080/00224499.2023.2225176
11. US Department of Health and Human Services. Sexual and Gender Minority Research Office: reports. July 1, 2024. Available at: https://dpcpsi.nih.gov/sgmro/reports. Accessed December 11, 2024.
12. Friedman MR, Chandler CJ, Adams BJ, et al. Toward a new framework for equity in epidemic allocations: implications of HIV-prevention-allocation misalignment. *Am J Public Health*. 2021;111(1):12–14. https://doi.org/10.2105/AJPH.2020.306032

Expanding Access, Elevating Equity: Lessons From Utah's Family Planning Elevated Contraceptive Access Program

Halley E. M. Riley, PhD, MPH

ABOUT THE AUTHOR

Halley E. M. Riley is with the Research Data Services Department, Georgia State University, Atlanta.

See also Simmons et al., p. 387.

Equitable, patient-centered contraceptive access can help individuals accomplish reproductive goals, maintain bodily autonomy and health, and control key aspects of their lives. In the post–*Dobbs v Jackson Women's Health Organization* era, contraceptive access is vital for people in the United States who do not wish to be pregnant, given increasingly restrictive abortion policies across the country.[1] Many people seek contraception for noncontraceptive benefits. Depending on the method, contraception can help people regulate menstruation, treat acne, and ease symptoms of premenstrual syndrome, premenstrual dysphoric disorder, endometriosis, and polycystic ovary syndrome.[2] Long-term use of some hormonal methods can decrease risks of certain cancers.[2] When people can plan pregnancies, risks of maternal morbidity and mortality decrease.[3] The evidence is clear: contraception can be a great tool for people who make freely informed decisions to use contraception.

Despite the availability of about 18 different contraceptive options in the United States, barriers to access remain, necessitating policies and programs that put contraception in the hands of those seeking it. In this issue of *AJPH*, Simmons et al. (p. 387) report findings from Utah's Family Planning Elevated (FPE) contraceptive access program (2018–2023), a statewide contraceptive access initiative (SCAI). The FPE program aimed to improve Utah's health care system capacity to (1) expand high-quality comprehensive contraceptive care for individuals newly eligible for Medicaid and (2) provide free contraceptive access for people who were uninsured or without contraceptive coverage.

The FPE program enrolled federally qualified health centers, county health departments, and rural clinics that met eligibility criteria (e.g., were able to bill Medicaid, served low-income patients, and had a provider who could be trained to insert long-acting reversible contraceptives [LARCs]). Participating clinics received staff training, technical assistance, financial support via grant funding and reimbursement for devices and services, and support for a media campaign.

The authors used a comparative interrupted time series analysis to assess changes to contraceptive provision before, during, and after FPE program implementation. Using electronic health records, they compared nine intervention clinics with nine matched controls over 48 months. They found that, compared with control sites, intervention clinics provided significantly more contraceptive-related visits during the intervention period (approximately 1.76 times more contraceptive-related visits per month). The proportion of contraceptive-related visits relative to all visits was also higher in intervention clinics. Although contraceptive provision ebbed after the intervention, decreases were not statistically significant and contraceptive provision remained higher at intervention clinics. The FPE program's success is impressive, especially given the significant challenges it faced. These included the COVID-19 pandemic and changes to Title X funding, which left Utah without any Title X–funded clinics.

The Simmons et al. article adds to the literature on the effectiveness of SCAIs. Broadly, SCAIs are programs designed to expand access to a range of contraceptive methods by addressing barriers such as cost, provider training and availability, and education. SCAIs generally involve collaboration between government, nonprofit, and private stakeholders, with the goal of building a framework to sustain ongoing, equitable contraceptive care.[4,5] Over the past two decades, about 30 SCAIs have been implemented across the United States.[6] Across contexts, SCAIs like Utah's FPE can increase contraceptive use.[5]

AJPH March 2025, Vol. 115, No. 3

Yet the implementation of SCAIs, as with all efforts to expand and promote contraceptive use, must be contextualized in the broader, often dark history of contraceptive provision. This history (and, all too often, the present) includes systemic reproductive coercion toward people of color, people with disabilities, and people with low income in the United States and globally. SCAIs have the potential to continue this legacy of harm by overemphasizing LARC uptake and pregnancy prevention. Alternatively, these programs could change the field by focusing on patient autonomy, well-being, and whole health.[7–10]

In recognition of the importance of these issues, *AJPH* published a supplement entitled *Reshaping Contraceptive Access Efforts by Centering Equity, Justice, and Autonomy* in June 2022. In this collection, authors outlined the principles and frameworks that should form the foundation of SCAIs to prevent harm. Key points include the following:

- SCAIs must reimagine their purpose, shifting focus away from pregnancy avoidance and LARC uptake to the promotion of sexual and reproductive health equity (SRHE), and patient satisfaction, well-being, and autonomy.[4,8–10]
- Programs should be designed using principles of reproductive justice and SRHE, with reproductive justice leaders, community stakeholders, and end users involved in program development, implementation, and evaluation.[8–11]
- Program success should be defined according to these goals, with patient-centered measures of satisfaction, well-being, and comfort incorporated as key outcomes. Such metrics should replace (or at least supplement) previously used metrics like LARC uptake and pregnancy prevention.[7,11]
- Sustainability should be prioritized and evaluated to create long-term change.[12]

Importantly, Simmons et al. demonstrate that SCAIs can be effective while adhering to principles of patient-centeredness and SRHE. The authors explain that their program was not specifically designed to reduce unintended pregnancies, promote contraceptive continuation, or increase LARC uptake. Instead, clients were encouraged to choose any method they preferred (including no method), switch methods if their preferences changed, and discontinue LARC methods at no cost if they so desired. This demonstrates a marked shift away from previous program priorities and toward the goals outlined in the 2022 *AJPH* supplement and other key documents, such as the Coalition to Expand Contraceptive Access's 2024 report, *State Contraceptive Access Initiatives: Recommendations Report*.[6] The authors took a broad approach to defining contraceptive-related visits, categorizing any encounter with a diagnostic or procedural code linked to contraception as such. Thus, visits that included contraceptive counseling, management, or discontinuation were considered contraceptive-related. Although this may seem like a subtle shift in focus, decisions like this may incentivize ongoing patient–provider communication about contraception and disincentivize directive contraceptive counseling.

Simmons et al. also recognize opportunities to continue advancing measurement in SCAI evaluations. For example, because they used electronic health record data from individuals aged 18 to 50 years who were assigned female at birth, they did not capture data on adolescent services or vasectomies. The authors acknowledge that additional metrics, including appointment wait time, would help evaluators more fully understand access. SCAI evaluations should also incorporate patient-centered measures related to equity, autonomy, satisfaction, and choice.[6] Qualitative work can allow patients and providers to describe their own complex experiences using their own words. Emphasizing such measures will help evaluators understand if SCAIs are advancing SRHE and ensure that measurement decisions are aligned with program goals.[6]

At the time of publication, many people in the United States are concerned about potential changes to family planning access under a second Trump presidential administration. Despite (or perhaps because of) this, it is important to reiterate the goals described here. As rights to bodily autonomy are threatened by restrictive policies (e.g., post-*Dobbs* restrictive abortion laws), informed decision-making and prioritization of patient autonomy in SCAIs are more important than ever. Simmons et al.'s article represents an encouraging shift in focus. As we envision and work toward a future in which people make supported, informed, and autonomous decisions about their sexual and reproductive health, interventions like Utah's FPE mark an important step toward achieving these goals. AJPH

CORRESPONDENCE

Correspondence should be sent to Halley E. M. Riley, PhD, MPH, 100 Decatur St SE, Atlanta, GA 30303 (e-mail: hriley@gsu.edu). Reprints can be ordered at https://www.ajph.org by clicking the "Reprints" link.

PUBLICATION INFORMATION

Full Citation: Riley HEM. Expanding access, elevating equity: lessons from Utah's Family Planning Elevated contraceptive access program. *Am J Public Health*. 2025;115(3):259–261.

Acceptance Date: December 14, 2024.
DOI: https://doi.org/10.2105/AJPH.2024.307987
ORCID iD:
Halley E. M. Riley https://orcid.org/0009-0008-7027-7482

ACKNOWLEDGMENTS

I thank the Coalition to Expand Contraceptive Access team and collaborators, as well as the authors featured in the 2022 *AJPH* supplement *Reshaping Contraceptive Access Efforts by Centering Equity, Justice, and Autonomy* for their leadership in envisioning the future of contraceptive access efforts.

CONFLICTS OF INTEREST

The author has no conflicts of interest to report.

REFERENCES

1. Guttmacher Institute. Abortion policy in the absence of Roe. 2024. Available at: https://www.guttmacher.org/state-policy/explore/abortion-policy-absence-roe. Accessed December 9, 2024.
2. ACOG Practice Bulletin No. 110: noncontraceptive uses of hormonal contraceptives. *Obstet Gynecol.* 2010;115(1):206–218. https://doi.org/10.1097/AOG.0b013e3181cb50b5
3. Askew I, Raney L, Kerrigan M, Sridhar A. Family planning saves maternal and newborn lives: why universal access to contraception must be prioritized in national maternal and newborn health policies, financing, and programs. *Int J Gynecol Obstet.* 2024;164(2):536–540. https://doi.org/10.1002/ijgo.15127
4. Malcolm NM, Patterson KV, Pliska ES, Akbarali S, Moskosky SB, Hart J. A prologue to the AJPH supplement: using evidence to expand contraceptive access. *Am J Public Health.* 2022;112(suppl 5):S470–S472. https://doi.org/10.2105/AJPH.2022.306927
5. Malcolm N, Danaux J, Parikh A, et al. Statewide contraceptive access initiatives: updated environmental scan report. 2024. Available at: https://static1.squarespace.com/static/5d35f1b39760f8000111473a/t/6668a4ef0dbae922c6663516/1718134000802/4.+SCAI+Environmental+Scan_Update_June+2024.pdf. Accessed December 9, 2024.
6. Danaux J, Malcolm N, Wilson J, et al. Statewide contraceptive access initiatives: recommendations report. 2024. Available at: https://static1.squarespace.com/static/5d35f1b39760f8000111473a/t/66e0b98a5d18a67c51963f09/1726003599318/1.+SCAI+Recommendations+Report_June+2024+v2.pdf. Accessed December 9, 2024.
7. Malcolm NM, Patterson KV, Pliska ES, Akbarali S, Moskosky SB, Hart J. Scaling up evidence-based practices in contraceptive access initiatives. *Am J Public Health.* 2022;112(suppl 5):S473–S477. https://doi.org/10.2105/AJPH.2022.306824
8. Axelson SM, Sealy GA, McDonald-Mosley RE. Reproductive well-being: a framework for expanding contraceptive access. *Am J Public Health.* 2022;112(suppl 5):S504–S507. https://doi.org/10.2105/AJPH.2022.306898
9. Hart J. Reshaping contraceptive access efforts by centering equity, justice, and autonomy. *Am J Public Health.* 2022;112(suppl 5):S468. https://doi.org/10.2105/AJPH.2022.306926
10. Cadena DS, Chaudhri A, Scott C. Contraceptive care using reproductive justice principles: beyond access. *Am J Public Health.* 2022;112(suppl 5):S494–S499. https://doi.org/10.2105/AJPH.2022.306915
11. Lassar M, Tao K, Thiede K. Advancing reproductive health equity through a new contraceptive access initiative. *Am J Public Health.* 2022;112(suppl 5):S500–S503. https://doi.org/10.2105/AJPH.2022.306899
12. Gavin LE. Steps needed to scale up statewide contraceptive access initiatives. *Am J Public Health.* 2022;112(suppl 5):S515–S517. https://doi.org/10.2105/AJPH.2022.306925

Parental Involvement Laws and the Best Interests of Minors: A Need for Reform

Joanne D. Rosen, JD, MA

ABOUT THE AUTHOR

Joanne D. Rosen is with the Department of Health Policy and Management, Johns Hopkins Bloomberg School of Public Health, Baltimore, MD.

See also Fulcher et al., p. 397.

State legislatures have long played a role in pregnant minors' access to abortion care. After the US Supreme Court first recognized a constitutionally protected right to abortion in *Roe v Wade* in 1973, many states enacted laws to ensure parental involvement in minors' abortion decisions.[1] Although the precise content of these laws varied by state, most laws required the notification, consent, or notification and consent of at least one parent or guardian 24 or 48 hours before the abortion procedure.[2] Currently, 35 states continue to mandate parental notice or consent as a condition of minors' access to abortion, and these laws are often accompanied by onerous requirements to demonstrate compliance.[3]

Most minors choose to involve a parent in their abortion decisions.[2] For these adolescents, parental involvement laws do not interfere with confidential abortion access. However, for the minority of adolescents who wish to seek abortion care without parental involvement—for reasons that include a fear of violence if the pregnancy is disclosed, harm to the parental relationship, forced continuation of an unwanted pregnancy, or logistical barriers[4,5]—mandatory parental involvement laws impose a significant burden on abortion access.

Six years after the *Roe* decision, the Supreme Court set the framework for permissible parental involvement laws in *Bellotti v Baird*.[6] In its decision, the court grappled with the competing considerations raised by these laws, many of which continue to ring true today: the laws' interference with minors' confidential and independent access to abortion; the particular burden of unwanted pregnancy on minors in light of their limited financial resources, education, and employment skills; the "guiding role" parents play in rearing their children to maturity; and the state's legitimate role in protecting youths and encouraging parental involvement in important decisions. Ultimately, the court upheld the power of states to enact parental notification laws as long as they were accompanied by a confidential, expeditious, alternative authorization proceeding that could be used by minors who did not wish to involve their parents.

ABORTION ACCESS AFTER *BELLOTTI*

Following the *Bellotti* decision, many states incorporated a judicial bypass option into their parental involvement laws. Judicial bypass proceedings enable a minor to go directly to a judge, instead of a parent or guardian, to obtain authorization for an abortion.[6] In theory, the judicial bypass option facilitates abortion access for minors who reside in parental involvement states and who do not want to notify a parent. In practice, parental involvement laws significantly impede abortion access for these adolescents. As documented by numerous studies of parental involvement laws over several decades, adolescents who reside in parental involvement states often go out of state to obtain abortions in states where parental involvement is not required, often traveling long distances to do so; they experience longer delays in access to abortion; and they obtain abortion at later gestational durations.[2,4]

For minors who do use the judicial bypass option, the process is intimidating, stressful, unpredictable, and difficult to navigate.[7,8] Minors must meet with an attorney, take time away from school or work to attend court, and arrange transportation to the hearing.[8] The judicial bypass process may also delay access to in-state abortion and result in abortions taking place at later gestational durations.[9] Finally, judges may deny judicial bypass petitions and withhold authorization.[8,10] One study found that judicial bypass denials in Florida rose from 6% to 13% over a three-year period.[10] Moreover, judicial bypass petitions may be denied for reasons that are unrelated to whether

AJPH March 2025, Vol. 115, No. 3

the adolescent is informed and mature enough to make this decision or whether abortion would be in the adolescent's best interests (the criteria permitted under the *Bellotti* framework).[8]

In December 2020, the Massachusetts legislature removed its parental consent and judicial bypass requirement for those aged 16 to 17 years as part of a larger legislative initiative to broaden abortion access. In this issue of *AJPH*, Fulcher at al. (p. 397) examine the impact of this change on the timeliness of abortion access. Using a comparative interrupted time series model, the authors compared the mean gestational duration at time of abortion for those aged 16 to 17 years before and after the removal of the requirement with a control group of older young adults who were not subject to the requirement. They found that removal of the parental consent requirement resulted in those aged 16 to 17 years receiving abortions an average of 5.6 days earlier than when parental consent was required. These findings reinforce and expand on what is known about the effects of parental involvement laws on the timing of abortion access. The authors note that, although their study does not establish a causal relationship between the legislative change and earlier access to abortion, it indicates that abortion access may be influenced by legislative measures.

IMPACT OF *DOBBS* ON MINORS' ABORTION ACCESS

Fulcher et al. examined minors' abortion access before *Dobbs v Jackson Women's Health Organization* was decided (June 24, 2022), which overturned *Roe v Wade* and extinguished the federal constitutional abortion right. With the removal of this right, and states' near-unfettered ability to ban or severely restrict abortion, abortion access is now substantially more challenging for all persons, but especially for minors and other marginalized groups.[8,11] Recent studies on abortion access after the *Dobbs* decision have documented an increase in out-of-state travel for abortion care, an increase in clinic volume in states that allow abortion, and an increase in the mean gestational duration at time of abortion.[11]

The *Dobbs* decision has particular implications for parental involvement laws. The Supreme Court's reasoning in *Bellotti*, and its requirement that parental involvement laws include a judicial bypass alternative, built directly on the constitutional scaffolding in *Roe v Wade*. Specifically, because parental involvement laws could allow a parent or guardian to veto a minor's abortion decision, an alternative authorization process was necessary to protect the minor's constitutional right to decide whether to terminate a pregnancy. With the reversal of *Roe* and the removal of this right, states with parental involvement laws are no longer required to offer a judicial bypass alternative to minors.

Following the *Dobbs* decision, Idaho enacted an "abortion trafficking law" to tighten its parental consent requirement and restrict minors' ability to travel out of state for abortion care.[12] Four other states with strict abortion bans have followed suit and enacted or introduced similar laws.[12] Under these laws, it is a crime for an adult to assist a minor in obtaining an abortion without parental consent, either in that state or by traveling to another state where abortion remains legal. These novel and aggressive measures may be the next wave in impeding minors' access to abortion.

NEED FOR REFORM OF PARENTAL INVOLVEMENT LAWS

The inequities that have long hindered abortion access for minors, and that are documented by Fulcher et al. in this issue, can be expected to worsen in the post-*Dobbs* legal landscape. Consequently, the repeal of existing parental involvement laws, which would ease abortion access for both minors in those states and minors who live in proximate states and can travel to those states for abortion care, is especially critical now. However, repeal may not be feasible in states where lawmakers and residents support some degree of parental involvement in minors' abortion decisions, where lawmakers have other reproductive health care priorities, or where lawmakers regard repeal efforts as a "political liability" in the current parental rights political climate.[13] In these states, the Massachusetts model, in which the state's parental involvement requirement was removed for those aged 16 to 17 years but retained for younger adolescents, may offer a more viable reform option. Although falling short of full repeal, the data generated by Fulcher et al. demonstrate that this is a significant step forward in protecting minors' abortion access. AJPH

CORRESPONDENCE

Correspondence should be sent to Joanne D. Rosen, Johns Hopkins Bloomberg School of Public Health, 615 N. Wolfe St, Room E6009, Baltimore, MD 21205 (e-mail: jrosen55@jhu.edu). Reprints can be ordered at https://www.ajph.org by clicking the "Reprints" link.

PUBLICATION INFORMATION

Full Citation: Rosen JD. Parental involvement laws and the best interests of minors: a need for reform. *Am J Public Health*. 2025;115(3):262–264.

Acceptance Date: December 14, 2024.

DOI: https://doi.org/10.2105/AJPH.2024.307988

ORCID iD:
Joanne D. Rosen https://orcid.org/0000-0002-7177-7832

CONFLICTS OF INTEREST

The author has no conflicts of interest to disclose.

REFERENCES

1. Merz JF, Klerman JA, Jackson CA. A chronicle of abortion legality, Medicaid funding, and parental involvement laws, 1967–1994. RAND Labor and Population Program Working Paper Series 96-08. May 1996. Available at: https://www.rand.org/content/dam/rand/pubs/drafts/2008/DRU1415.pdf. Accessed January 3, 2025.
2. Dennis A, Henshaw SK, Joyce TJ, Finer LB, Blanchard K. The impact of laws requiring parental involvement for abortion: a literature review. March 2009. Available at: https://www.guttmacher.org/sites/default/files/report_pdf/parentalinvolvementlaws.pdf. Accessed November 30, 2024.
3. Kaiser Family Foundation. Parental consent/notification for minors seeking abortion by state. September 2024. Available at: https://www.kff.org/womens-health-policy/state-indicator/parental-consentnotification. Accessed November 30, 2024.
4. Kramer A, Ti A, Travis L, Laboe A, Ochieng WO, Young MR. The impact of parental involvement laws on minors seeking abortion services: a systematic review. *Health Aff Sch*. 2023;1(4):1–13. https://doi.org/10.1093/haschl/qxad045
5. Henshaw SK, Kost K. Parental involvement in minors' abortion decisions. *Fam Plann Perspect*. 1992;24(5):196–207, 213. https://doi.org/10.2307/2135870
6. US Supreme Court. *Bellotti v Baird*. July 2, 1979. *US Rep U S Supreme Court*. 1979;443:622–657.
7. Coleman-Minahan K, Stevenson AJ, Obront E, Hays S. Young women's experiences obtaining judicial bypass for abortion in Texas. *J Adolesc Health*. 2019;64(1):20–25. https://doi.org/10.1016/j.jadohealth.2018.07.017
8. Horvath S, Frietsche S. Judicial bypass for minors post-*Dobbs*. *Womens Health (Lond)*. 2023;19:17455057231219601. https://doi.org/10.1177/17455057231219601
9. Janiak E, Fulcher IR, Cottrill AA, et al. Massachusetts' parental consent law and procedural timing among adolescents undergoing abortion. *Obstet Gynecol*. 2019;133(5):978–986. https://doi.org/10.1097/AOG.0000000000003190
10. Stevenson AJ, Coleman-Minahan K. Use of judicial bypass of mandatory parental consent to access abortion and judicial bypass denials, Florida and Texas, 2018–2021. *Am J Public Health*. 2023;113(3):316–319. https://doi.org/10.2105/AJPH.2022.307173
11. Riley T, Fiastro AE, Benson LS, Khattar A, Prager S, Godfrey EM. Abortion provision and delays to care in a clinic network in Washington State after *Dobbs*. *JAMA Netw Open*. 2024;7(5):e2413847. https://doi.org/10.1001/jamanetworkopen.2024.13847
12. Vollers AC. Helping a minor travel for an abortion? Some states have made it a crime. *Idaho Capital Sun*. August 26, 2024. Available at: https://idahocapitalsun.com/2024/08/26/helping-a-minor-travel-for-an-abortion-some-states-have-made-it-a-crime. Accessed January 3, 2025.
13. Messerly M, Ollstein AM. Dems split on whether parents must know their child is having an abortion. *Politico*. May 17, 2023. Available at: https://www.politico.com/news/2023/05/16/democrats-gop-parental-notification-abortion-laws-00097245. Accessed January 3, 2025.

Health Care Stereotype Threat: The Danger and Damage of Stigma and Discrimination in Health Care

Rodman E. Turpin, PhD, MS

ABOUT THE AUTHOR

Rodman Turpin is an assistant professor in the Department of Global and Community Health, College of Public Health, at George Mason University, Fairfax, VA.

See also Manning et al., p. 425.

In this issue of *AJPH*, Manning et al. (p. 425) describe a study on health care stereotype threat: a measure of anticipated stigma and discrimination in health care settings. Their findings highlight how health care stereotype threat remains prevalent among minoritized groups in the COVID-19 pandemic, including sexual, gender, and racial/ethnic minorities, demonstrating the importance of identity-based stigma and discrimination as a barrier to accessing and utilizing care. Racism, homophobia, and cisgenderism are among the greatest threats to health equity efforts in the United States. Effective health promotion and delivery require not only understanding how stigma and discrimination operate at several levels of health care but also prioritizing antidiscrimination and antibias efforts at these levels. Eliminating health care stereotype threat for sexual, gender, and racial/ethnic minorities requires significant systemic changes in our health care institutions.

SEXUAL/GENDER MINORITY STIGMA AND DISCRIMINATION

Extant research consistently demonstrates that sexual and gender minority people are more likely to have unmet medical needs and less likely to receive routine medical care compared with their heterosexual counterparts.[1] When they do receive care, they are more likely to face substantial stigma and discrimination in these settings, including experiencing slurs, violence, sexual harassment, and microaggressions.[2] This aligns with the research by Manning et al., where, compared with heterosexual and cisgender individuals, gay, lesbian, bisexual, other sexual minority, and transgender individuals had greater health care stereotype threat. In addition, increased health care stereotype threat among sexual and gender minorities persisted after adjustment for socioeconomic measures, various health conditions, and health insurance.

While sexual minority adults are more likely to face socioeconomic barriers to care, including a lack of health insurance and difficulty affording care even when insured, discrimination toward sexual minority people extends beyond socioeconomics.[1,2] As such, efforts to achieve equitable health care for sexual and gender minorities must include both socioeconomic and access intervention, as well as addressing additional institutional factors such as cultural competency training on sexual and gender minority populations. Understanding differences in specific sexual and gender identities is a core component of competent care for these communities. For example, bisexual people can experience very different forms of stigma and discrimination in health care settings compared with gay and lesbian people.[3] Similarly, people with sexual identities such as same-gender–loving and pansexual may have differing experiences in and outside these settings as well. Understanding the differences among these identities is important for informing both health care practice and research efforts, with implications for health equity goals.

RACIAL/ETHNIC STIGMA AND DISCRIMINATION

Manning et al. also found that health care stereotype threat was higher among non-Hispanic Black participants compared with any other racial or ethnic group, and that individuals with a health condition reported more health care stereotype threat, irrespective of health insurance status. Black individuals anticipating racism when seeking care is

AJPH March 2025, Vol. 115, No. 3

rooted in a litany of abuses by the health care system, both past and present.[4,5] This is reflected in the increased medical mistrust among many Black communities. The reality is, in our current health care systems, this mistrust is entirely justified. It is well-documented that racial/ethnic minorities receive a lower standard of health care compared with their White counterparts, even when controlling for several other socioeconomic and demographic differences.[5] This lower standard of care is largely driven by both racial biases and structural health care discrimination.[5,6]

For these reasons, addressing anticipated racism in health care cannot happen simply at the individual level because the anticipation is based on an accurate assessment of a structural threat. Intervening on this threat has to happen through several institutional-level changes; this is especially urgent given the concurrent impact racism has on health disparities. Racial health disparities include several adverse health outcomes influenced both directly and indirectly by racism at multiple levels. Structural and interpersonal racism are psychobiological stressors that have a direct impact on health, such as a greater risk of incident hypertension.[7] Structural racism also marginalizes people of color, particularly Black people, through discrimination in employment and wages, unequal education access, and residential segregation such as redlining.[8] This leads to not only greater vulnerability to several acute and chronic illnesses but also more difficulty accessing effective care. This means that, much like sexual and gender minorities, racial/ethnic minorities are also faced with having greater health care needs yet more barriers to competent care. Racism further exacerbates systemic harms toward the most vulnerable people.

INTERSECTIONALITY

In tandem, the findings related to both race and sexual/gender identity underscore the need for intersectional approaches in understanding discrimination among minoritized communities. These approaches explore interlocking systems of power that minoritize individuals along multiple axes of identity; this large-scale social–structural oppression ultimately produces adverse individual-level outcomes.[9] People are multifaceted, and so are their experiences in health care settings. Understanding stigmatizing and discriminatory experiences through an intersectional lens is necessary for providing relevant nuance and context. And just as intersectionality should inform our understanding of discrimination, it should also inform approaches to address discrimination in these settings.

Proactively, cultural competency trainings need to incorporate understanding the lived experiences of intersectional minorities because the context at these intersections is often different. For instance, Black queer men face unique stigmatizing experiences both within and outside health care settings when seeking health services.[10] Representation along these overlapping identities is important as well, as many people with multiple minoritized identities can be more comfortable engaging with care services when they see themselves represented in their health care setting. In addition, policies must allow for safe reporting of experiences of discrimination and provide accountability when said discrimination is identified.

Finally, it is critical that health care providers at every level understand the seriousness of identity-based stigma and discrimination in health care settings. Stigma and discrimination are not merely about vague feelings or mild offenses; they translate directly into numerous adverse health outcomes, including prolonged and incident illness, substandard treatment, and mortality.[1,7,11] Stigma and discrimination kill.[7,11] And, like any lethal disease, we need to aggressively address stigma and discrimination in health care at every level. AJPH

CORRESPONDENCE

Correspondence should be sent to Rodman Turpin, 4400 University Blvd, Fairfax, VA 22030 (e-mail: rturpin@gmu.edu). Reprints can be ordered at https://www.ajph.org by clicking the "Reprints" link.

PUBLICATION INFORMATION

Full Citation: Turpin RE. Health care stereotype threat: the danger and damage of stigma and discrimination in health care. *Am J Public Health*. 2025;115(3):265–267.

Acceptance Date: December 14, 2024.

DOI: https://doi.org/10.2105/AJPH.2024.307989

ORCID iD:

Rodman E. Turpin https://orcid.org/0000-0003-0457-5584

ACKNOWLEDGMENTS

R. Turpin acknowledges the continued support from the George Mason University College of Public Health, Department of Global and Community Health. R. Turpin is also supported by the National Institute on Minority Health and Health Disparities (K01MD016346); the National Heart, Lung, and Blood Institute (R01HL165686); and the National Institute of Mental Health (UG3MH133258).

Note. Any interpretations and opinions expressed herein are solely those of the author and may not reflect those of the National Institutes of Health.

CONFLICTS OF INTEREST

The author has no competing interests to declare that are relevant to the content of this article.

REFERENCES

1. Fish JN, Turpin RE, Williams ND, Boekeloo BO. Sexual identity differences in access to and satisfaction with health care: findings from nationally representative data. *Am J Epidemiol.* 2021;190(7): 1281–1293. https://doi.org/10.1093/aje/kwab012
2. Casey LS, Reisner SL, Findling MG, et al. Discrimination in the United States: experiences of lesbian, gay, bisexual, transgender, and queer Americans. *Health Serv Res.* 2019;54(suppl 2): 1454–1466. https://doi.org/10.1111/1475-6773.13229

3. Sileo KM, Baldwin A, Huynh TA, et al. Assessing LGBTQ+ stigma among healthcare professionals: an application of the health stigma and discrimination framework in a qualitative, community-based participatory research study. *J Health Psychol.* 2022; 27(9):2181–2196. https://doi.org/10.1177/13591053211027652
4. Nuriddin A, Mooney G, White AIR. Reckoning with histories of medical racism and violence in the USA. *Lancet.* 2020;396(10256):949–951. https://doi.org/10.1016/S0140-6736(20)32032-8
5. Yearby R, Clark B, Figueroa JF. Structural racism in historical and modern US health care policy. *Health Aff (Millwood).* 2022;41(2):187–194. https://doi.org/10.1377/hlthaff.2021.01466
6. Vela MB, Erondu AI, Smith NA, Peek ME, Woodruff JN, Chin MH. Eliminating explicit and implicit biases in health care: evidence and research needs. *Annu Rev Public Health.* 2022;43(1):477–501. https://doi.org/10.1146/annurev-publhealth-052620-103528
7. Forde AT, Sims M, Muntner P, et al. Discrimination and hypertension risk among African Americans in the Jackson Heart Study. *Hypertension.* 2020; 76(3):715–723. https://doi.org/10.1161/HYPERTENSIONAHA.119.14492
8. Braveman PA, Arkin E, Proctor D, Kauh T, Holm N. Systemic and structural racism: definitions, examples, health damages, and approaches to dismantling. *Health Aff (Millwood).* 2022;41(2):171–178. https://doi.org/10.1377/hlthaff.2021.01394
9. Bowleg L. The problem with the phrase women and minorities: intersectionality—an important theoretical framework for public health. *Am J Public Health.* 2012;102(7):1267–1273. https://doi.org/10.2105/AJPH.2012.300750
10. Turpin R, Camp AD, Mandell CJ, et al. PrEP stigma as a minority stressor among Black sexual minority men: a mixed-methods study. *AIDS Behav.* 2024; epub ahead of print September 17, 2024. https://doi.org/10.1007/s10461-024-04481-1
11. Hatzenbuehler ML, Bellatorre A, Lee Y, Finch BK, Muennig P, Fiscella K. Structural stigma and all-cause mortality in sexual minority populations [erratum in *Soc Sci Med.* 2018;200:271. https://doi.org/10.1016/j.socscimed.2017.11.043]. *Soc Sci Med.* 2014;103:33–41. https://doi.org/10.1016/j.socscimed.2013.06.005

Measurement Matters for Transgender Veterans' Visibility in the Electronic Health Record

Joanne G. Patterson, PhD, MPH, MSW

ABOUT THE AUTHOR

Joanne G. Patterson is with the Division of Health Behavior and Health Promotion, The Ohio State University College of Public Health and the Center for Tobacco Research, The Ohio State University Comprehensive Cancer Center, Columbus.

See also Leder et al., p. 403.

In the United States, an estimated 21.4% of transgender and gender diverse (TGD) adults have served in the US armed forces, twice that of the general population (10.4%).[1] Whereas a growing literature documents physical[2] and mental[3] health disparities among TGD adults generally, data describing TGD veterans' health are limited.

Accurate measurement of transgender-inclusive gender identity is critical for understanding health disparities among TGD veterans. Although electronic health record (EHR) systems traditionally use sex measures in the patient record, gender identity questions have been integrated in EHR packages over the past decade. Until 2021, the Veteran's Health Administration (VHA) included only legal sex measures (i.e., assigned sex at birth or, more recently, sex reflected in current legal documents). As such, researchers applied diagnostic codes for gender identity disorder[4,5] and related issues (e.g., transsexualism,[5,6] transvestic fetishism[6]) from the *International Classification of Diseases* (*ICD*) to identify TGD veterans. I believe these terms are derogatory and stigmatizing, as they pathologize gender variance as a mental health condition. However, in the absence of self-reported gender identity data, *ICD* codes have produced the most accurate method for identifying TGD veterans to date.[7]

Using *ICD* classifications, researchers have documented disparities in physical and mental health among TGD veterans, including cardiovascular disease,[8] diabetes,[8] HIV,[8] disability,[9] depression,[8] and suicidality.[8] Yet, this method cannot comprehensively identify TGD veterans in the VHA. Not all TGD veterans seek nonsurgical gender-affirming care (e.g., hormone replacement therapy, permanent hair removal, voice training), which are the only services available through the VHA. And even for those interested, knowledge about available gender-affirming services is lacking among VHA patients and providers.[10] Consequently, TGD veterans not receiving gender-affirming care through the VHA may be invisible in studies reliant on *ICD* codes.

In this issue of *AJPH*, Leder et al. (p. 403) examine how adding a self-reported gender identity field to the EHR affects estimates of health conditions among TGD veterans receiving services in the VHA. Using EHR data from fiscal years 2017 to 2023, the authors compare sociodemographic characteristics and estimate the odds of diagnosed physical and mental health conditions among TGD veterans across three groups: (1) TGD veterans identified only via *ICD* diagnoses indicating TGD experience ("*ICD* Group"), (2) self-identified TGD veterans without a TGD-related *ICD* diagnosis ("GI Group"), and (3) self-identified TGD veterans with a TGD-related *ICD* diagnosis ("Both Group").

Of 12 745 TGD participants, over two thirds self-reported TGD identity but did not have TGD-related *ICD* codes. This GI Group was younger, more racially diverse, majority urban-residing, and had higher rates of service-connected disability. When sociodemographic differences were accounted for, the GI Group reported lower odds of all physical health conditions than the *ICD* Group, including hypertension, ischemic heart disease, diabetes, HIV, and traumatic brain injury, among others. They also reported lower odds of all mental health conditions than the *ICD* Group, including anxiety, depression, posttraumatic stress disorder (PTSD), and suicide. By contrast, the Both Group and the *ICD* Group demonstrated few differences in physical health conditions, but the Both Group reported higher odds of some mental health conditions, including anxiety, PTSD, and suicidal ideation.

The variance in mental and physical health conditions experienced across these groups underscores that researchers must be cautious in applying diagnostic methods alone in population health studies of TGD veterans. That said, researchers cannot simply throw out diagnostic methods. In this sample, 23% of veterans with TGD experience did not self-report gender identity and would be excluded from samples based on gender identity alone.

AJPH March 2025, Vol. 115, No. 3

Future research utilizing VHA data should use multiple methods, as outlined by Leder et al., to identify TGD subgroups that may experience health differences. Failure to do so limits our capacity to identify these veterans' unique needs.

In addition to using self-reported gender identity and *ICD* codes, the authors also applied a two-step approach, which assesses discordance between self-reported assigned sex at birth and current gender identity to identify TGD individuals. However, for VHA data, this approach is problematic. In 2011, the VHA began allowing veterans to change their legal sex in the EHR, but did not track any changes until 2022. As such, TGD veterans who changed their sex would not have been included in this cohort unless they self-identified as transgender or had TGD-related *ICD* codes. As the two-step approach is the gold standard for identifying TGD individuals in population health surveillance,[11] future studies should examine how classification of TGD veterans via the two-step method, self-reported gender identity, and diagnostic codes affects sample demography and health estimates.

Multiple factors may explain the prevalence of chronic health conditions experienced by TGD veterans in Leder et al.'s study, which are likely cumulative and multilevel. Although the impact of social determinants on health among this population is understudied, TGD veterans are at increased risk of housing instability, financial strain, and violence. Using Department of Veterans Affairs (VA) administrative data from the years 1997 to 2014, Blosnich et al. determined that these factors were associated with poor health outcomes among TGD veterans, including mood disorders, PTSD, and suicidality.[6]

Structural stigma likely compounds these factors. Although the Department of Defense (DoD) operates separately from the VA, the historical treatment of TGD military personnel within the DoD engenders a culture of minority stress. While the US Congress repealed "Don't Ask Don't Tell" in 2011, this policy decision only benefitted sexual minority military personnel, as DoD considered TGD experience a mental health disorder or medical condition. Only when President Obama's administration rescinded the transgender ban in 2016 could TGD military personnel openly serve. This win was short-lived, as in 2017 President Trump barred TGD individuals from serving in the US military (effective in 2019). The Biden Administration overturned this ban in 2021; however, reports suggest that President Trump is planning an expanded Executive Order that would medically discharge active TGD military personnel and prevent new TGD military recruits—once again treating TGD experience as a medical condition. Given President Trump's historical treatment of TGD military members, rhetoric about "woke" military policies, and campaign promises to "cease the promotion of sex or gender transition at any stage," it is wholly unsurprising that TGD veterans fear that disclosing their TGD experience might affect their personal safety, including access to VHA benefits and services.[12] Accordingly, Leder et al. surmise that *ICD* Group members may be less willing to self-report TGD identity because of structural stigma and negative health care experiences. They also suggest that veterans identified by *ICD* codes may experience greater gender dysphoria and internalized stigma, exacerbating poor mental and physical health.

From a health equity perspective, Leder et al.'s study is a critical first step toward reducing health disparities among TGD veterans. In 2011, a landmark Institute of Medicine report highlighted TGD health and demography as priority research areas. Subsequently, the National Institutes of Health has strengthened infrastructure to support TGD research. The reality of a second Trump Administration threatens these advancements, especially for vulnerable populations for whom population-level data are lacking. Leder at al. underscore that methods matter—such that self-reported TGD-inclusive measures are critical for comprehensively documenting TGD veterans' health. For public health researchers, advocating for sex and gender identity data collection must be a continued priority. We need rigorous, population-based research to identify how social determinants, and their behavioral sequelae, account for mental and physical health conditions among TGD veterans. Only then can we identify intervention points to effectively protect and promote TGD veterans' health. AJPH

CORRESPONDENCE

Correspondence should be sent to Joanne G. Patterson, PhD, 1841 Neil Ave, Cunz 352, Columbus OH 43210 (e-mail: Patterson.1191@osu.edu). Reprints can be ordered at https://www.ajph.org by clicking the "Reprints" link.

PUBLICATION INFORMATION

Full Citation: Patterson JG. Measurement matters for transgender veterans' visibility in the electronic health record. *Am J Public Health*. 2025;115(3):268–270.

Acceptance Date: December 14, 2024.

DOI: https://doi.org/10.2105/AJPH.2024.307990

ORCID iD:
Joanne G. Patterson https://orcid.org/0000-0002-3125-2839

ACKNOWLEDGMENTS

The author has no conflicts of interest to declare.

CONFLICTS OF INTEREST

The author has no conflicts of interest to disclose.

REFERENCES

1. Gates GJ, Herman JL. Transgender military service in the United States. The Williams Institute, UCLA. 2014. Available at: https://williamsinstitute.law.ucla.edu/publications/trans-military-service-us. Accessed December 5, 2024.
2. Rich AJ, Scheim AI, Koehoorn M, Poteat T. Non-HIV chronic disease burden among transgender populations globally: a systematic review and narrative synthesis. *Prev Med Rep.* 2020;20:101259. https://doi.org/10.1016/j.pmedr.2020.101259
3. Valentine SE, Shipherd JC. A systematic review of social stress and mental health among transgender and gender non-conforming people in the United States. *Clin Psychol Rev.* 2018;66:24–38. https://doi.org/10.1016/j.cpr.2018.03.003
4. Blosnich JR, Brown GR, Shipherd JC, et al. Prevalence of gender identity disorder and suicide risk among transgender veterans utilizing Veterans Health Administration care. *Am J Public Health.* 2013;103(10):e27–e32. https://doi.org/10.2105/AJPH.2013.301507
5. Kauth MR, Shipherd JC, Lindsay J, Blosnich JR, Brown GR, Jones KT. Access to care for transgender veterans in the Veterans Health Administration: 2006–2013. *Am J Public Health.* 2014;104(suppl 4):S532–S534. https://doi.org/10.2105/AJPH.2014.302086
6. Blosnich JR, Marsiglio MC, Dichter ME, et al. Impact of social determinants of health on medical conditions among transgender veterans. *Am J Prev Med.* 2017;52(4):491–498. https://doi.org/10.1016/j.amepre.2016.12.019
7. Wolfe HL, Reisman JI, Yoon SS, et al. Validating data-driven methods for identifying transgender individuals in the Veterans Health Administration of the US Department of Veterans Affairs. *Am J Epidemiol.* 2021;190(9):1928–1934. https://doi.org/10.1093/aje/kwab102
8. Brown GR, Jones KT. Mental health and medical health disparities in 5135 transgender veterans receiving healthcare in the Veterans Health Administration: a case-control study. *LGBT Health.* 2016;3(2):122–131. https://doi.org/10.1089/lgbt.2015.0058
9. Downing J, Conron K, Herman JL, Blosnich JR. Transgender and cisgender US veterans have few health differences. *Health Aff (Millwood).* 2018;37(7):1160–1168. https://doi.org/10.1377/hlthaff.2018.0027
10. Boyer TL, Wolfe HL, Littman AJ, Shipherd JC, Kauth MR, Blosnich JR. Patient experiences and provider perspectives on accessing gender-affirming surgical services in the Veterans Health Administration. *J Gen Intern Med.* 2023;38(16):3549–3557. https://doi.org/10.1007/s11606-023-08389-9
11. National Academies of Sciences, Engineering, and Medicine. *Measuring Sex, Gender Identity, and Sexual Orientation.* Bates N, Chin M, Becker T, eds. Washington, DC: National Academies Press; 2022. https://doi.org/10.17226/26424
12. Wolfe HL, Boyer TL, Rodriguez KL, et al. Exploring research engagement and priorities of transgender and gender diverse veterans. *Mil Med.* 2023;188(5-6):e1224–e1231. https://doi.org/10.1093/milmed/usab460

Building a Representative Local Public Health Workforce: Progress, Promise, and Looming Challenges

Leah E. Masselink, PhD

ABOUT THE AUTHOR

Leah E. Masselink is with the Department of Health Policy and Management and the Mullan Institute for Health Workforce Equity at the Milken Institute School of Public Health, The George Washington University, Washington, DC.

See also Balio et al., p. 333.

Local health departments (LHDs) are on the front lines of delivering public health services to their communities, including disease prevention and surveillance, health education, and advocacy. The success of LHD activities often depends on public trust and community responsiveness, so it is critical to understand factors that foster positive relationships between LHDs and their communities. As the United States population becomes more diverse, one factor that has been discussed extensively as a possible facilitator of trust and responsiveness in public health agencies (and in health care organizations more broadly) is the degree to which the racial and ethnic composition of the workforce aligns with that of the communities they serve.[1]

MEASURING LOCAL HEALTH DEPARTMENT REPRESENTATIVENESS

The overall diversity of the governmental public health workforce (including state and local public health agencies) has been estimated before,[1] but less is known about how closely LHD employees reflect the racial and ethnic composition of their local communities. Balio et al. (p. 333) address this question by using LHD workforce race and ethnicity data from the 2021 Public Health Workforce Interests and Needs Survey and community race and ethnicity data from the 2019 National Association of City and County Health Officials Profile to estimate the representativeness of LHD workforces relative to their communities' Black, American Indian or Alaska Native, Asian, Native Hawaiian or Pacific Islander, Hispanic, and Black, Indigenous, and People of Color (BIPOC—a combination of all non-White groups) populations.

The authors' overall findings are somewhat encouraging: Balio et al. found that about 60% of LHDs in their sample had workforces that were representative of their communities' BIPOC populations—that is, the percentage of their workforce that was BIPOC was at least equal to the percentage of the community population. They also used bivariate analyses to identify several factors that were associated with higher likelihood of representativeness including serving a midsized population, being accredited, and having a decentralized governance structure. A few measures of community disadvantage were also associated with higher representativeness, including higher uninsurance rates for Black/African American and BIPOC populations and health professional shortage area designation for BIPOC populations. Multivariate analyses showed that LHDs serving larger populations were more likely to have representative workforces for BIPOC populations and most individual race and ethnicity groups. Having a shared governance structure and higher population uninsured rates were also associated with higher BIPOC representativeness.

DEVELOPING A DIVERSE PUBLIC HEALTH WORKFORCE

In interpreting their findings, Balio et al. called for LHDs and public health training programs to adopt "evidence-based practices to promote diversity, equity, and inclusion," (p. 341) with the hope that these activities will continue to increase the number of LHDs whose workforces are representative of the communities they serve. Diversity, equity, and inclusion (DEI) efforts in public health training have been ongoing for many years, including several "pipeline" programs funded by the Centers for Disease Control and Prevention that seek to increase representation of racial and ethnic minority groups in the public health workforce through early exposure and mentorship for interested undergraduate and graduate students.[2] Pipeline programs that have

AJPH March 2025, Vol. 115, No. 3

been evaluated show that most participants view them as instrumental in shaping their career goals, and high numbers of participants end up pursuing advanced degrees or careers in public health or health care.[3]

The diversity of roles pursued by alumni of public health pipeline programs also highlights a challenge for all public health employers, but especially governmental health agencies: the pipeline for the public health workforce is much less clearly defined than it is in other fields like medicine. Thousands of students earn undergraduate and graduate degrees in public health every year, and the number of undergraduate public health education programs in particular has grown in the past 20 years.[4] Undergraduate public health students are also more likely to be racial and ethnic minorities compared with public health graduate students.[5] However, most public health graduates work in roles other than governmental public health, and most governmental public health employees have degrees in fields other than public health.[4] While the presence of a growing and diverse talent pool with public health training is likely beneficial for public health employers in general, it may not be especially helpful for LHDs—especially given the range of opportunities available to public health graduates in sectors such as health care or academia.

LHDs have long faced significant challenges recruiting and retaining qualified employees because of competition with employers that offer higher salaries and more opportunities for career growth.[6] In addition to low salaries, governmental public health jobs are sometimes less appealing to applicants because of heavy workloads and complex hiring processes.[6] The consequences of these obstacles can be dire for governmental public health agencies: the governmental public health workforce lost about one in six employees between 2008 and 2019, and turnover accelerated further during the COVID-19 pandemic, when nearly half of all governmental public health employees left their jobs.[7] Turnover of governmental public health employees has been attributed to high levels of job dissatisfaction, pay dissatisfaction, and burnout, and younger and BIPOC employees are significantly more likely than others to say they plan to leave their jobs.[8]

INCREASING ACCESS IN A HOSTILE ENVIRONMENT

At the same time, public health programs (and higher education institutions in general) in many states have been forced to make major changes to their admissions processes and campus activities that could make it more difficult for them to recruit and support minority students. A recent Supreme Court decision forbade colleges and universities from considering applicants' race and ethnicity in admissions decisions,[9] and colleges and universities around the country have also curtailed campus activities focused explicitly on racial and ethnic diversity (e.g., DEI-focused job roles, identity-focused centers or courses).[10] The impact of the admissions rule changes for public health programs will take longer to track, but it is critical for colleges and universities to find new ways to increase access (e.g., need-based aid or tuition-free education based on income, closer collaboration with community colleges[11]) even in an environment that is hostile to DEI efforts—and to continue tracking student characteristics and outcomes over time to understand their impact.

LHDs and public health education programs already face distinct challenges in heeding the call by Balio et al. to implement DEI efforts to increase the racial and ethnic representativeness of LHD employees, and it is likely that funding crunches for LHDs and legal wrangling over DEI efforts in higher education will continue as the new administration takes office in 2025. In such an uncertain environment, it will be critical for LHDs and public health programs to continue and improve data collection to track the impact of DEI policy changes on public health education programs, LHD recruitment and hiring processes,[6] workforce characteristics, and outcomes. The next round of the Public Health Workforce Interests and Needs Survey was conducted in 2024, and organizers hoped it would include the largest and most comprehensive sample of LHDs yet.[12] This and other efforts to monitor LHD workforce training, diversity, and performance will be vital to improving understanding of factors that contribute to the success and sustainability of the local public health workforce. AJPH

CORRESPONDENCE

Correspondence should be sent to Leah E. Masselink, Department of Health Policy and Management, Milken Institute School of Public Health, The George Washington University, 950 New Hampshire Ave NW, Suite 600, Washington, DC 20052 (e-mail: lmasselink@gwu.edu). Reprints can be ordered at https://www.ajph.org by clicking the "Reprints" link.

PUBLICATION INFORMATION

Full Citation: Masselink LE. Building a representative local public health workforce: progress, promise, and looming challenges. *Am J Public Health*. 2025;115(3):271–273.

Acceptance Date: December 17, 2024.

DOI: https://doi.org/10.2105/AJPH.2024.307994

ORCID iD:

Leah E. Masselink https://orcid.org/0000-0001-5276-1037

CONFLICTS OF INTEREST

The author has no conflicts of interest to report.

REFERENCES

1. Coronado F, Beck AJ, Shah G, Young JL, Sellers K, Leider JP. Understanding the dynamics of diversity in the public health workforce. *J Public Health Manag Pract.* 2020;26(4):389–392. https://doi.org/10.1097/PHH.0000000000001075
2. Bouye KE, McCleary KJ, Williams KB. Increasing diversity in the health professions: reflections on student pipeline programs. *J Healthc Sci Humanit.* 2016;6(1):67–79.
3. Young KH, Liburd L, Penman-Aguilar A. An evaluation of a pipeline program to support diversity in the public health workforce: CDC Undergraduate Public Health Scholars (CUPS) Program. *Pedagogy Health Promot.* 2021;7(1, suppl): 23S–35S. https://doi.org/10.1177/237337992 11047522
4. Leider JP, Resnick B, Erwin P. Educated citizenry or workforce pipeline development? Questions for the future of undergraduate public health in the United States. *Am J Public Health.* 2022;112(4): 582–585. https://doi.org/10.2105/AJPH.2022. 306742
5. Vichare A, Park YH, Plepys CM. Diversity of the US public health workforce pipeline (2016–2020): role of academic institutions. *Am J Public Health.* 2023;113(9):1000–1008. https://doi.org/10.2105/ AJPH.2023.307352
6. Yeager VA, Krasna H. When money is not enough: reimagining public health requires systematic solutions to hiring barriers. *Health Aff (Millwood).* 2024;43(6):840–845. https://doi.org/ 10.1377/hlthaff.2024.00020
7. Leider JP, Castrucci BC, Robins M, et al. The exodus of state and local public health employees: separations started before and continued throughout COVID-19. *Health Aff (Millwood).* 2023;42(3):338–348. https://doi.org/10.1377/ hlthaff.2022.01251
8. Leider JP, Shah GH, Yeager VA, Yin J, Madamala K. Turnover, COVID-19, and reasons for leaving and staying within governmental public health. *J Public Health Manag Pract.* 2023;29(suppl 1):S54–S63. https://doi.org/10.1097/PHH.0000000000001634
9. Aaron DG, Bajaj SS, Stanford FC. Supreme Court cases on affirmative action threaten diversity in medicine. *Proc Natl Acad Sci USA.* 2023;120(17): e2220919120. https://doi.org/10.1073/pnas. 2220919120
10. Gretzinger E, Hicks M, Dutton C, Smith J. Tracking higher ed's dismantling of DEI. *Inside Higher Education.* November 15, 2024. Available at: https:// www.chronicle.com/article/tracking-higher-eds-dismantling-of-dei. Accessed November 20, 2024.
11. Lohrmann DK, Auld ME, Hawkins MI, Hicks ER, Hutton-Rogers LS. Foundational courses in health education: pathways for linking community colleges to baccalaureate programs in health education. *Pedagogy Health Promot.* 2016;2(1): 34–47. https://doi.org/10.1177/2373379916 628881
12. de Beaumont Foundation. About PH WINS: frequently asked questions. Available at: https://debeaumont.org/phwins/faqs. Accessed November 18, 2024.

The Effects of Racial Exclusion and Racial Othering on South Asian American Identity and Population Health

Ritika Rastogi, PhD, Vaishali V. Raval, PhD, Tiffany Yip, PhD, Justin A. Chen, MD, MPH, and Cindy H. Liu, PhD

ABOUT THE AUTHORS

Ritika Rastogi is with the Department of Pediatrics, Brigham and Women's Hospital, Boston, MA. Vaishali V. Raval is with the Department of Psychology, Miami University, Oxford, OH. Tiffany Yip is with the Department of Psychology, Fordham University, New York, NY. Justin A. Chen is with the Department of Psychiatry, Weill Cornell Medicine/New York–Presbyterian, New York, NY. Cindy H. Liu is with the Departments of Pediatrics and Psychiatry, Brigham and Women's Hospital, and Harvard Medical School, Boston, MA.

Asian Americans are the fastest-growing racial group in the United States,[1] yet public health research to address unique population needs is severely underfunded.[2] South Asian Americans (SAAs)—with ancestry from Bangladesh, Bhutan, India, Maldives, Nepal, Pakistan, and Sri Lanka[3]—represent a significant segment of the Asian American population: Indian Americans constitute the largest Asian national origin group in the United States, and Nepali Americans are the fastest growing.[4] As a racially marginalized group, Asian Americans and SAAs are subject to disproportionate health risks via social-structural determinants such as racism and discrimination.[5] In-depth exploration of these experiences and their role in SAA health is warranted.

SAAs face an urgent public health crisis with regard to cardiometabolic dysfunction and health risks (e.g., high blood pressure, atherosclerosis, insulin resistance, high visceral fat), exhibiting greater disease burden, earlier age of onset, and higher rates of hospitalization and mortality from these causes than Whites and other racially marginalized groups.[6] Similar to other racially marginalized groups, SAAs face barriers to mental health, including cultural stigma, access to culturally sensitive care, and sociocultural stressors.[7] Increasing evidence underscores discrimination as a driver of mental and cardiovascular health risks across populations.[8] By directly intervening on discrimination exposure in SAAs, it may be possible to disrupt the health disparities in this population.

To address this need, we advance a hypothesis of South Asian American dual racial/ethnic exclusion, specifically that SAAs experience marginalization both from broader US society and within the Asian American community. We conceive of race/ethnicity-based exclusion as a form of discrimination, or differential treatment on the basis of racial/ethnic background. We propose that these dual exclusions exacerbate health risks for SAAs and may therefore in part drive the observed disparities affecting this population. We first synthesize national survey data on the standing of SAAs within the Asian American community. To make sense of the trends, we then elaborate on the unique race/ethnicity-based experiences of SAAs, their divergence from the "prototypical Asian American experience," and the implications for within-group exclusion of SAAs from the Asian American community. We conclude by outlining an agenda for future research to disentangle race/ethnicity- and identity-based processes on health in diverse SAA communities.

GROUP-LEVEL RACIAL/ETHNIC EXCLUSION AND NONBELONGING

Asian Americans are one of the most heterogeneous racial/ethnic groups in the United States, boasting diversity in national origin, citizenship and documentation status, religion, caste, skin color, socioeconomic status, and more.[9] Nevertheless, East Asian Americans (EAAs)—with ancestry from China, Japan, Mongolia, North Korea, South Korea, and Taiwan—are overwhelmingly considered in the United States as prototypical, or representative, of the Asian American population as a whole.[10–12] Although communities of color may already face substantial disinvestment and marginalization in US society, the positioning of EAAs as normative contributes to the further erasure of SAA communities. This EAA prototypicality stereotype masks the unique sociocultural needs and barriers to health facing SAAs.

Diverse sources highlight the public prevalence of the EAA prototypicality stereotype. Using 2016 data, Lee and Ramakrishnan[13] demonstrate a significant racial/ethnic assignment incongruity: whereas 92% of Indian Americans and 94% of Pakistani Americans consider their national origin group as "somewhat" or "very likely" to be Asian American, only 74% of all Asian American adults, and 46% of all US adults, endorsed the same regarding Indian Americans. An even fewer proportion of Asian American adults (57%) and of all US adults (37%) endorsed Pakistani Americans as Asian Americans. Similar data from the Pew Research Center show that only 67% of Asian American adults perceive SAAs as part of the Asian American umbrella, relative to EAAs (89%) and Southeast Asian Americans (88%).[1] Upon disaggregation, a significant 91% of Indian Americans labeled SAA as Asian American whereas a smaller fraction of other Asian groups—ranging from 48% of Vietnamese Americans to 64% of Chinese Americans—endorsed the same. More generally, the Asian American Foundation shows that US adults surveyed on the diverse national origins of Asian Americans are least likely to identify a South Asian country as a possible place of origin.[14] These data highlight the racial/ethnic exclusion of SAAs from the Asian American community, by Asian Americans and non-Asian Americans alike.

Colorism—discrimination and erasure on the basis of skin tone—may be a potential contributor to the prototypicality of EAAs and erasure of SAAs. Although skin tone diversity spans the Asian continent, Asian Americans are largely represented as having a lighter skin tone on the basis of stereotypic depictions of EAAs.[12] By contrast, SAAs are racialized as "brown." Early and contemporary Asian American political organizing has relied on the reclamation of "Yellow Peril" rhetoric, which results in the centering of EAA experiences at the expense of others.[15] By constructing Asian American experiences of racial marginalization as synonymous with the Yellow Peril violence, Asian Americans effectively exclude as "other" the members of their community for whom such experiences do not resonate.

Racial/ethnic discrimination and colorism toward SAAs is likely exacerbated by religious discrimination, Islamophobia, and the racialization of SAAs as terrorists.[11] SAAs boast significant religious diversity, including Bahaism, Buddhism, Christianity, Hinduism, Islam, Jainism, Judaism, Sikhism, Zoroastrianism, and various Indigenous and folk traditions. Religious discrimination toward SAAs may reflect their personal faith, evidenced by Islamophobic harassment after September 11, 2001, hate crimes targeting Sikh Americans and *gurdwaras* (Sikh places of worship), and rioting and "Dotbuster" gangs against "Hindoos" throughout the 20th century.[11] Simultaneously, SAAs face Islamophobic violence regardless of religious background: the terrorist stereotype evokes the image of an ambiguously brown-skinned, bearded, or turbaned man[11,16]—characteristics spanning SAA cultures beyond religious boundaries. Spiritual practices such as wearing a *hijab* or *pagri* (turban) or keeping a beard have been construed as markers of terrorists in mainstream US culture and media, and data show that SAA men are perceived as more threatening than their East Asian American counterparts, particularly when they keep facial hair.[17] Such perceptions may reify the racial/ethnic exclusion of SAAs from other Asian American groups. Pakistani Americans appear to face greater racial/ethnic exclusion from Asian Americans than Indian Americans,[13] highlighting important within-group heterogeneity. It may be that Islamophobic attitudes drive the further distancing of Pakistanis—who are largely Muslim—from the Asian American community relative to Indians.

Thus, although SAAs overwhelmingly classify their group as belonging to Asian America, other Asian Americans are less likely to consider SAAs as members of their in-group. Non-Asian US adults are particularly unlikely to view SAAs as Asian American. Important variation appears to exist in external perceptions and classifications of SAAs, with non-SAAs classifying Indian Americans as Asian American at higher rates than Pakistani Americans. The SAA diaspora can trace their ancestry to diverse countries of origin beyond just India and Pakistan[3]; it remains to be understood whether the dual racial/ethnic exclusion extends to, or manifests differently for, other SAAs such as Bangladeshi Americans, as well as twice-migrated groups such as Indo-Guyanese or Indo-Mauritian Americans.

INDIVIDUAL RACIAL/ETHNIC SELF-IDENTIFICATION

Societal classifications of SAAs must be juxtaposed against individual self-identifications, as a survey of (dis)concordance in racial/ethnic classification holds insights for future research on multilevel mechanisms to health. Although the group-level data show that SAAs overwhelmingly classify their racial/ethnic group as belonging to the

Asian American community, important discrepancies emerge in the individual-level self-identification of SAAs. Almost two thirds (62%) of Indian adults self-identify using a national origin label (i.e., "Indian" or "Indian American") whereas only 15% use a pan-racial/ethnic label (i.e., "Asian" or "Asian American").[1] By contrast, 51% of all Asian American adults use a national origin label whereas 28% use a pan-racial/ethnic label. Among Chinese Americans, who more closely align with the Asian American prototype, 51% use a national origin label whereas one third (36%) use a pan-racial/ethnic label. Our own analysis of a large young adult sample, the 2022 American College Health Association-National College Health Assessment III,[18] revealed 830 respondents who self-identified as "other race," of whom 187 provided a write-in response indicating Asian heritage. The majority of "other race" Asians (74%) self-identified as South Asian.

Together, the data reveal a complicated picture: among individual SAAs, there is a tendency to self-identify with a national origin label (e.g., Indian, Pakistani) as opposed to the pan-racial/ethnic "Asian American" classification. Yet, when these same SAA individuals are asked about their group's overall racial standing, they strongly classify SAAs as members of the Asian American community. There may be implications for how the discrepancies in individual-level, group-level, and societal-level racial classifications of SAAs shape identity, belonging, and health processes among SAA communities.

HEALTH CONSEQUENCES OF EXCLUSION AND MISCLASSIFICATION

We propose that the dual racial/ethnic exclusion and discrimination toward SAAs from Asian Americans and non-Asian Americans contributes to either the lack of detection of poor health or direct impacts to poor health in this population. A concrete manifestation of the dual racial/ethnic exclusion of SAAs is racial/ethnic aggregation and racial misclassification in government health data. Investigating county data on suicide rates among SAAs in northern Illinois, Jha et al.[19] determined that 55% of SAAs were racially misclassified as "White" or "other race." The misclassification resulted in the gross underestimation of suicidality in this population; once corrected, suicide rates among SAAs surpassed national rates for White, Black/African American, and Asian American populations overall. Similarly, although nationwide data during the COVID-19 pandemic suggested low rates of disease burden and mortality among Asian Americans, disaggregation highlighted particularly high rates of disease positivity in SAAs.[20] As illustrated, population-level misclassification and aggregation have severe consequences for disease burden, morbidity, and mortality. Underestimates of these figures are fatal, as they mask urgent health disparities. This furthers the structural neglect of marginalized communities by deterring intervention and prevention efforts.

At the individual level, the racial/ethnic ambiguity and misclassification are likely to detrimentally affect mental health via feelings of nonbelonging and social isolation. These processes have not been explicitly examined in SAAs, yet research in American Indian/Alaska Native and multiracial individuals shows that miscategorization confers increased life stress, anxiety symptoms, depressive symptoms, and suicidal ideation.[21] As miscategorization may originate as a distinct form of racial discrimination, these experiences may further distinguish risk of discrimination-driven health outcomes in SAAs relative to "prototypical" Asian American groups.

There are competing hypotheses according to which being othered or excluded from the Asian American category may help or hinder SAA well-being. On the one hand, the exclusion of SAAs from Asian America may compound the effects of the general exclusion Asian Americans experience as racial minorities in the United States. Social exclusion—and the more subtle lack of inclusion—are harmful to mental health as they may prompt feelings of loneliness and disconnection, and this may lead to long-term declines in mental and physical well-being among SAAs.[22] Alternatively, one might view the exclusion of SAAs as protective, particularly in the context of increasing Sinophobic violence targeting Chinese Americans and Asian Americans phenotypically similar to Chinese Americans. COVID-19–related anti-Asian racism has been associated with increased depressive, anxiety, and posttraumatic stress symptomatology[23]; thus, exclusion from the Asian American umbrella and COVID-19–related anti-Asian hate may be protective for SAAs. Puzzlingly, SAAs have been found to report greater rates of COVID-19–related anti-Asian discrimination, and greater worry about future incidents of discrimination, than EAAs.[24] This preliminarily suggests that the racial/ethnic exclusion of SAAs may not be protective.

A CALL TO ACTION

Despite burgeoning evidence of the consequential effects of social determinants on health, the discussed sociocultural processes have been largely ignored in contemporary health research. To advance this area of study, we suggest that multilevel investigation of identity, race/ethnicity, and discrimination processes on SAA mental and physical health outcomes be conducted. We specifically outline two strands of inquiry that must be conducted: (1) SAA individuals' racial/ethnic self-identification and (2) SAA individuals' experiences with non-SAAs' racial (mis)classification of SAA. With respect to individual self-identifications, examples of relevant research questions include the following:

- How do individual self-identifications shape health? Are there health differences between SAAs using a national origin label (e.g., Indian, Indian American), regional label (South Asian, South Asian American), or pan-racial/ethnic label (Asian, Asian American)?
- What factors predict the likelihood of using each label? Might these factors explain observed differences in health on the basis of self-identification?

To understand SAA individuals' experiences with other Asian Americans and non-Asian Americans, relevant research questions might include the following:

- How do SAA individuals' experiences with other Asian Americans affect health? Might we observe differences in health or functioning between
  - Someone using only a national origin label experiencing exclusion from Asian Americans and
  - Someone using both a national origin label and a pan-racial/ethnic label experiencing exclusion from Asian Americans?
- How do SAA individuals' experiences with other Asian Americans and non-Asian Americans affect health? For instance, are there differences in health between
  - Someone who identifies only with a national origin label experiencing exclusion from Asian Americans and non-Asian Americans and
  - Someone using only a national origin label experiencing inclusion from Asian Americans but exclusion from non-Asian Americans?

Critically, we note that the dynamics of prototypicality and erasure present in the Asian American community at large may also plague SAAs. Individuals who fit a distinct "well-educated, English proficient" profile of Indian Americans, who demonstrate greater academic success and socioeconomic mobility,[9] may be viewed as prototypical and representative of all SAAs, masking important experiences of marginalization and oppression within SAA communities. Indeed, extant data on individual-, group-, and societal-level racial/ethnic classifications of SAAs largely represent the voices of Indian Americans, and occasionally Pakistani Americans.[1,13] It is critical to extend Asian American disaggregation efforts to SAAs, as community experiences and health may vary on the basis of national origin, skin color, religious background, socioeconomic status, caste location, migration history (e.g., once- vs twice-migrated groups, first- vs second-generation immigrants, undocumented or refugee status), and linguistic capital (e.g., English proficiency).

Future research must investigate whether the dual racial/ethnic exclusion manifests similarly for other SAAs as it does for Indian and Pakistani Americans. We also underscore the urgency of understanding the within-SAA community dynamics and whether prototypicality of Indian American affects identity and health for non-Indian American groups. Marginalization within the SAA community might exacerbate the marginalization of SAAs from Asian Americans, placing these multiply marginalized groups at elevated health risk. For instance, on the one hand, Bhutanese American individuals identifying as both SAA and Asian American may face particularly high levels of racial/ethnic exclusion and associated poor health. On the other hand, a Bhutanese American who does not identify as SAA or Asian American may not experience the same level of individual health risk.

To reach multiply marginalized individuals and communities, it is critical to use community-engaged and participatory approaches. Without intentional community building, it is likely that research on SAAs will predominantly include samples of high-income, highly educated, caste-privileged North Indian Americans. Rubin et al. outline a comprehensive plan for sensitive and rigorous study design, data collection, and analysis of health in "small and hard-to-reach communities,"[25(p20)] including those plagued by issues of racial misidentification and misclassification. It is imperative to invest in efforts to develop methodologically rigorous approaches that adequately contend with the limits posed by small sample sizes. To advance population health equity, it is necessary to disentangle the roles of identity, race/ethnicity, and discrimination processes on, and within, SAA communities. AJPH

CORRESPONDENCE

Correspondence should be sent to Cindy H. Liu, PhD, Brigham and Women's Hospital, 221 Longwood Ave, BLI 341, Boston, MA 02215 (e-mail: chliu@bwh.harvard.edu). Reprints can be ordered at https://www.ajph.org by clicking the "Reprints" link.

PUBLICATION INFORMATION

Full Citation: Rastogi R, Raval VV, Yip T, Chen JA, Liu CH. The effects of racial exclusion and racial othering on South Asian American identity and population health. *Am J Public Health*. 2025;115(3): 274–278.

Acceptance Date: November 11, 2024.

DOI: https://doi.org/10.2105/AJPH.2024.307938

ORCID iDs:

Ritika Rastogi https://orcid.org/0000-0002-1998-7795

Vaishali V. Raval https://orcid.org/0000-0002-8790-7953

Tiffany Yip https://orcid.org/0000-0001-7488-533X

Justin A. Chen https://orcid.org/0000-0002-1504-0094

CONTRIBUTORS

R. Rastogi was involved in conceptualization, data curation, formal analysis, investigation, methodology, project administration, writing the original draft, and writing review and editing. V. V. Raval was involved in writing review and editing. T. Yip and J. A. Chen contributed to writing review and editing. C. H. Liu contributed to conceptualization, data curation, methodology, project administration, and writing review and editing.

ACKNOWLEDGMENTS

R. Rastogi, T. Yip, and C. H. Liu were supported by the National Institute of Mental Health (1R01 MH129360-01). C. H. Liu was additionally supported by the Family Health and Resilience Fund.

We thank the members of the Developmental Risk and Cultural Resilience Laboratory for their feedback and support in completing this project. We also thank the American College Health Association (ACHA) for providing and approving the use of the American College Health Association-National College Health Assessment III (ACHA-NCHA III) spring 2022 data set.

Note. The opinions, findings, and conclusions reported in this article are those of the authors and do not represent in any way the opinions, views, or policies of the ACHA. The ACHA does not warrant nor assume any liability or responsibility for the accuracy, completeness, or usefulness of any information presented in this article/presentation.

CONFLICTS OF INTEREST

The author has no conflicts of interest to disclose.

HUMAN PARTICIPANT PROTECTION

This analysis was exempt from human subjects review according to the institutional review board of Mass Brigham General.

REFERENCES

1. Ruiz NG, Noe-Bustamante L, Shah S. Diverse cultures and shared experiences shape Asian American identities. Pew Research Center. 2023. Available at: https://www.pewresearch.org/race-and-ethnicity/2023/05/08/diverse-cultures-and-shared-experiences-shape-asian-american-identities. Accessed May 10, 2024.
2. Yip T, Lorenzo K, Bae J, et al. Anti-Asian biases in federal grant reviews: commentary on Yip et al. (2021). *Am Psychol*. 2024;79(5):770–776. https://doi.org/10.1037/amp0001337
3. Kandula NR, Islam N, Needham BL, et al. A multi-level framework to investigate cardiovascular health disparities among South Asian immigrants in the United States. *Ann Epidemiol*. 2023;81: 24–30.e1. https://doi.org/10.1016/j.annepidem.2023.02.012
4. Rico B, Hahn JK, Spence C. Chinese, except Taiwanese, was the largest Asian alone or in any combination group; Nepalese population grew fastest. US Census Bureau. 2023. Available at: https://www.census.gov/library/stories/2023/09/2020-census-dhc-a-asian-population.html. Accessed November 4, 2024.
5. Paradies Y, Ben J, Denson N, et al. Racism as a determinant of health: a systematic review and meta-analysis. *PLoS One*. 2015;10(9):e0138511. https://doi.org/10.1371/journal.pone.0138511
6. Volgman AS, Palaniappan LS, Aggarwal NT, et al. Atherosclerotic cardiovascular disease in South Asians in the United States: epidemiology, risk factors, and treatments: a scientific statement from the American Heart Association [erratum in *Circulation*. 2018;138(5):e76]. *Circulation*. 2018;138(1):e1–e34. https://doi.org/10.1161/CIR.0000000000000580
7. Karasz A, Gany F, Escobar J, et al. Mental health and stress among South Asians. *J Immigr Minor Health*. 2019;21(suppl 1):7–14. https://doi.org/10.1007/s10903-016-0501-4
8. Williams DR, Lawrence JA, Davis BA, Vu C. Understanding how discrimination can affect health. *Health Serv Res*. 2019;54(suppl 2):1374–1388. https://doi.org/10.1111/1475-6773.13222
9. Budiman A, Ruiz NG. Key facts about Asian Americans, a diverse and growing population. Pew Research Center. 2021. Available at: https://www.pewresearch.org/short-reads/2021/04/29/key-facts-about-asian-americans. Accessed June 12, 2023.
10. Goh JX, McCue J. Perceived prototypicality of Asian subgroups in the United States and the United Kingdom. *J Exp Soc Psychol*. 2021;97: 104201. https://doi.org/10.1016/j.jesp.2021.104201
11. Kurien P, Purkayastha B. Why don't South Asians in the US count as "Asian"? Global and local factors shaping anti-South Asian racism in the United States. *Sociol Inq*. 2024;94(2):351–368. https://doi.org/10.1111/soin.12592
12. Ma DS, Koltai K, McManus RM, Bernhardt A, Correll J, Wittenbrink B. Race signaling features: identifying markers of racial prototypicality among Asians, Blacks, Latinos, and Whites. *Soc Cogn*. 2018;36(6):603–625. https://doi.org/10.1521/soco.2018.36.6.603
13. Lee J, Ramakrishnan K. Who counts as Asian. *Ethn Racial Stud*. 2020;43(10):1733–1756. https://doi.org/10.1080/01419870.2019.1671600
14. Asian American Foundation. Attitudes towards Asian Americans and Pacific Islanders. 2023. Available at: https://www.staatus-index.org. Accessed June 12, 2023.
15. Nadal KL. The Brown Asian American movement: advocating for South Asian, Southeast Asian, and Filipino American communities. *Asian Am Policy Rev*. 2019;29:2–11. Available at: https://studentreview.hks.harvard.edu/the-brown-asian-american-movement-advocating-for-south-asian-southeast-asian-and-filipino-american-communities. Accessed November 4, 2024.
16. Thangaraj S. "They said 'Go back to Afghanistan'": South Asian American basketball culture and challenging the "terrorist" stereotype. *Amerasia J*. 2015;41(2):25–46. https://doi.org/10.17953/aj.41.2.25
17. Goh JX, Trofimchuk V. Gendered perceptions of East and South Asian men. *Soc Cogn*. 2023;41(6): 537–561. https://doi.org/10.1521/soco.2023.41.6.537
18. Lederer AM, Hoban MT. The development of the American College Health Association-National College Health Assessment III: an improved tool to assess and enhance the health and well-being of college students. *J Am Coll Health*. 2022;70(6): 1606–1610. https://doi.org/10.1080/07448481.2020.1834401
19. Jha A, Ahuja M, Wani RJ. Suicide among South Asians in the United States: a growing public health problem. *SAGE Open*. 2022;12(4). https://doi.org/10.1177/21582440221140378
20. Marcello RK, Dolle J, Tariq A, et al. Disaggregating Asian race reveals COVID-19 disparities among Asian American patients at New York City's public hospital system. *Public Health Rep*. 2022;137(2): 317–325. https://doi.org/10.1177/00333549211061313
21. Laster Pirtle WN, Brown TN. Inconsistency within expressed and observed racial identifications: implications for mental health status. *Sociol Perspect*. 2016;59(3):582–603. https://doi.org/10.1177/0731121415602133
22. Valtorta NK, Kanaan M, Gilbody S, Ronzi S, Hanratty B. Loneliness and social isolation as risk factors for coronary heart disease and stroke: systematic review and meta-analysis of longitudinal observational studies. *Heart*. 2016;102(13):1009–1016. https://doi.org/10.1136/heartjnl-2015-308790
23. Ibrahim A, Wong SHM, Kim SE, et al. A scoping review of mental health and discrimination of Asian Americans and Pacific Islanders in the United States during the COVID-19 pandemic. *Nat Ment Health*. 2024;2(2):244–253. https://doi.org/10.1038/s44220-023-00177-y
24. Okazaki S, Lee CS, Prasai A, Chang DF, Yoo N. Disaggregating the data: diversity of COVID-19 stressors, discrimination, and mental health among Asian American communities. *Front Public Health*. 2022;10:956076. https://doi.org/10.3389/fpubh.2022.956076
25. Rubin V, Ngo D, Ross Á, Butler D, Balaram N. Counting a diverse nation: disaggregating data on race and ethnicity to advance a culture of health. PolicyLink. 2018. Available at: https://www.policylink.org/sites/default/files/Counting_a_Diverse_Nation_08_15_18.pdf. Accessed November 4, 2024.

Public Health Data to Action: Reframing Surveillance to Build Trust in Public Health

Thomas J. Stopka, PhD, MHS, Jack Cordes, PhD, MS, Dana Bernson, MPH, Ric Bayly, MS, MPH, and Cici Bauer, PhD, MS

ABOUT THE AUTHORS

Thomas J. Stopka, Jack Cordes, and Ric Bayly are with the Department of Public Health and Community Medicine, Tufts University School of Medicine, Boston, MA. Dana Bernson is with the Office of Population Health, Department of Public Health, Commonwealth of Massachusetts, Boston, MA. Cici Bauer is with the Department of Biostatistics and Data Science and the Center for Spatial-Temporal Modeling for Applications in Population Sciences, School of Public Health, University of Texas Health Science Center at Houston.

If one searches for definitions of "surveillance" online, various options are found, including "close observation, especially of a suspected spy or criminal"[1]; "the monitoring of behavior . . . or information for the purpose of information gathering, influencing, managing, or directing"[2]; "close watch kept over someone or something (as by a detective)"[3]; and "the act of watching a person or a place, especially a person believed to be involved with criminal activity."[4] Except for the second definition, there is a nefarious element to these descriptions, often tied to criminal activity. By contrast, in public health and epidemiology, surveillance is meant to define "the ongoing systematic collection, analysis, and interpretation of data, closely integrated with the timely dissemination of these data to those responsible for preventing and controlling disease and injury."[5(p164)] Considering the unintended negative connotations commonly associated with the term, public health leaders have questioned whether the use of "surveillance" should be abandoned, especially considering the declining trust in public health institutions in the United States since the COVID-19 pandemic.[6,7]

"Public health data monitoring" may be a better alternative to surveillance, but as Morabia et al. point out, "monitoring" also carries connotations of supervision, overseeing, or regulation.[6] They note that "public health data" alone avoids the negative connotations of "surveillance" or "monitoring." However, this term may be too broad, as it encompasses all types of public health data. Additionally, "public health data" may overlook the importance of the data collection process and the need to interpret data to inform public health or clinical actions.

We advocate using the term "public health data to action" to supplant the term "surveillance." The term "data to action" eschews the negative connotations of "surveillance" or "monitoring" while remaining active and specific to conducting ongoing evaluation of public health data. Furthermore, "data to action" suggests the idea of "translating knowledge to action," promoting public health data collection and analysis that strives to be unbiased, systematic, and essential to data-informed decision-making and interventions.

A data-to-action framework, as described by Zakocs et al., is a rapid program improvement process that aims to "guide evaluators and practitioners in using rapid-feedback cycles to generate actionable data for improving implementation of ongoing multicomponent programs."[8(p472)] This framework appears to embody all the attributes of surveillance, in its traditional public health and epidemiological sense, but without the nefarious subtexts. We suggest a modified and enhanced rendition of this data-to-action framework, incorporating the following key elements and flow: data collection, measurement, cleaning, analysis, interpretation, planning, and action. Each subsequent element builds on the previous constituent step, ultimately enabling opportunities for data-informed action and helping to prioritize public health responses. We provide examples and contemplations herein on the role that public health data to action has played and can play to inform our work.

The Massachusetts Department of Public Health (MDPH), where coauthor Bernson helps lead statewide epidemiological efforts, adopted the term "Public Health Data Warehouse" in 2017 to describe a large public health data system. This system includes more than 35 linked administrative data sets, including data from most of the Massachusetts population.[9] The MDPH Public Health Data Warehouse was initially developed, following a state legislative mandate, to help public health practitioners, policymakers, and researchers better understand the opioid-related overdose epidemic.

Although initially referred to as a "surveillance system," MDPH recognized the challenges associated with this term. Input from a community advisory board, which expressed concerns about the term "surveillance" similar to those we have noted, ultimately led to MDPH's decision to call the Public Health Data Warehouse a "public health data analysis tool."

The term "public health data" was believed to remove references to connotations of devious behavior, crime, sleuthing, and detectives. It plainly stated what the data represented: data from and for the masses used to protect the public's health writ large. However, "public health data" lost the active components of the surveillance definition (e.g., analysis, interpretation, planning, and action through dissemination and guidance), a challenge that MDPH addressed by adding "analysis tool."

In our fieldwork, we often contemplate the public health jargon we use, aiming to communicate clearly and effectively with a broad audience. When conducting studies on opioid-related morbidity and mortality, we have noticed confusion and hesitancy among potential participants who use drugs when we use terms such as "syndromic surveillance," "investigations," and "monitoring and evaluation." Such terms, sometimes frightening for lay community members and study participants, evoke connotations of suspicion and criminality, cultivating mistrust between researchers and participants. This mistrust is compounded by the appalling historical missteps of studies that failed to follow ethical research standards, such as the untreated syphilis study at Tuskegee—which fostered long-lasting skepticism toward public health and clinical agencies and hesitation to participate in subsequent reputable and ethically conducted research.[10] To address and diminish such skepticism, we believe that use of the term "public health data to action" in the screening, consent, and data collection steps of research and in documents tied to research can help to better set the stage for the important work of assessing and responding to public health challenges.

A significant portion of public health data are subject to structures of power because governments, corporations, academic institutions, or other organizations ultimately have control over what data are collected and how they are used. Moving away from the term "surveillance" and toward "data to action" may take us one step closer to the democratization of public health and public health data, as aspired to in Nancy Krieger's *Epidemiology and the People's Health*.[11] "Public health data to action," a term that is devoid of jargon, can help to broaden understanding of public health data and data systems without reference to surveillance, monitoring, and evaluation. Using this terminology can help us get closer to making public health data more accessible and equitable, broadening the understanding that data benefit all stakeholders through analysis, interpretation, dissemination, planning, and action. AJPH

CORRESPONDENCE

Correspondence should be sent to Thomas J. Stopka, PhD, MHS, Department of Public Health and Community Medicine, Tufts University School of Medicine, 136 Harrison Ave, Boston, MA 02111 (e-mail: Thomas.Stopka@tufts.edu). Reprints can be ordered at https://www.ajph.org by clicking the "Reprints" link.

PUBLICATION INFORMATION

Full Citation: Stopka TJ, Cordes J, Bernson D, Bayly R, Bauer C. Public health data to action: reframing surveillance to build trust in public health. *Am J Public Health*. 2025;115(3):279–281.

Acceptance Date: November 18, 2024.

DOI: https://doi.org/10.2105/AJPH.2024.307947

ORCID iDs:

Thomas J. Stopka https://orcid.org/0000-0003-2314-8924

Jack Cordes https://orcid.org/0000-0003-2706-615X

Dana Bernson https://orcid.org/0000-0003-1510-4489

Ric Bayly https://orcid.org/0009-0008-3295-1704

Cici Bauer https://orcid.org/0000-0002-2337-7965

CONTRIBUTORS

T. J. Stopka and C. Bauer acquired funding. All authors wrote, reviewed, and edited the editorial.

ACKNOWLEDGMENTS

This editorial was supported by the National Institute on Drug Abuse, National Institutes of Health ([NIH] award R01DA054267; multiple principal investigators: T. J. S., C. B.).

Note. The content of this editorial is solely the responsibility of the authors and does not necessarily represent the official views of the NIH.

CONFLICTS OF INTEREST

The authors do not have any conflicts of interest to report.

REFERENCES

1. Oxford University Press. *Oxford English Dictionary*, s.v. "surveillance." 2024. Available at: https://languages.oup.com/research/oxford-english-dictionary. Accessed December 3, 2024.
2. Surveillance. *Wikipedia*. August 3, 2024. Available at: https://en.wikipedia.org/w/index.php?title=Surveillance&oldid=1238446293. Accessed August 13, 2024.
3. *Merriam-Webster Dictionary*, s.v. "surveillance." 2024. Available at: https://www.merriam-webster.com/dictionary/surveillance. Accessed August 13, 2024.
4. Cambridge University Press. *Cambridge English Dictionary*, s.v. "surveillance." 2024. Available at: https://dictionary.cambridge.org/us/dictionary/english/surveillance. Accessed August 13, 2024.
5. Thacker SB, Berkelman RL. Public health surveillance in the United States. *Epidemiol Rev*. 1988;10(1):164–190. https://doi.org/10.1093/oxfordjournals.epirev.a036021
6. Morabia A, Dasgupta N, Thorpe L. Public health surveillance, monitoring, or data? Time to decide. *Am J Public Health*. 2024;114(7):661–662. https://doi.org/10.2105/AJPH.2024.307709
7. SteelFisher GK, Findling MG, Caporello HL, et al. Trust in US federal, state, and local public health agencies during COVID-19: responses and policy implications. *Health Aff (Millwood)*. 2023;42(3):328–337. https://doi.org/10.1377/hlthaff.2022.01204

8. Zakocs R, Hill JA, Brown P, Wheaton J, Freire KE. The data-to-action framework: a rapid program improvement process. *Health Educ Behav.* 2015;42(4):471–479. https://doi.org/10.1177/1090198115595010
9. Massachusetts Department of Public Health. Public Health Data Warehouse (PHD). 2024. Available at: https://www.mass.gov/public-health-data-warehouse-phd. Accessed August 13, 2024.
10. Centers for Disease Control and Prevention. The untreated syphilis study at Tuskegee timeline. September 4, 2024. Available at: https://www.cdc.gov/tuskegee/about/timeline.html. Accessed August 13, 2024.
11. Krieger N. *Epidemiology and the People's Health: Theory and Context.* New York, NY: Oxford University Press; 2011. https://doi.org/10.1093/acprof:oso/9780195383874.001.0001

Real-Time Linkage of Public-Facing Jail Registers and Syphilis Testing and Treatment Monitoring Data, Washington State, 2023–2024

Steven J. Erly, PhD, MPH, Leighton O. Hill, MPH, Kiara B. Gavigan, Kari L. Haecker, BS, and Rachel M. Amiya, PhD

Between June 22, 2023, and January 22, 2024, we implemented scripts to collect public-facing correctional facility rosters and used a matching algorithm to link these data to unresolved syphilis investigations in Washington state. We reviewed the results and sent alerts to the assigned disease intervention specialist. We captured data from 60 of Washington's 69 correctional facilities and linked 54 individuals to testing or treatment. Fifty-eight percent of individuals had been unlocated for 60 days or more and may not have been found otherwise. (*Am J Public Health*. 2025;115(3):282–286. https://doi.org/10.2105/AJPH.2024.307911)

AJPH March 2025, Vol. 115, No. 3

Syphilis diagnoses have increased dramatically nationally and in Washington state over recent years. In the absence of additional funding and staff, new tools are needed to improve the efficiency and reach of disease intervention specialists (DISs), particularly in populations disproportionately affected by syphilis.

INTERVENTION AND IMPLEMENTATION

We developed an automated linkage process between Washington state's surveillance reporting system Public Health Issue Management System–Sexually Transmitted Diseases and publicly available correctional rosters. Using the Rvest and HTTR packages in R software version 4.3.2 (RStudio, Boston, MA), we accessed and parsed jail and prison rosters on local government Web sites, then we used a simple deterministic linkage algorithm to match them to all unresolved syphilis investigations since the beginning of 2023. The algorithm blocks on first and last name Soundex and compares first and last name (weighted by 2010 census name frequency),[1] middle name, date of birth, year of birth, and county of incarceration or residence. Because Soundex matches by sound, it allows phonetic matches even if names are spelled slightly differently, which may happen, as case reports are manually entered. The results of the match were output as a daily report containing matched identifiers from the STI surveillance and corrections data systems and the name of the facility where the person was being held.

Surveillance staff manually reviewed the report to check the quality of the matches and to ensure that no free-text notes indicated successful contact or knowledge of the person's incarceration. For the remaining matches, we sent an e-mail alert to the assigned DIS containing the individual's unique identifier and the facility of incarceration. An overview of the data-processing steps can be found in Figure 1.

PLACE, TIME, AND PERSONS

We describe results from our linkage process performed between June 22, 2023, and January 22, 2024, in Washington state. The linkage and alert process occurred three times a week (Monday, Wednesday, and Friday) from June 22, 2023, through October 20, 2023, and daily after this.

PURPOSE

In the United States, the number of primary and secondary syphilis diagnoses increased by 68% between 2018 and 2022.[2] Along with this, there has been

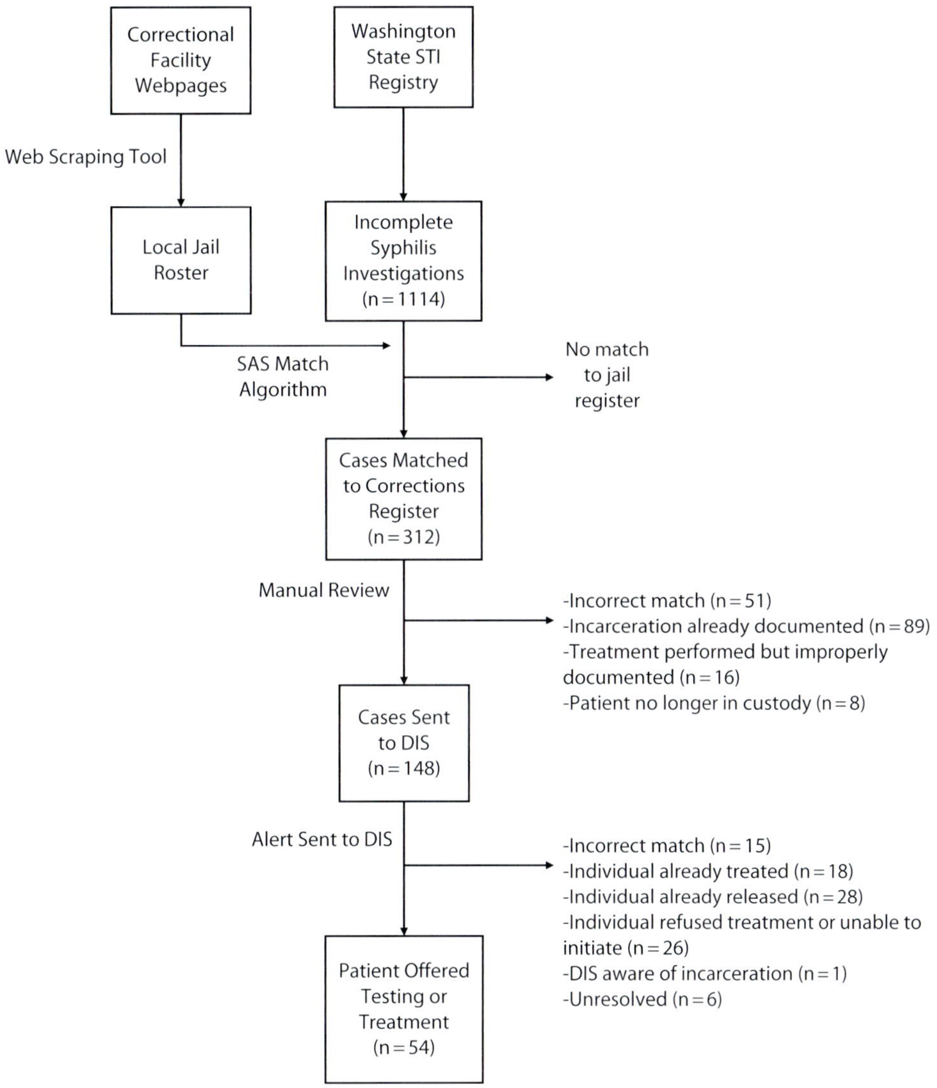

FIGURE 1— Process Map of Syphilis–Jail Record Linkage: Washington State, June 22, 2023–January 22, 2024

Note. DIS = disease intervention specialist; SAS = statistical analysis system; STI = sexually transmitted infection.

declining success in locating index patients and partners for syphilis partner services.[3,4] One reason for this may be a shift in the demographics of individuals with syphilis; there have been large increases in the proportion of primary and secondary syphilis patients reporting methamphetamine use in the past 12 months among women (168% increase in 2013–2017) and men who have sex with women (166% increase in 2013–2017).[2,5,6] More than ever, the epidemic continues to concentrate among populations experiencing poor access to health services, social marginalization, or low socioeconomic status.[7]

The factors that make these populations difficult to find via traditional means also increase their chances of criminal–legal involvement.[8,9] For DISs, this presents an opportunity for locating individuals when they appear in correctional facilities. However, the information shared by these facilities in many cases is decentralized and spread across individual facility Web sites. This makes monitoring these rosters for unlocated individuals prohibitively time consuming, especially when individuals appear in jail or prison weeks or months after their syphilis exposure or diagnosis. Jail-based syphilis screening is not offered in all facilities and may be logistically difficult for individuals who are incarcerated for a short time.

Automated collection and linkage may be an opportunity to make this information more available and actionable for DISs. Web-scraping tools have been used in other public health settings to collect information about incarcerated populations and could increase public health's ability to make services accessible to people with a syphilis diagnosis or exposure, especially among populations that are difficult to reach via traditional means.

EVALUATION AND ADVERSE EFFECTS

We tabulated the number of matches generated, the number of e-mail alerts sent, and the outcome of each alert as of January 22, 2024. We stratified these results by whether the identified person had syphilis or was a named partner of someone with syphilis (Table 1).

We described the population successfully tested and treated by age, gender identity, race/ethnicity, coinfection with gonorrhea or chlamydia, and time from infection to documentation of treatment by health department staff. We compared these demographics to those of other successful syphilis investigations in Washington state in this time frame using the Fisher exact test.

We successfully collected data from 60 of 69 adult correctional facilities in Washington state. We identified 312 individuals with potential matches between these registries. We sent data for 148 (47%) individuals to DISs for investigation: 54 (36%) individuals were successfully tested, treated, or both. Of the remainder, we found that 18 (12%) had already been treated and this documentation was then updated appropriately in our surveillance system, 26 (18%) were individuals for whom treatment could not be initiated or verified or was refused by the patient, information on 15 (10%) individuals sent for investigation ultimately involved incorrect matches, and information on 28 (19%) were true matches but the individual was released from custody before follow-up could be initiated. Information on 6 (4%) individuals was unresolved as of January 22, 2024, and will continue to be monitored.

Among the incorrect matches (16% of all matches), most were among people with common first and last names that exactly matched but whose county or year of birth did not match. This was intentional in our match code, as patients may move between counties, and years are sometimes misentered by one digit. Given that there were several true matches under these conditions, we felt it was important to initially include all possible matches to avoid missing potential patients. It typically took us less than five minutes per day to manually review incorrect matches.

Compared with individuals with syphilis found through traditional means, the individuals found through the corrections match were more likely to identify

TABLE 1— Outcome of Record Linkages Between Public Jail Registers and Unresolved Syphilis Investigations: Washington State, June 22, 2023–January 22, 2024

Outcome	Index Cases, No. (%)	Partners, No. (%)	Total, No. (%)
All matches	102 (100)	210 (100)	312 (100)
Incorrect match[a]	12 (12)	39 (19)	51 (16)
DIS aware of incarceration[a]	44 (43)	45 (21)	89 (29)
Individual already treated[a]	5 (5)	11 (5)	16 (5)
Patient not in custody[a]	2 (2)	6 (3)	8 (3)
Sent for investigation[a]	39 (38)	109 (52)	148 (47)
Individual found, tested, and/or treated[b]	13 (33)	41 (38)	54 (36)
Patient already treated[b]	6 (15)	12 (11)	18 (12)
Unable to initiate/verify treatment or treatment refused[b]	8 (20)	18 (17)	26 (18)
DIS aware of incarceration[b]	0 (0)	1 (< 1)	1 (< 1)
Incorrect match[b]	1 (3)	14 (13)	15 (10)
Individual released before contact[b]	8 (21)	20 (18)	28 (19)
Unresolved[b]	3 (8)	3 (3)	6 (4)

Note. DIS = disease intervention specialist. We collected corrections rosters from public-facing registers for 60 of 69 correctional institutions in Washington state and linked them to the Washington state sexually transmitted infection surveillance registry via a deterministic match process. We defined unresolved syphilis investigations as syphilis diagnoses or exposures reported to the Washington State Department of Health that did not have documented testing and treatment (if necessary).

[a]We computed percentages based on the number of all matches.

[b]We computed percentages based on the number of matches that were sent for investigation.

as American Indian/Alaska Native (17% vs 5%; $P < .01$) and more likely to have been unlocated for 60 or more days (58% vs 3%; $P < .01$). The distribution of gender identity, age group, stage of syphilis at diagnosis, and likelihood of having a coinfection with another STI was similar between groups. For located patients found via record linkage or other means, cisgender men represented 63%. Cisgender women represented 37% of individuals found via the record linkage and 33% found via other means ($P = .16$). Although the gender distribution was similar among located patients, it was different from the overall distribution of incarcerated people. From 2020 to 2022, more than 92% of people in state or federal correctional authorities were men.[10] Syphilis stage of diagnosis was comparable for individuals found via the record linkage (60% early syphilis, 40% late or unknown) and those found via other means (63% early syphilis, 37% late or unknown; $P = .73$). Age at diagnosis was comparable for individuals found via record linkage and other means, with those aged 25 to 54 years making up 80% and 78% of located patients, respectively ($P = .08$). Among individuals found through the record linkage, 83% were incarcerated in a jurisdiction that matched the jurisdiction of their documented case, and 17% were not.

The 39 individuals with syphilis matched to the rosters and sent for investigation during this time represented 4% of the 1114 individuals with syphilis who were unlocated during the project and eligible for our match. This information was not available for partners, as partner testing data are not automatically date stamped in the Washington STI surveillance registry. There were no adverse outcomes related to this program.

SUSTAINABILITY

After the initial establishment of the scripts, the process we developed took very little time to run and is significantly faster than the previous process of manually searching a limited number of local jail rosters. Because this automation improved the efficiency of processes the DIS was already undertaking manually, we did not need to hire additional surveillance staff or reallocate work. We estimated that the daily amount of time spent on this effort was 15 minutes (5 minutes to perform the linkage and 10 minutes to review the results and send alerts). Approximately 60 minutes per month were spent on maintaining the Web-scraping programs.

PUBLIC HEALTH SIGNIFICANCE

Our program was successful at identifying when individuals with incomplete syphilis investigations entered a correctional facility and linking them to care. The relatively large amount of time that most of the individuals we found went unlocated (58% of individuals were unlocated for ≥ 60 days) strongly suggests, based on common syphilis investigation protocols, that they were no longer being actively pursued and would not have otherwise been found. A meaningful number of individuals (17%) was in a jurisdiction different from that of the original case and would have been difficult for investigators to find even if they were actively monitoring the original county's jail roster. Finally, we have received positive feedback from DISs involved in this project, with staff indicating that it both saved time and helped them find individuals that they had considered lost.

As syphilis continues to concentrate in marginalized populations, enhanced monitoring of jail rosters can be a useful tool for ensuring that all people are aware of their syphilis infections and have access to appropriate treatment. Public health programs looking to bolster their STI services should consider a similar approach. AJPH

ABOUT THE AUTHORS

Steven J. Erly is with the Washington State Department of Health, Tumwater, and the Department of Epidemiology, University of Washington, Seattle. Leighton O. Hill, Kiara B. Gavigan, Kari L. Haecker, and Rachel M. Amiya are with the Office of Infectious Disease, Washington State Department of Health, Tumwater.

CORRESPONDENCE

Correspondence should be sent to Leighton Hill, 101 Israel Rd S.E., Tumwater, WA 98501 (e-mail: leighton.hill@doh.wa.gov). Reprints can be ordered at https://www.ajph.org by clicking the "Reprints" link.

PUBLICATION INFORMATION

Full Citation: Erly SJ, Hill LO, Gavigan KB, Haecker KL, Amiya RM. Real-time linkage of public-facing jail registers and syphilis testing and treatment monitoring data, Washington state, 2023–2024. *Am J Public Health*. 2025;115(3):282–286.

Acceptance Date: October 28, 2024.

DOI: https://doi.org/10.2105/AJPH.2024.307911

ORCID iDs:

Steven J. Erly https://orcid.org/0000-0001-5477-9660

Leighton O. Hill https://orcid.org/0009-0009-9070-8275

Kari L. Haecker https://orcid.org/0009-0006-6582-2728

CONTRIBUTORS

S. J. Erly and L. O. Hill developed the automated match process, analyzed the data, and drafted the article. S. J. Erly and K. L. Haecker developed the idea for this record linkage. K. B. Gavigan led the manual match review and data collection. K. L. Haecker, K. B. Gavigan, and R. M. Amiya contributed to the writing.

ACKNOWLEDGMENTS

The authors would like to thank all disease intervention specialists in Washington state who supported linkage to care efforts for individuals located through this program.

CONFLICTS OF INTEREST

The authors have no conflicts of interest to disclose.

HUMAN PARTICIPANT PROTECTION

This project was performed as a program evaluation using surveillance data and is exempt from institutional review board review in Washington state.

REFERENCES

1. Comenetz J. Frequently occurring surnames in the 2010 census. October 2016. Available at: https://www2.census.gov/topics/genealogy/2010surnames/surnames.pdf. Accessed December 13, 2024.
2. Centers for Disease Control and Prevention. Sexually transmitted infections surveillance, 2023. November 12, 2024. Available at: https://www.cdc.gov/sti-statistics/annual/index.html. Accessed December 13, 2024.
3. Cope AB, Bernstein K, Matthias J, et al. Unnamed partners from syphilis partner services interviews, 7 jurisdictions. *Sex Transm Dis.* 2020;47(12):811–818. https://doi.org/10.1097/OLQ.0000000000001269
4. Rowlinson E, Goings S, Minnerly S, Surita K, Pogosjans S. Differences in partner services outcomes for men who have sex with men diagnosed with primary and secondary syphilis by HIV serostatus. *Sex Transm Dis.* 2018;45(3):152–157. https://doi.org/10.1097/OLQ.0000000000000710
5. Schmidt R, Carson PJ, Jansen RJ. Resurgence of syphilis in the United States: an assessment of contributing factors. *Infect Dis (Auckl).* 2019;12:1178633719883282. https://doi.org/10.1177/1178633719883282
6. Centers for Disease Control and Prevention. Increased methamphetamine, injection drug, and heroin use among women and heterosexual men with primary and secondary syphilis—United States, 2013–2017. *MMWR Morb Mortal Wkly Rep.* 2019;68(6):144–148. https://doi.org/10.15585/mmwr.mm6806a4
7. Fenton KA, Breban R, Vardavas R, et al. Infectious syphilis in high-income settings in the 21st century. *Lancet Infect Dis.* 2008;8(4):244–253. https://doi.org/10.1016/S1473-3099(08)70065-3
8. Harmon JL, Dhaliwal SK, Burghardt NO, et al. Routine screening in a California jail: effect of local policy on identification of syphilis in a high-incidence area, 2016–2017. *Public Health Rep.* 2020;135(1 suppl):57S–64S. https://doi.org/10.1177/0033354920928454
9. Wiehe SE, Barai N, Rosenman MB, Aalsma MC, Scanlon ML, Fortenberry JD. Test positivity for chlamydia, gonorrhea, and syphilis infection among a cohort of individuals released from jail in Marion County, Indiana. *Sex Transm Dis.* 2015;42(1):30–36. https://doi.org/10.1097/OLQ.0000000000000224
10. Carson EA. Prisoners in 2022—statistical tables. 2024. Available at: https://bjs.ojp.gov/document/p22st.pdf. Accessed October 6, 2024.

Improving Participation in HIV Preexposure Prophylaxis via an Informatics Approach—a Process-Improvement Project

Jeremy J. Mandia, MD, MPH, MSHI, Case H. Keltner, MD, MPH, MS, Robert C. Haynes III, DO, MPH, Lisa Cruz, MD, Keith Solveson, and Luke E. Mease, MD, MPH

With this project, we aimed to re-engage military health care beneficiaries with expired HIV preexposure prophylaxis prescriptions at Madigan Army Medical Center (Tacoma, WA). We identified prescriptions expired between August 2022 and August 2023 via electronic health records, then called patients to assess HIV risk and arrange follow-up. Of those with clinical indications, 80% agreed to re-engage with preexposure prophylaxis services, increasing the number of patients receiving preexposure prophylaxis at our institution by 30%. Systematic electronic health records query can reduce nonadherence when active case management is not feasible. (*Am J Public Health*. 2025;115(3):287–291. https://doi.org/10.2105/AJPH.2024.307919)

AJPH March 2025, Vol. 115, No. 3

Adherence to preexposure prophylaxis (PrEP) for HIV prevention is essential for averting incident infections, but many patients fall out of services. The Joint Base Lewis McChord Department of Public Health (Tacoma, WA) underwent a process improvement project after two service members with new HIV diagnoses were found to have been lost to follow-up and nonadherent with preexposure prophylaxis at Madigan Army Medical Center. Madigan is the premier medical center serving Military Health System (MHS) beneficiaries in the Puget Sound region.

INTERVENTION AND IMPLEMENTATION

The primary goal was to proactively identify and re-engage individuals disengaged from care and promote PrEP continuation during periods with HIV exposure. Objectives included identifying patients with expired PrEP prescriptions using the MHS Genesis electronic health record (EHR), assessing PrEP indications, and offering services if indicated. We proactively identified patients disengaged from PrEP care and aimed to reduce barriers to access.

Levine et al. found underutilization of preventive treatments, such as PrEP, was the result of an implementation, rather than information, gap.[1] Qualitative and quantitative research on PrEP retention has underscored limited flexibility in the settings, timing, and nature of appointments as a key barrier.[2,3] Current practice is for MHS patients to make all appointments themselves. Choice architecture, a behavioral economics concept, suggests that how choices are presented significantly impacts decision-making; individuals will follow the path of least resistance.[4,5] Adjusting default options to proactively contact patients and "nudge" them toward preventive care services can increase engagement.[6]

PrEP-nonadherent patients were defined as anyone prescribed oral emtricitabine-tenofovir (T/FTC; Truvada or Descovy) who still had an indication for PrEP but had not renewed their prescription after their last clinical encounter. We designed a custom algorithm to identify expired oral T/FTC prescriptions in MHS Genesis. This algorithm pulled all prescriptions dispensed in the Puget Sound in one year. Dispensing date, the number of pills dispensed, and patient demographic information were collectively logged as unique observations.

Expired prescriptions were defined as the most recent prescription dispensed more than 14 days after its effective date (e.g., for 30-day supplies,

> 44 days). Indication for T/FTC prescriptions was ascertained by chart review. If HIV PrEP was the indication, and the patient was prescribed a daily regimen, then the record was reviewed to see if PrEP was prescribed outside the region or was discontinued by a medical provider. Patients with no active prescription or records showing discontinuation were classified as having expired prescriptions.

These patients were then contacted via telephone to discuss their current HIV prevention needs, reasons for discontinuation, and interest in resuming PrEP therapy. Patients were screened for indications using 2021 Centers for Disease Control and Prevention (CDC) PrEP guidelines. Patients were also asked if they received PrEP from another location, had any sexually transmitted infection (STI) since discontinuing or in the last 6 months, or ever had syphilis. Patients with continued indication and no active prescription were assisted in scheduling an appointment in the MHS, with the Department of Veterans Affairs, or with a civilian health care provider. Chart review was conducted six months after the initial interview to determine persistence of this intervention.

PLACE, TIME, AND PERSONS

The intervention took place at Madigan Army Medical Center, a large military hospital located in Tacoma, Washington, providing inpatient and outpatient services to more than 100 000 beneficiaries. The project covered August 31, 2022, to August 31, 2023. The population subject to the intervention comprised military personnel and their dependents who received oral T/FTC prescriptions for HIV PrEP within the Puget Sound Marketplace.

This group included individuals with previous PrEP indications but expired prescriptions, indicating potential nonadherence or discontinuation of the medication. Expired PrEP prescriptions were identified via a custom EHR algorithm. The focus was on patients with continued indications for PrEP, based on CDC guidelines, who had not actively renewed their prescription.

PURPOSE

Oral PrEP is about 99% effective in preventing the transmission of HIV.[7] Growing PrEP use, in conjunction with improved HIV testing, has contributed to a 12% decline in HIV incidence from 2017 to 2021.[8] Despite its effectiveness and increasing popularity, only 30% of the 1.2 million Americans who could benefit from PrEP received prescriptions in 2021.[9]

PrEP adherence is required to effectively prevent transmission,[10] as protection wanes with inconsistent use.[8] Despite the high efficacy, optimal use is difficult in real-world settings. Hojilla et al. found that 52% of patients discontinued PrEP after initiating, with 60% of these individuals subsequently reinitiating PrEP.[11]

Current CDC guidelines recommend providers monitor and offer support to address factors preventing adherence. Identifying and removing barriers to PrEP adherence is an active area of research.[12] For example, the PrEP Optimization Intervention centralized PrEP coordination to guide patients through the health care system. The authors concluded that their PrEP optimization intervention was feasible to implement and acceptable to providers.[13] More than 300 000 people are prescribed PrEP annually in the United States, so providers need efficient systems to flag patients at risk for nonadherence. EHRs provide an opportunity to proactively identify this population.

EVALUATION AND ADVERSE EFFECTS

We identified 469 T/FTC prescriptions for 192 patients. Forty prescriptions were for conditions other than PrEP. Of 152 HIV PrEP prescriptions, 52% had expired. Ninety percent (71/79) of patients with expired medications were contacted and consented to participate in the project, with 80% (57/71) endorsing a continued indication for PrEP. Twenty-one percent (12/57) of those with indications had received PrEP and STI screening outside of the Puget Sound marketplace (Figure 1). The physician who contacted patients obtained informed consent from all contacted persons.

Of the 45 patients with PrEP indications without active prescriptions, 24% had a previous diagnosis of syphilis. Fifty-three percent (24/45) of the nonadherent group had not received STI or HIV testing after discontinuing PrEP. Twenty-four percent (5/21) of patients screened had an STI since PrEP discontinuation, with 80% (4/5) of those infections occurring within the past 6 months. When offered proactive assistance with scheduling an appointment, 80% (36/45) of patients agreed to restart PrEP and STI screening (Figure 1). Seventy-eight percent (28/36) of these patients obtained care in the MHS; of these, 64% (18/28) had a clinical encounter and filled their prescription. Seventy-two percent of these (13/18) completed a 3-month follow-up appointment and had an active prescription at 6 months. Overall, the rate of re-engagement in PrEP care was 40% (18/45) with 29% retention in care (13/45).

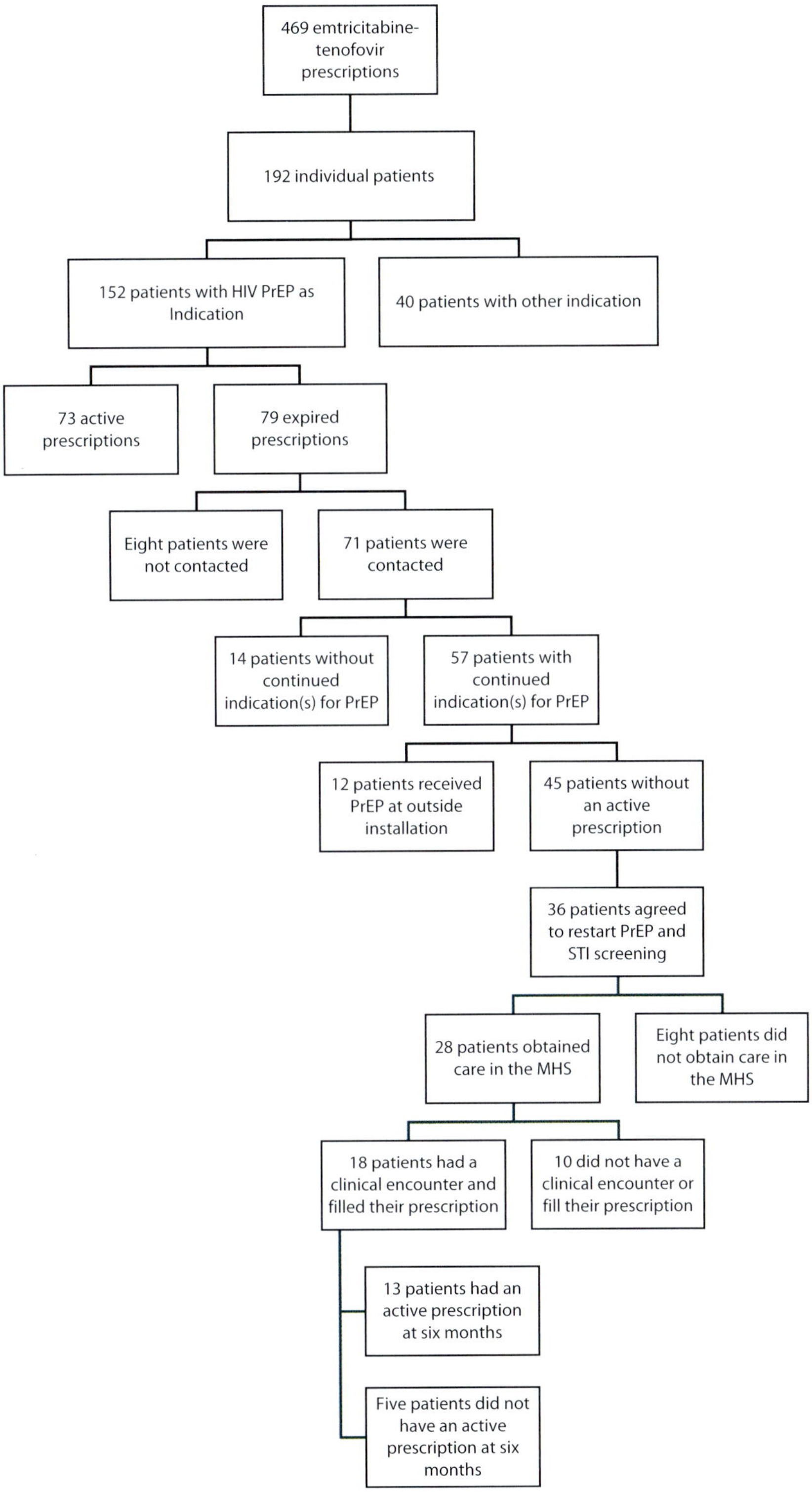

FIGURE 1— Breakdown of Military Health System (MHS) Puget Sound Marketplace Patients With Documented Emtricitabine-Tenofovir Prescription by Continued Need, Desire, and Completed Follow-up for HIV Preexposure Prophylaxis (PrEP) Care: Tacoma, WA, September 2022–August 2023

Note. No patients endorsed taking preexposure prophylaxis as a nondaily regimen.

SUSTAINABILITY

The EHR algorithm was an efficient method to search a large patient population with minimal resources. We prioritized sensitivity in the tool's design. As a consequence, the algorithm exhibited a 20% false-positive rate. Most of these false positives could be prevented by code refinement to exclude HIV postexposure prophylaxis and treatment.

Although patient EHR utilization is increasing nationwide, 43% of patients were not offered or did not access their online medical record or patient portal in 2022.[14] The use of automated EHR reminders improves follow-up across clinical settings, but those without patient portal access cannot view such reminders. Phone calls are an effective and sustainable way to remind patients of follow-up care, and 97% of Americans own a cell phone.[15] One full-time physician with various clinical and research obligations outside the scope of this project contacted all 71 patients in less than 10 cumulative hours. Most health care clinics should have the time and personnel capacity to execute similar telephone interventions. Ideally, health systems employ active patient portal enrollment strategies to ensure most beneficiaries access their portal. The proportion of eligible MHS beneficiaries utilizing the patient portal needs to be clarified. Therefore, employing telephone, rather than automated patient portal, reminders may be advantageous assuming significant gaps in patient portal utilization exist.

PUBLIC HEALTH SIGNIFICANCE

This project offers a novel approach to identify and re-engage nonadherent PrEP patients using EHR prescribing data. More than half of nonadherent patients had an indication for PrEP and were not obtaining care. This finding highlights a gap in the opt-in nature of health care delivery systems, which require consumers to engage without clear instructions or mechanisms for interfacing with care. Our strategy contacted 90% of patients with an expired medication, and 72% of individuals who reentered care had active prescriptions 6 months after the intervention.

This method increased preventive care utilization. At the Joint Base Lewis McChord Department of Public Health, this project increased the total number of PrEP patients managed in the system by 20%. Potential increased revenues from higher health care utilization produced from this intervention would more than offset the development and operational costs. Despite the intervention being a single phone call, it had a sustained effect with a substantial minority having persistent adherence to PrEP at 6 months. All patients we were unable to contact had left military service by the time the project was conducted.

Future work should focus on enhancing the effectiveness and applicability of EHR-based approaches. Refining the query to decrease false-positive rates and alert care teams of nonadherence would improve its utility. Further research should examine cost-effectiveness, whether nonphysician team members can achieve the same effect, and whether other means of communication (e.g., EHR messages, text reminders, mobile applications) yield different results. This intervention can be tailored to nonmilitary EHR systems, and civilian clinics should consider implementing similar strategies. In addition, this technique could be expanded to other medications with critical adherence requirements, improving the management of prevalent chronic diseases like hypertension and diabetes. AJPH

ABOUT THE AUTHORS

At the time of project completion, all authors were with Madigan Army Medical Center, Tacoma, WA. Jeremy Mandia, Case Keltner, Robert Haynes, and Luke Mease were with the Department of Preventive Medicine; Lisa Cruz is with the Department of Family Medicine; and Keith Solveson is with the Department of Informatics.

CORRESPONDENCE

Correspondence should be sent to Robert Haynes, Unit 8900 Box 330, DPO, AE 09831 (e-mail: robert.c.haynes53.mil@health.mil). Reprints can be ordered at https://www.ajph.org by clicking the "Reprints" link.

PUBLICATION INFORMATION

Full Citation: Mandia JJ, Keltner CH, Haynes RC III, Cruz L, Solveson K, Mease LE. Improving participation in HIV preexposure prophylaxis via an informatics approach—a process-improvement project. *Am J Public Health*. 2025;115(3):287–291.

Acceptance Date: November 6, 2024.

DOI: https://doi.org/10.2105/AJPH.2024.307919

ORCID iD:
Robert C. Haynes III https://orcid.org/0000-0002-0823-8537

CONTRIBUTORS

J. Mandia, C. Keltner, and R. Haynes conceptualized the project. J. Mandia and K. Solveson collected data and conducted field work. J. Mandia and L. Cruz wrote the first draft. J. Mandia, C. Keltner, R. Haynes, L. Cruz, and L. Mease contributed to editing and review of the article.

ACKNOWLEDGMENTS

All authors are US federal employees or uniformed personnel, and this project was completed as part of their official duties. No external funding was used in the completion of this project.

Results were previously presented at the Preventive Medicine 2024 conference in Washington, DC.

Authors would like to acknowledge Jeanne Slusher and Terra Forward for their clinical oversight.

Note. Material has been reviewed by the Walter Reed Army Institute of Research, Eisenhower Army Medical Center, and Kimbrough Ambulatory Care Center. There is no objection to its presentation and/or publication. The opinions or assertions contained herein are the private views of the authors and do not reflect the official policy of the Department of the Army, the Defense Health Agency, the Department of Defense, or the US government.

CONFLICTS OF INTEREST

All authors have no conflicting affiliations to disclose.

HUMAN PARTICIPANT PROTECTION

Project was determined "not research" and granted exempt status by the Madigan Army Medical Center institutional review board and was registered under the institutional record of process improvement projects. The investigators have adhered to the policies for protection of human participants as prescribed in AR 70-25 and 45 CFR, Part 46.

REFERENCES

1. Levine S, Malone E, Lekiachvili A, Briss P. Health care industry insights: why the use of preventive services is still low. *Prev Chronic Dis*. 2019;16:E30. https://doi.org/10.5888/pcd16.180625
2. MacDonald J, Estcourt CS, Flowers P, et al. Improving HIV pre-exposure prophylaxis (PrEP) adherence and retention in care: process evaluation and recommendation development from a nationally implemented PrEP programme. *PLoS One*. 2023;18(10):e0292289. https://doi.org/10.1371/journal.pone.0292289
3. Sidebottom D, Ekström AM, Strömdahl S. A systematic review of adherence to oral pre-exposure prophylaxis for HIV—how can we improve uptake and adherence? *BMC Infect Dis*. 2018;18(1):581. https://doi.org/10.1186/s12879-018-3463-4
4. Johnson EJ, Shu SB, Dellaert BGC, et al. Beyond nudges: tools of a choice architecture. *Marketing Letters*. 2012;23(2):487–504. https://doi.org/10.1007/s11002-012-9186-1
5. Adkisson R. *Nudge: Improving Decisions About Health, Wealth and Happiness*. *Soc Sci J*. 2008; 45(4):700–701. https://doi.org/10.1016/j.soscij.2008.09.003
6. Chapman GB, Li M, Colby H, Yoon H. Opting in vs opting out of influenza vaccination. *JAMA*. 2010; 304(1):43–44. https://doi.org/10.1001/jama.2010.892
7. Mayer KH, Molina JM, Thompson MA, et al. Emtricitabine and tenofovir alafenamide vs emtricitabine and tenofovir disoproxil fumarate for HIV pre-exposure prophylaxis (DISCOVER): primary results from a randomised, double-blind, multicentre, active-controlled, phase 3, non-inferiority trial. *Lancet*. 2020;396(10246):239–254. https://doi.org/10.1016/S0140-6736(20)31065-5
8. Centers for Disease Control and Prevention. PrEP for HIV prevention in the US. 2021. Available at: https://web.archive.org/web/20220620104046/https://www.cdc.gov/nchhstp/newsroom/fact-sheets/hiv/PrEP-for-hiv-prevention-in-the-US-factsheet.html. Accessed June 15, 2022.
9. Centers for Disease Control and Prevention. How do I prescribe PrEP? 2023. Available at: https://web.archive.org/web/20230628215957/https://www.cdc.gov/hiv/images/clinicians/prevention/cdc-hiv-nexus-prevention-assessing-sexually-active-patients-1800x1550.png. Accessed August 1, 2023.
10. Cottrell ML, Yang KH, Prince HM, et al. A translational pharmacology approach to predicting

outcomes of preexposure prophylaxis against HIV in men and women using tenofovir disoproxil fumarate with or without emtricitabine. *J Infect Dis*. 2016;214(1):55–64. https://doi.org/10.1093/infdis/jiw077

11. Hojilla JC, Hurley LB, Marcus JL, et al. Characterization of HIV preexposure prophylaxis use behaviors and HIV incidence among US adults in an integrated health care system. *JAMA Netw Open*. 2021;4(8):e2122692. https://doi.org/10.1001/jamanetworkopen.2021.22692
12. Garrison LE, Haberer JE. Pre-exposure prophylaxis uptake, adherence, and persistence: a narrative review of interventions in the US. *Am J Prev Med*. 2021;61(5, suppl 1):S73–S86. https://doi.org/10.1016/j.amepre.2021.04.036
13. Saberi P, Berrean B, Thomas S, Gandhi M, Scott H. A simple pre-exposure prophylaxis (PrEP) optimization intervention for health care providers prescribing PrEP: pilot study. *JMIR Form Res*. 2018;2(1):e2. https://doi.org/10.2196/formative.8623
14. Strawley C, Richwine C. Individuals' access and use of patient portals and smartphone health apps, 2022. ONC Data Brief No. 69. October 2023. Assistant Secretary for Technology Policy/Office of the National Coordinator for Health IT. Available at: https://www.healthit.gov/data/data-briefs/individuals-access-and-use-patient-portals-and-smartphone-health-apps-2022. Accessed March 2, 2024.
15. Pew Research Center. Mobile fact sheet. 2024. Available at: https://www.pewresearch.org/internet/fact-sheet/mobile. Accessed July 17, 2024.

Medical Care or Deportation: Examining Interior Border Checkpoints and Access to Higher-Level Medical Care for Undocumented Immigrants in South Texas

Christine Crudo Blackburn, PhD, Mayra Rico, MPH, Jessica Hernandez, MPH, and Miryoung Lee, PhD

We examined the impacts of interior border checkpoints on access to higher-level medical care via ground ambulance for undocumented immigrants in South Texas. Using purposive sampling, we conducted interviews (n = 30) with ground ambulance personnel in the lower Rio Grande Valley, Texas. Procedures implemented in 2018 mandate that hospitals notify Border Patrol of a patient's legal status before transfer. Undocumented immigrants cannot access higher-level medical care through ground ambulance transport without notifying Border Patrol. (*Am J Public Health*. 2025;115(3):292–295. https://doi.org/10.2105/AJPH.2024.307927)

AJPH March 2025, Vol. 115, No. 3

Enforcing immigration laws has increased in both scale and funding,[1] and related policies have been shown to decrease access to health care and result in poorer health outcomes for undocumented immigrants in the United States.[2–4] One relevant form of immigration law enforcement is the establishment and maintenance of interior border checkpoints (IBCs). IBCs are located in the interior of the United States, and motorists are required to verify their legal status at these locations.[5] There are 18 IBCs in Texas[6] (Figure 1), and their presence can prevent undocumented immigrants' access to necessary health care services.[7,8]

STUDY OBJECTIVES

We examined the impacts of IBCs on access to necessary higher-level medical care via ground ambulance for undocumented immigrants in South Texas. To our knowledge, this study is the first to examine the medical transport process for undocumented immigrants in South Texas who are seeking necessary higher-level medical care.

PARTICIPANTS, SAMPLE, GEOGRAPHIC LOCATION, SETTING, AND YEAR OF STUDY

The demographics of participants are captured in Appendix A (available as a supplement to the online version of this article at http://www.ajph.org). We chose participants for study inclusion who were currently employed as medical personnel on ambulances for an emergency medical service organization in Texas's Rio Grande Valley.

The study took place in the lower Rio Grande Valley: Cameron, Hidalgo, Starr, and Willacy counties. We conducted all interviews from November to December 2023 at the organization's administration building in Cameron County.

METHODS

We used naturalistic inquiry,[9] which allowed us to capture the subjective experiences and perceptions of the

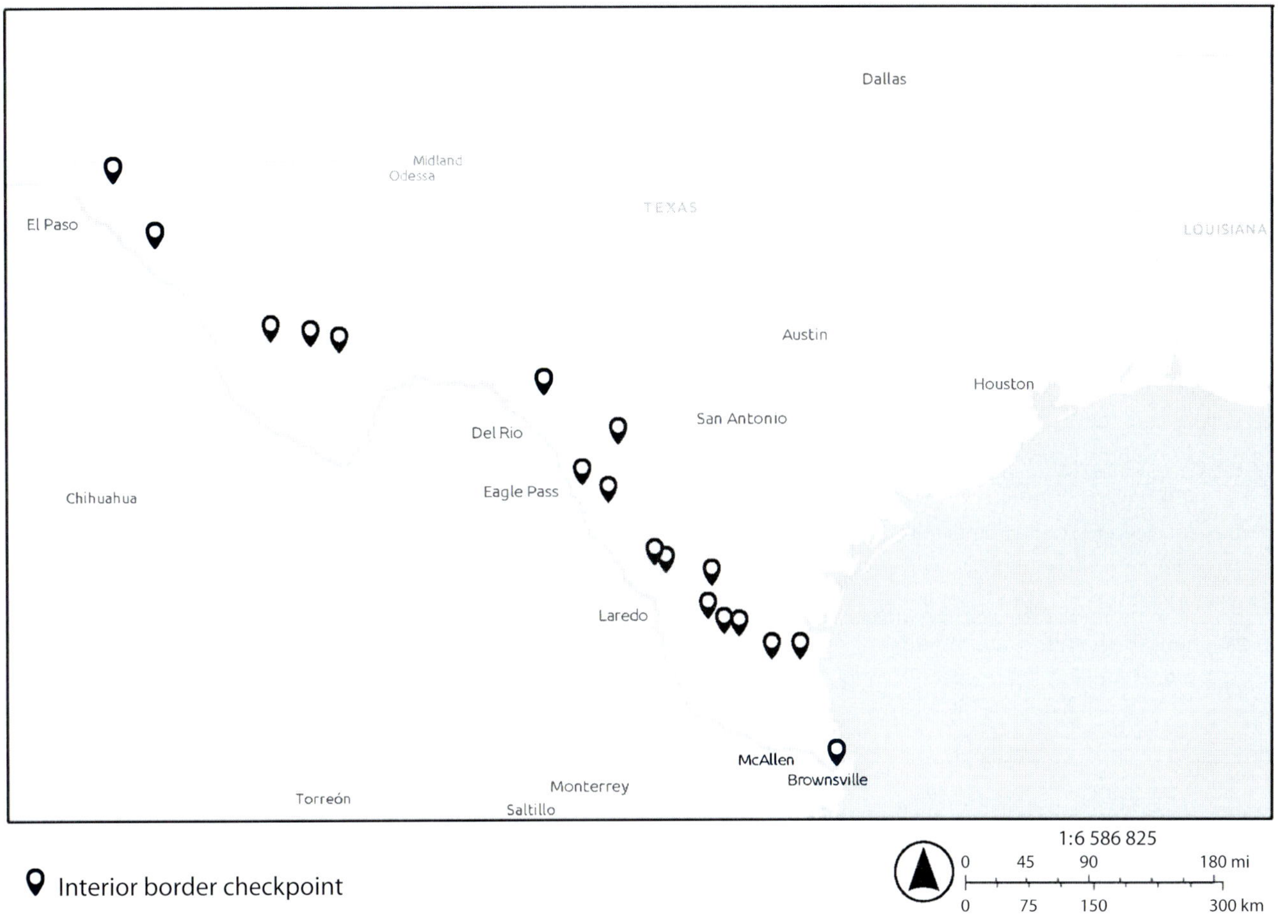

FIGURE 1— Map of Interior Border Checkpoint Locations: Rio Grande Valley, Texas, November–December 2023

personnel participating in the interviews. We collected data from participants (n = 30) in one-on-one interviews. We selected participants using purposive sampling, focusing on individuals who had experience transporting undocumented patients through IBCs.

We conducted semistructured interviews in which we asked participants about their experiences transporting undocumented individuals in South Texas to higher-level care located beyond IBCs (Appendix B, available as a supplement to the online version of this article at http://www.ajph.org). We also asked participants about experiences in which they transported a pediatric patient who was a citizen but had one or more undocumented parents.

We audio recorded all interviews and transcribed them using NVivo Transcription version 14 (QSR International, Burlington, MA).

Three members of the research team coded the transcripts using NVivo 14. We undertook coding using a descriptive qualitative approach, which is a methodology that aims to understand a process or event directly from the individuals experiencing it.[10] This descriptive approach resulted in the development of parent codes and child codes to reflect the experiences of participants in transporting undocumented patients and minors from mixed-status families from IBCs to higher-level medical care. Mixed-status families are those in which some members do not have legal status in the United States whereas others do. When the coding process was complete, one member of the research team reviewed all codes to ensure that coded segments accurately reflected code names. Finally, using thematic analysis,[11] we examined the codes to identify the primary themes evident in the data as they related to IBCs and access to higher-level health care for undocumented immigrants in South Texas.

KEY FINDINGS

We found that the process of transferring undocumented patients was streamlined in 2018 to avoid long delays at IBCs. Additionally we found that, because of this change, hospitals notify Border Patrol when an undocumented patient needs transfer, which leads Border Patrol to accompany the patient to their higher-level medical care location and can result in undocumented parents being unable to accompany their minor children. Participant quotations exemplifying these findings can be found in Appendix C (available as a supplement to the online version of this article at http://www.ajph.org).

Participants with more than five years of experience reported that, before the 2018 changes in transfer procedures, ambulances would be held at IBCs if the patient or the patient's family member was undocumented. The delays could last as long as 45 minutes to many hours. Delays caused significant stress for emergency responders responsible for caring for the patients during the delays. Over time, ground ambulance delays at the checkpoints became such a significant problem that emergency medical service representatives, hospital administrators, and Border Patrol came together to develop a new process that would reduce the delays. The changes made to the patient transfer process for undocumented patients or patients with undocumented family members have eliminated delays at IBCs.

The new transfer process for undocumented patients or pediatric patients with undocumented family members requires hospitals to notify Border Patrol of a patient's immigration status before the patient is allowed to be transferred to a hospital beyond an IBC. Across all interviews, there was consensus that the hospital plays the primary role of making sure Border Patrol is notified of the patient's immigration status before patient transfer. Participants frequently saw this procedural change as increasing their ability to provide timely, high-quality care to their patients.

Participants explained that after Border Patrol was notified of a patient's undocumented status, Border Patrol agents took custody of the patient. Most of the time, taking custody of the patient meant that Border Patrol was required to accompany the ambulance from the transferring hospital to the receiving hospital and to stay with the patient throughout their medical care. For some participants, the presence of Border Patrol on these transports had a positive impact. Participants worked regularly with Border Patrol agents, and most discussed a positive working relationship.

Participants stated that the requirement that the hospital notify Border Patrol of a parent's undocumented status to allow the parent to accompany their minor child to their medical care beyond an IBC meant that many parents choose to send their children alone or to have a relative beyond the IBC meet their child at the receiving hospital. In some cases, however, undocumented parents decide to accompany their child, knowing that it means Border Patrol will be notified of their undocumented status. Some participants said that it was emotionally difficult for them to transport pediatric patients when the parents could not accompany them. These participants explained that they did their best to make the children feel comfortable, but it was often still a traumatic experience for the child.

EVALUATION, TRANSFERABILITY, AND ADVERSE EFFECTS

Our results provide rich information on IBCs' impacts on access to necessary higher-level medical care via ground ambulance for undocumented immigrants in South Texas. We found that the process of transporting undocumented patients in the Rio Grande Valley to higher-level medical care beyond IBCs has changed over time. These changes have shortened delays at IBCs.

Our findings show, however, that as transport processes have been streamlined, disclosure of a patient's immigration status has become mandatory for that patient to receive care beyond IBCs. If a patient refuses to disclose their undocumented status or if they do not want the hospital to notify Border Patrol of their undocumented status, they are not allowed to be transported via ambulance to needed higher-level medical care. The requirement forces the choice between health care and freedom for the patient or their family members. Such a choice may become increasingly difficult for undocumented patients or parents with the passage of Texas's Senate Bill 4, which makes entry into the United States between ports of entry a state crime.

Our findings have suggested new research questions regarding whether the transfer process is unique to South Texas or has been implemented in other southern border states. Additionally, questions remain as to whether the changes made to the ground ambulance transfer process have increased access to higher-level medical care or whether the requirement to notify Border Patrol leads more undocumented patients to refuse transfer.

SCALABILITY

This study could be scaled up into a large, multistate survey of emergency medical service personnel in border communities across the four southern border states of Texas, New Mexico, Arizona, and California. A study of this scale would provide increased insight into whether South Texas's procedures are unique or notification to Border Patrol of a patient's or parent's undocumented status is required for ground ambulance transfer in other southern border states.

PUBLIC HEALTH IMPLICATIONS

Transferring undocumented patients or pediatric patients with undocumented parents in need of higher-level medical care in the lower Rio Grande Valley has been streamlined over time. The current process has lessened the stress on emergency medical service personnel by eliminating uncertainty about whether they will be able to pass through IBCs with undocumented patients or minor citizens with undocumented caregivers. The procedures have also helped ensure that patient transfer is timely and guarantee access to health care not available in the Rio Grande Valley once the transfer process is initiated. Thus, these procedural changes have eliminated uncertainty about a patient's ability to access health care once they make a transfer decision.

The process, however, requires health care professionals to report their patients' immigration status to provide them with necessary medical care—medical care that is sometimes life or death. Such a requirement may deter some undocumented immigrants from seeking health care for themselves or their children. This barrier to health care access may contribute to health disparities among immigrants in South Texas. AJPH

ABOUT THE AUTHORS

Christine Crudo Blackburn is with the Department of Health Policy and Management and USA Center for Rural Public Health Preparedness, School of Public Health, Texas A&M University, College Station. Mayra Rico is with the USA Center for Rural Public Health Preparedness, School of Public Health, Texas A&M University. Jessica Hernandez is a masters of public health student in the Department of Health Behavior, School of Public Health, Texas A&M University. Miryoung Lee is with the Department of Epidemiology, University of Texas Health Science Center at Houston, Brownsville.

CORRESPONDENCE

Correspondence should be sent to Christine Crudo Blackburn, Department of Health Policy and Management, School of Public Health, Texas A&M University, 212 Adriance Lab Rd, College Station, TX 77843-1266 (e-mail: ccblackburn@tamu.edu). Reprints can be ordered at https://www.ajph.org by clicking the "Reprints" link.

PUBLICATION INFORMATION

Full Citation: Blackburn CC, Rico M, Hernandez J, Lee M. Medical care or deportation: examining interior border checkpoints and access to higher-level medical care for undocumented immigrants in South Texas. *Am J Public Health*. 2025;115(3):292–295.

Acceptance Date: November 5, 2024.

DOI: https://doi.org/10.2105/AJPH.2024.307927

ORCID iDs:

Mayra Rico https://orcid.org/0009-0005-9895-6047

Jessica Hernandez https://orcid.org/0009-0000-8867-2159

Miryoung Lee https://orcid.org/0000-0003-4088-304X

CONTRIBUTORS

C. C. Blackburn conceptualized the study, developed data collection instruments, collected interview data, led data analysis, curated the data, wrote the first draft of the article, and supervised the study. C. C. Blackburn, M. Rico, and J. Hernandez performed the formal analysis and the investigation. C. C. Blackburn and M. Lee administered the project. M. Rico and M. Lee contributed to the writing of and reviewed and edited the article.

ACKNOWLEDGMENTS

We would like to thank our community partners for their guidance and insight during the study.

CONFLICTS OF INTEREST

The authors have no conflicts of interest to report.

HUMAN PARTICIPANT PROTECTION

The Texas A&M University institutional review board considered this study exempt from human participant review (reference IRB2023-0842M). All participants provided written consent.

REFERENCES

1. Akkerman M. Global spending on immigration enforcement is higher than ever and rising. May 31, 2023. Available at: https://www.migrationpolicy.org/article/immigration-enforcement-spending-rising. Accessed January 10, 2024.
2. Koball H, Kirby J, Hartig S. The relationship between states' immigrant-related policies and access to health care among children of immigrants. *J Immigr Minor Health*. 2022;24(4):834–841. https://doi.org/10.1007/s10903-021-01282-9
3. Young MDT, Chen L, Sudhinaraset M, Saadi A, Kietzman KG, Wallace SP. Cumulative experiences of immigration enforcement policy and the physical and mental health outcomes of Asian and Latinx immigrants in the United States. *Int Migr Rev*. 2023;57(4):1537–1568. https://doi.org/10.1177/01979183221126726
4. Đoàn LN, Chon SK, Misra S, Kwon SC, Yi SS. Immigrant communities and COVID-19: strengthening the public health response. *Am J Public Health*. 2021;111(suppl 3):S224–S231. https://doi.org/10.2105/AJPH.2021.306433
5. American Civil Liberties Union. US Border Patrol interior checkpoints: frequently asked questions. Available at: https://www.aclu-sdic.org/sites/default/files/border-patrol-checkpoint-faqs.pdf. Accessed January 19, 2024.
6. Government Accountability Office. Border Patrol: actions needed to improve checkpoint oversight and data. June 2022. Available at: https://www.gao.gov/assets/gao-22-104568.pdf. Accessed January 17, 2023.
7. Martinez O, Dodge B, Reece M, et al. Sexual health and life experiences: voices from behaviourally bisexual Latino men in the Midwestern USA. *Cult Health Sex*. 2011;13(9):1073–1089. https://doi.org/10.1080/13691058.2011.600461
8. Castañeda H, Melo MA. Geographies of confinement for immigrant youth: checkpoints and immobilities along the US/Mexico border. *Law Policy*. 2019;41(1):80–102. https://doi.org/10.1111/lapo.12115
9. Lincoln YS, Guba EG, Pilotta JJ. *Naturalistic Inquiry*. Beverly Hills, CA: Sage; 1985. https://doi.org/10.1016/0147-1767(85)90062-8
10. Sandelowski M. Whatever happened to qualitative description? *Res Nurs Health*. 2000;23(4):334–340. https://doi.org/10.1002/1098-240x(200008)23:4<334::aid-nur9>3.0.co;2-g
11. Braun V, Clarke V. *Thematic Analysis: A Practical Guide*. Los Angeles, CA: Sage; 2022.

Increasing Access Through Integration: Behavioral Health Services and Beyond

Della Hughes Carter, DNP, MSN, APRN, GNP-BC, Mary Claire Meimers, DNP, RN, and Emily Fowler Bemben, DNP, MSN, APRN, PMHNP-BC

An academic health center (AHC) that provides primary care to an urban, underresourced population recognized the need for an integrated model of care to address behavioral health needs. The Ambulatory Integration of the Medical and Social (AIMS) Collaborative Care Model's five pillars provided the framework and enhanced outcomes through tailored initiatives at the AHC, expanding to onsite satellite locations in senior subsidized housing, and through telehealth services. The results showed increased access to behavioral health care and improved depression and anxiety symptoms. (*Am J Public Health*. 2025;115(3):296–300. https://doi.org/10.2105/AJPH.2024.307939)

AJPH March 2025, Vol. 115, No. 3

Equitable access to quality mental health care services remains a crucial public health priority, with barriers causing undue suffering and premature death in our most vulnerable populations.[1,2] This growing national problem unfairly affects racial and ethnic minorities; those with disabilities; lesbian, gay, bisexual, transgender, queer, intersex, and asexual (LGBTQIA+) individuals; and those underinsured, economically disadvantaged, and incarcerated.[1] Nearly 96% of US adults face one or more barriers to accessing health care, an issue that disproportionately affects individuals experiencing psychological distress, with depression and anxiety being the most common.[1–3] The COVID-19 pandemic further illuminated the burden of untreated behavioral health conditions. During the pandemic, 12.8% of US adults reported an unmet mental health need, nearly double that of prepandemic trends.[4] Dawes et al. estimate that the complex and significant cost of premature mental and behavioral health–related deaths among US racial and ethnic minorities is $278 billion over four years.[1] They advocate smaller-scale, integrated physical and mental health services customized to meet the specific needs of individual communities rather than implementing one-size-fits-all solutions.[1,2] Despite policymakers and scholars promoting integrated care models to improve access and quality, integrated care is not the mainstay.[1,5] This article shares the journey of a nurse-led team that applied an integrated model of care in a community-based academic health center (AHC). The project's central mission was to bridge the gap between medically underserved adults' need for behavioral health care and limited access to these essential services.

INTERVENTION AND IMPLEMENTATION

This project centered on creating an integrated model of care by incorporating a behavioral health team (BHT) within an AHC. A full-time psychiatric mental health nurse practitioner (PMHNP), a master of social work (MSW), a part-time registered nurse (RN) case manager, a peer support advocate, and a graduate assistant were fully integrated into daily practice. The work involved incorporating the AIMS Collaborative Care Model (CoCM),[6,7] expanding services within an existing practice, and measuring outcomes.

The AHC team was introduced to the CoCM early during information sessions. After onboarding the BHT, two separate day-long retreats were organized to enhance the implementation of the CoCM and integrate systems, fostering collegiality. The five pillars of the CoCM established at the practice included the following (Figure 1).

1. Patient-centered care. The primary care provider and BHT collaborated to create shared care plans. Communication was enhanced through shared nomenclature, daily preshift huddles, weekly joint

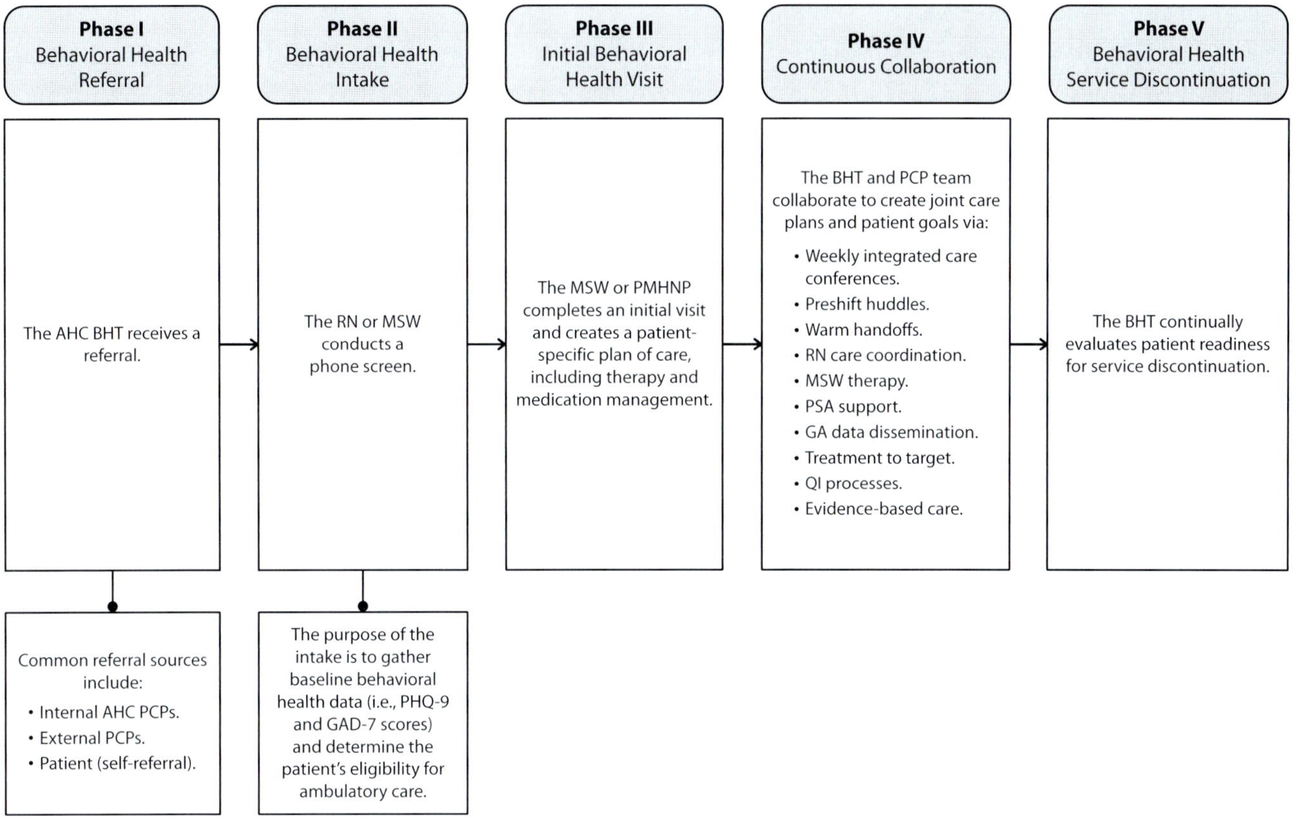

FIGURE 1— Patient Throughput Flowchart Using the Collaborative Care Model

Note. AHC = community-based academic health center; BHT = behavioral health team; GA = graduate assistant; GAD-7 = General Anxiety Disorder-7; MSW = master of social work; PCP = primary care provider; PHQ-9 = Patient Health Questionnaire-9; PMHNP = psychiatric mental health nurse practitioner; PSA = patient support advocate; QI = quality improvement RN = registered nurse.

care planning conferences, and standardization of report giving and warm handoffs,[8] allowing for efficient patient throughput. The peer support advocate, working under the direction of the RN and PMHNP, provided individual and small discussion groups.

2. Population-based care. The MSW provided an initial assessment, triage, and nonmedical care planning. The RN proactively contacted patients to address follow-up issues and care management and to offer therapeutic communication.
3. Measurement-based treatment to target. The PMHNP used the Patient Health Questionnaire-9 (PHQ-9) and the General Anxiety Disorder-7 (GAD-7) to assess treatment progress.[9]
4. Evidenced-based care. The integrated team continuously adjusted care plans, provided patient and family education, implemented motivational interviewing, prescribed and managed psychotropic medications, facilitated individual and small group therapy, and made appropriate referrals.
5. Accountable care. The graduate assistant collected and analyzed data to provide outcomes at the provider and program levels.

PLACE, TIME, AND PERSONS

The grant-funded project, co-led by faculty from a university, operated from January 2021 to April 2023. It was implemented in a nurse-managed AHC, seeing about 3500 child and adult patients annually, in a midwestern city that included satellite locations in senior subsidized housing and telehealth. The urban population that was served faced vulnerabilities because of low income, social determinants of health, limited political prioritization, and marginalization based on race, ethnicity, sexual orientation, or disabilities. Outreach included meet-and-greet events at senior housing, newsletters, university marketing, local news coverage, and self-referral flyers.

PURPOSE

An AHC providing primary care to a disproportionately underresourced population recognized the need for an integrated model of care to address co-occurring physical and behavioral health needs.[6] This project aimed to improve access to mental health care, thus improving behavioral health outcomes, through small-scale initiatives tailored to the population served.[2]

EVALUATION AND ADVERSE EFFECTS

The PMHNP treated 217 adults during the grant period, 98 of whom received three or more visits, allowing for the evaluation of the CoCM pillar Measurement-Based Treatment to Target.[6,7] The remaining 119 patients were seen once by patient choice or clinical judgment. Some were referred to primary care, RN care management, outside referral, or emotional support for issues like grief and relationship stress. Five patients required acute care for psychiatric emergencies.

Of the 98 patients, most were women (73%), single (49%), and White (79%); the average age was 39 years, and the oldest was aged 79 years. Notably, 18% of patients self-identified as disabled, in contrast to the county's disabled population of 11.2%.[7] Similarly, whereas the local county had a 4.4% unemployment rate,[10] 21% of the patients were unemployed. Seven percent of patients identified as homeless or reported housing instability, higher than county statistics of 1.4% and 3.5%, respectively.[10] Consistent with existing literature, 96% of the patients reported a history of mental illness. Likewise, 19% of the patients self-reported having received substance use treatment in the past. This included a wide range, from acute care admission to outpatient treatment. This is clinically significant because nationally, over one calendar year, 16% of US persons aged 12 years and older had an indication for substance use treatment, yet less than 2% received related care.[11] These statistics provide evidence of the AHC population's vulnerability.

Measurement-based care involves gathering patient data using validated outcome scales such as PHQ-9 and GAD-7 and using the findings to inform decision-making, which leads to efficient treatment.[9] The PHQ-9 and GAD-7 are fluid measures that were consistently assessed, comparing the initial score (on intake) and the last score recorded by the BHT. The last score was recorded when the patient completed treatment, transferred, did not return, or the project ended. The time between the initial and last score varied depending on follow-up recommendations, patient choice, and scheduling. The PHQ-9 initial and last scores ($n = 81$) improved by 2.48 points ($P < .001$; $t = 3.80$; 95% confidence interval [CI] = 1.817, 3.781). The median score for the highest PHQ-9 recorded was 15, and the lowest was 7. When initial and subsequent GAD-7 scores ($n = 77$) were compared, an average improvement of 2.31 points ($P < .001$; $t = 3.50$; 95% CI = 0.9953, 3.6281) was noted. The median score for the highest recorded GAD-7 was 14, and the lowest was 7.

Evidence-based care is evident in the high number of patients (77%) participating in pharmacotherapy and psychotherapy, likely contributing to improved mental health outcomes. Evidence suggests that the concurrent use of both modalities is more effective for treating conditions like depression than monotherapy.[12] Thus, clinicians encouraged all patients to participate in psychotherapy, with 79% of patients receiving therapy.

Population-based care is exemplified by the MSW conducting a multifactorial, hour-long behavioral assessment and developing an integrated care plan for each patient seen by the BHT. The MSW also prepared the agenda for the weekly joint planning conference. Regarding care coordination, the RN facilitated community support, with 58% of patients receiving assistance, as detailed in Table 1. Additionally, care was adapted by tailoring the behavioral assessment to include the CAGE-AID, a valid screening tool for substance use disorders.[13] The adaptation improved screening rates from 32% to 71%.

The addition of the integrated BHT and the elimination of transportation barriers significantly increased access to mental health services for hundreds who otherwise would have gone untreated. Although reimbursement and technical difficulties may present challenges, telehealth services can increase access and utilization in underresourced behavioral health populations.[14] In this project, 59% of patients completed one or more behavioral telehealth appointments. Although the satellite locations in senior subsidized housing provided care where residents live, they also sometimes prefer telehealth.

SUSTAINABILITY

Universities with health education programs can enhance their communities by supporting academic community

TABLE 1— Common Care Coordination Activities at an Academic Health Center in a Midwestern US City: January 2021–April 2023

Care Coordination Activity	Patients Affected (n = 98), No. (%)
Referral to neuropsychology	18 (18.4)
Preventative care follow-up[a]	15 (15.3)
Resource coordination[b]	15 (15.3)
Housing	6 (6.1)

Note. This table outlines the four most common care coordination activities. This is not an exhaustive list of care coordination activities rendered. Some patients received other, less common forms of care coordination such as hypertension management, preventative care screening (needs for mammography, Papanicolaou test, or colonoscopy), and medication management. Some patients received more than one of the services listed.
[a]Including community-based mental health awareness and educational programs, workplace mental health initiatives, and university support services.
[b]Topics include alcohol use disorder, access to food, transportation services, home budgeting, insurance, dietary referrals, sleep specialists, area on aging, physical therapy, occupational therapy, and speech therapy.

health centers, distinct from student health centers.[15] They can partner with public housing authorities for rent-free satellite locations in senior housing. Faculty can lead the implementation of the CoCM, acquire grants, and provide care while training future health care professionals. Although Current Procedural Terminology billing codes for CoCM, approved by Medicare in January 2018, offer reimbursement potential for integrated care, maintaining budget neutrality remains challenging despite additional funding.[13]

PUBLIC HEALTH SIGNIFICANCE

Barriers to high-quality health care pose devastating problems for far too many, especially marginalized populations.[1,2] This project highlights improved access and outcomes through an integrated BHT in an AHC. The application of the CoCM's five pillars is discussed as a small-scale initiative specifically tailored to the unique needs of a highly vulnerable population. The project team successfully invested in behavioral health solutions in our community, reducing the economic burden of access for the underserved while addressing social determinants of health and behavioral health wellness.[2] AJPH

ABOUT THE AUTHORS

Della Hughes Carter, Mary Claire Meimers, and Emily Fowler Bemben are with the Kirkhof College of Nursing, Grand Rapids, MI.

CORRESPONDENCE

Correspondence should be sent to Della Hughes Carter, 458 Cook DeVos Bldg, 301 Michigan St NE, Grand Rapids, MI (e-mail: hughedel@gvsu.edu). Reprints can be ordered at https://www.ajph.org by clicking the "Reprints" link.

PUBLICATION INFORMATION

Full Citation: Carter DH, Meimers MC, Bemben EF. Increasing access through integration: behavioral health services and beyond. *Am J Public Health*. 2025;115(3):296–300.

Acceptance Date: November 11, 2024.

DOI: https://doi.org/10.2105/AJPH.2024.307939

ORCID iDs:
Della Hughes Carter https://orcid.org/0000-0001-7397-1594

Emily Fowler Bemben https://orcid.org/0009-0007-5468-5403

CONTRIBUTORS

D. Hughes Carter and M. C. Meimers performed material preparation, data collection, and analysis. All authors contributed to the project's conceptualization and design, contributed equally to the first draft of the manuscript, recommended edits, and prepared the final manuscript that was approved for submission.

ACKNOWLEDGMENTS

This project was supported by a grant from the Michigan Health Endowment Fund (#R-2004-146311).

We thank Katherine Moran, DNP, RN, for reviewing the manuscript.

CONFLICTS OF INTEREST

The authors declare no conflicts of interest relevant to this work.

HUMAN PARTICIPANT PROTECTION

The Grand Valley State University institutional review board issued a nonresearch determination.

REFERENCES

1. Dawes DE, Bhatt J, Dunlap N, Amador C, Gebreyes K, Rush B. The projected costs and economic impact of mental health inequities in the United States. Deloitte Center for Health Solutions. May 15, 2024. Available at: https://www2.deloitte.com/us/en/insights/industry/health-care/economic-burden-mental-health-inequities.html. Accessed October 27, 2024.
2. Dawes DE, Amador CM, Jha M, et al. The economic burden of mental health inequities in the United States report. Satcher Leadership Institute & Morehouse School of Medicine. September 2022. Available at: https://satcherinstitute.org/wp-content/uploads/2022/09/The-Economic-Burden-of-Mental-Health-Inequities-in-the-US-Report-Final-single-pages.V6.pdf. Accessed October 27, 2024.
3. National Institute of Mental Health. Major depression. US Dept of Health and Human Services. July 2023. Available at: https://www.nimh.nih.gov/health/statistics/major-depression. Accessed October 27, 2024.
4. Nagata JM, Ganson KT, Bonin SL, et al. Prevalence and sociodemographic correlates of unmet needs for mental health counseling among adults during the COVID-19 pandemic. *Psychiatr Serv*. 2022;73(2):206–209. https://doi.org/10.1176/appi.ps.202100111
5. Ko M, Murphy J, Bindman A. Integrating health care for the most vulnerable: bridging the difference in organizational cultures between US hospitals and health centers. *Am J Public Health*. 2015;105(suppl 5):S676–S679. https://doi.org/10.2105/AJPH.2015.302931
6. Rizzo VM, Rowe JM, Han W, et al. The effect of the ambulatory integration of the medical and social (AIMS) model on health risk and depression. *Soc Work Health Care*. 2022;61(5):353–368. https://doi.org/10.1080/00981389.2022.2092581
7. AIMS Center. About collaborative care. University of Washington Psychiatry & Behavioral Sciences. 2023. Available at: https://aims.uw.edu/collaborative-care. Accessed October 27, 2024.
8. Mitchell D, Olson A, Randolph N. The impact of warm handoffs on patient engagement with

behavioral health services in primary care. *J Rural Ment Health*. 2022;46(2):82–87. https://doi.org/10.1037/rmh0000199

9. Hong RH, Murphy JK, Michalak EE, et al. Implementing measurement-based care for depression: practical solutions for psychiatrists and primary care physicians. *Neuropsychiatr Dis Treat*. 2021;17:79–90. https://doi.org/10.2147/NDT.S283731
10. Brummel M. Kent County community health needs assessment. 2020. Available at: https://accesskent.com/Health/CHNA/pdf/FINAL-2020-CHNA-REPORT.pdf. Accessed February 21, 2024.
11. Substance Abuse and Mental Health Services Administration. Key substance use and mental health indicators in the United States: results from the 2021 national survey on drug use and health. US Dept of Health and Human Services. 2022. Available at: https://www.samhsa.gov/data/sites/default/files/reports/rpt39443/2021NSDUHFFRRev010323.pdf. Accessed February 07, 2024.
12. Cuijpers P, Noma H, Karyotaki E, Vinkers CH, Cipiani A, Furukawa TA. A network meta-analysis of the effects of psychotherapies, pharmacotherapies, and their combination in the treatment of adult depression. *World Psychiatry*. 2020;19(1):92–107. https://doi.org/10.1002/wps.20701
13. Gerrity M. Integrating primary care into behavioral health settings: what works for individuals with serious mental illness. The Reforming States Group & Milbank Memorial Fund. 2016. Available at: https://www.milbank.org/wp-content/uploads/2016/04/Integrating-Primary-Care-Report.pdf. Accessed February 26, 2024.
14. Lombardi BM, de Saxe Zerden L, Greeno C. Federally qualified health centers use of telehealth to deliver integrated behavioral health care during COVID-19. *Community Ment Health J*. 2024;60(2):215–223. https://doi.org/10.1007/s10597-022-01070-1
15. Wilkins CH, Alberti PM. Shifting academic health centers from a culture of community service to community engagement and integration. *Acad Med*. 2019;94(6):763–767. https://doi.org/10.1097/ACM.0000000000002711

Celebrating 115 Years of *AJPH*: Perspectives on Public Health in a New Political Era

Alfredo Morabia, MD, PhD, B. Ethan Coston, PhD, Paul Erwin, MD, DrPH, Laura Ferguson, PhD, Bisola Ojikutu, MD, MPH, Wendy E. Parmet, JD, and Julian Santaella Tenorio, DrPH

ABOUT THE AUTHORS

Alfredo Morabia is AJPH *editor in chief, and is with the Barry Commoner Center for Health and the Environment, Queens College, City University of New York, and the Department of Epidemiology, Mailman School of Public Health, Columbia University, New York, NY. B. Ethan Coston is with the Department of Gender, Sexuality and Women's Studies, Virginia Commonwealth University, Richmond. Paul Erwin is with the School of Public Health, University of Alabama at Birmingham. Laura Ferguson is with the Institute on Inequalities in Global Health, University of Southern California, Los Angeles, CA. Bisola Ojikutu is with the Boston Public Health Commission, the Infectious Disease Division, Massachusetts General Hospital, and the Division of Global Health Equity, Brigham and Women's Hospital, Boston, MA. Wendy Parmet is with the School of Law and the Center for Health Policy and Law, Northeastern University, Boston, MA. Julian Santaella Tenorio is with the Department of Public Health and Epidemiology, Pontificia Universidad Javeriana, Cali, Colombia.*

See also *AJPH* 115th Anniversary, pp. 304–325.

As we celebrate 115 years of *AJPH*, we reflect on its enduring mission: to advance public health knowledge and practice by publishing rigorous scientific research and serving as a platform for diverse perspectives on pressing issues and policies. This milestone invites us to look both backward and forward—to honor *AJPH*'s legacy while considering its role in addressing the challenges of an ever-evolving public health landscape.

To mark this anniversary, we asked a group of public health professionals to share their perspectives on what the shifting political climate means for *AJPH* and the broader field of public health. Their insights arrive at a critical juncture. We are navigating an era of deep societal division, in which public health itself is often politicized. Yet, public health has always been the art and science of bridging divides—protecting and promoting the health of all, even in the most challenging circumstances.

Since its first issue in 1911, *AJPH* has borne witness to history: wars, economic upheavals, pandemics, and polarized political landscapes. Through it all, the journal has steadfastly documented health inequities, championed environmental justice, and elevated the voices of marginalized communities. *AJPH* has also been unwavering in countering misinformation—whether about COVID-19 vaccines, climate change, or other crises—while ensuring its own contributions remain grounded in evidence.

The reflections we received underscore the complexities of the current moment, shaped by the 2024 presidential election and its implications for public health throughout the United States and around the world. Although the intersection of politics and public health is often indirect, the consequences can be tangible: rising risks of infectious diseases, worsening air quality, climate-related disasters, widening health inequities, weakened public health systems, retrogression of health-related human rights, and the persistent threats of misinformation and disinformation. This moment demands vigilance, resilience, and a renewed commitment to public health values—principles *AJPH* has upheld for more than a century and must continue to champion in the years to come.

Our contributors offer insight on how the current political climate relates to public health and what it may portend for the future of public health. They also offer a roadmap for *AJPH*—and for public health practitioners—to navigate these challenges. Their insights can be summarized under five overarching themes:

1. The need to research and disseminate information about possible and experienced harms resulting from policies that could undermine many vital institutions, such as the Department of Health and Human Services, the Centers for Disease Control and Prevention, the Environmental Protection Agency, the Food and Drug Administration, the US Agency for International Development, the National Institutes of Health, and the US President's Emergency Plan for AIDS Relief.
   - *Sound the Alarm:* Mary Bassett, former commissioner of public health for both New York City and New York State, currently director of the

François-Xavier Bagnoud Center for Health and Human Rights at Harvard University, in "Threats to Democracy and the Right to Health" (p. 307), emphasizes the need to sound the alarm, collaborate with state and local stakeholders, and document harms to mitigate expected adverse health impacts.
- *Bear Witness:* David Michaels, professor at the George Washington University Milken Institute School of Public Health and assistant secretary of labor for the Occupational Safety and Health Administration from 2009 to 2017, and Gregory R. Wagner, adjunct professor of environmental health, Department of Environmental Health, Harvard T. H. Chan School of Public Health, in "Bearing Witness and Spurring Action for Worker Safety and Health" (p. 316) highlight *AJPH*'s historic and ongoing role in advancing occupational health and safety and call on the journal to build on that role as new threats arise.
- *Ensure Accountability:* Nancy Krieger, professor of social epidemiology at Harvard T. H. Chan School of Public Health, in "Buyer's Remorse, Betrayal, and Blame: Who Will Be Held Responsible for the Adverse Health Impacts of the US Elections?" (p. 324), warns against scapegoating vulnerable populations for future harms to health, while calling for clarity on the structural roots of public health challenges.

2. The need to emphasize the relationship between political engagement and public health and support increased civic engagement by public health professionals and those who care about public health.
   - *Promote Civic Engagement:* Jerome Adams, 20th US Surgeon General and Presidential Fellow and executive director of the Center for Community Health Enhancement and Learning at Purdue University, in "The Imperative Link Between Civic Engagement and Public Health: Insights from a Former US Surgeon General" (p. 313), underscores the critical role of civic engagement, from voter registration to community advocacy, in advancing public health.
   - *Speak Truth*: Georges Benjamin, executive director of the American Public Health Association, in "Speaking Truth to Power: Making Optimal Health a Top National Priority" (p. 304), affirms the necessity of organizations such as the American Public Health Association to defend and advance public health and the importance of *AJPH*'s independence and capacity to speak truth to power in the quest to "make optimal health a top national priority."
3. Ensure that public health education remains innovative and focused on equity to prepare the next generation of public health leaders.
   - *Foster Equity-Driven Education:* Laura Magaña, president and CEO of the Association of Schools and Programs of Public Health, in "*AJPH*'s Coverage of Education in Public Health in the Age of Democracy's Crisis" (p. 321), argues for equity-driven public health education as a cornerstone of democratic resilience and global health progress.
4. Address the risks posed to the current record high 92% health insurance coverage rate by rising premiums, reduced Medicare and Medicaid benefits, and restricted access to care.
   - *Protect Health Insurance Coverage:* Sherry Glied, dean of New York University's Robert F. Wagner Graduate School of Public Service, in "Four Distinct Dimensions Through Which Government Actions May Affect Health Insurance Coverage" (p. 319), outlines how policy changes could reshape health insurance, including shifts in coverage costs, Medicaid and Medicare benefits, and the range of services available.
5. Recognize that public health progress is built over time and cannot be reversed by a single election.
   - *Maintain Historical Perspective:* Daniel Dawes, founding dean of the School of Global Health at Meharry Medical College in Nashville, Tennessee, in "Wide Awake: The Movement for Health Equity Continues" (p. 310), reminds us that the fight for health equity transcends electoral cycles.

Together, these contributions mark the beginning of *AJPH*'s 115th anniversary reflections that we will continue throughout the year ahead. They offer a framework to confront uncertainty and inspire action. As we move into 2025, we will continue this conversation and deepen our exploration of the critical issues shaping public health. Stay tuned. AJPH

CORRESPONDENCE

Correspondence should be sent to Alfredo Morabia, Professor of Epidemiology, Queens College, Barry Commoner Center, 65-30 Kissena Blvd, Remsen #311, Flushing, NY 11367 (e-mail: editorajph@apha.org). Reprints can be ordered at https://www.ajph.org by clicking the "Reprints" link.

PUBLICATION INFORMATION

Full Citation: Morabia A, Coston BE, Erwin P, et al. Celebrating 115 years of *AJPH*: perspectives on public health in a new political era. *Am J Public Health*. 2025;115(3):301–303.

Acceptance Date: January 6, 2025.

DOI: https://doi.org/10.2105/AJPH.2025.308018

CONTRIBUTORS

The authors contributed equally to this editorial.

CONFLICTS OF INTEREST

The authors have no conflicts of interest to declare.

Speaking Truth to Power: Making Optimal Health a Top National Priority

Georges C. Benjamin, MD, MACP

ABOUT THE AUTHOR

Georges C. Benjamin is the executive director of the American Public Health Association and professorial lecturer, The Milken Institute School of Public Health, The George Washington University, Washington, DC.

See also *AJPH* 115th Anniversary, pp. 301–325.

The United States of America is a republic where the power of the government is derived by the people under its authority. Our republic is governed by our constitution, which is the supreme law of the land that defines the rights of the people. The US Constitution, unlike that in many other nations, does not explicitly guarantee the right to health; however, the preamble does indirectly define the conditions essential to good health. It states, "We the People of the United States, in Order to form a more perfect Union, establish Justice, ensure domestic Tranquility, provide for the common defense, promote the general Welfare, and secure the Blessings of Liberty to ourselves and our Posterity." It is impossible to achieve this vision without achieving optimal societal health, and there is a strong link between the health of a society and the health of its people. In addition, community safety, inclusion, community engagement, justice, and equity are societal attributes essential to strong social cohesion and a robust democratic society.

The American Public Health Association (APHA), since its founding in 1872, has striven to be the nation's chief health strategist to drive the attainment of achieving optimal health for all Americans. The association's current strategic plan states that the APHA will work to achieve optimal, equitable health, and well-being for all. The APHA will accomplish this by serving as a convenor, catalyst, and advocate to build capacity in the public health community to accomplish this vision. *The American Journal of Public Health* (*AJPH*) is celebrating its 115th anniversary as an independent component of the association's work to strengthen our knowledge base by advancing research, policy, practice, and education. The *Journal*'s strength is its editorial and programmatic independence from for-profit influence. This independence allows the *Journal* to seek the truth through its publication of high-quality research and insightful commentary.

The theme of this 115th anniversary issue, "Threats to Democracy Are Threats to Public Health," is timely, as the very foundation of our republic is threatened, and our democracy is at risk by political forces that are trying to undermine the historical role of public health. That role is to ensure that we, as a society, do what is necessary to ensure optimal health for all. This societal responsibility is being challenged like never before by parties that are working to tear apart the social cohesion of our communities by creating false conflict, articulating false equivalencies, and undermining the trust we have in institutions.

The national election of 2024 resulted in the Republican party scoring a trifecta: They won the Presidency and the Senate and maintained control of the House of Representatives. In addition, the majority on the US Supreme Court has recently shown a tendency to support more conservative positions that have been unfriendly to public health policy.[1] It remains to be seen how effective this governing majority will be, as many of the winning margins—on both sides of the political aisle—were tight. The narrowness of these victories means that the legislators will be more likely to compromise to maintain public support. This is especially true for members of the House, as these members must run again in two years. Several political pundits have proclaimed that President Trump has a mandate to move his political agenda, especially since he narrowly won the popular vote. However, like the 2020 election, this was a close race, and there is little evidence that he and his party have a mandate. Historically, all political parties overestimate their mandates, and it often forces them to overreach. President Trump is effectively in his second term and, as with other second-term presidents, it is unclear how long he will have significant influence. The core fundamentals of politics are still in play, and there are enormous opportunities to move a proactive pro-health agenda despite fears that the nation is going into a prolonged period of regression on the public's health.

The next administration and Congress start 2025 with a large health agenda that can only be addressed if they work in a collaborative way with their federal, state, local, and civil society partners. It includes the need to rein in health care costs and to fix the mismatch between what we spend for health care and the poor value we receive for this investment.[2,3] This year, the Centers for Medicare and Medicaid Services project that national health spending will exceed $5 trillion for the first time. If the current spending trends continue as projected, national health spending will exceed $7.7 trillion—more than 19.7% of GDP—by 2032.[4] This enormous spending, double that of the next high-income nation, shows we do not get the value for this investment. We continue to rank at the bottom of health systems compared with other high-income countries.[5,6] In fact, the United States ranks poorly in life expectancy, with a more than 5.6-year gap between the United States and the highest nation, Japan.[7] The list of some of the other public health issues we must address is shown in Box 1. This list demonstrates the depth of the current challenges already on our agenda to address. The *AJPH* has a long history of addressing these threats to health.[8]

We do not have room for distractions. The science as we understand it today does not support limiting access to vaccines[9] or breaking up the Centers for Disease Control and Prevention. Instituting policies that underfund or put requirements on Medicaid in ways that limit access to care is counterproductive to achieving health care for all. Reversing regulations that protect our air, water, or food is not in the public's interest. Finally, our ethical principles do not support using our health-monitoring systems for invasive and inappropriate purposes such as tracking women's menstrual periods and pregnancies. Policy initiatives like these that are being floated around are counterproductive to achieving optimal health for all.

BOX 1— A Short List of Current National Health Problems

- Reversing declines in life expectancy
- Access to care
  - Achieving universal coverage, defend ACA, prevention fund
  - 7.7% of the US population is still uninsured (25.3 million)
  - Growing number of underinsured
- Women's health care, reproductive health, family planning, maternal mortality
  - Gender-affirming care
  - Emergency Medical Treatment and Labor Act (EMTALA)
- Addressing social determinants of health
- Long-term care
  - Alzheimer's disease clinical research & care systems
- Infectious disease threats
  - COVID-19 now an endemic disease
  - Increase in respiratory & other infectious diseases
  - RSV & influenza
  - Measles, polio, & other vaccine-preventable diseases
  - Sexually transmitted diseases (neonatal syphilis up)
  - Malaria & vector-borne diseases
  - Hepatitis C & HIV control
  - PEPFAR reauthorization
- Vaccination enhancement: childhood & adult vaccine program
- Mis/disinformation
- Pandemic preparedness—reauthorization of PAHPA
- Environmental health
  - Climate change
  - Environmental issues (exposures, toxins, Clean Air Act, Clean Water Act)
  - Lead exposure—line replacement & dust
- Injury
  - Gun violence epidemic
  - Domestic violence
  - Violent extremism
  - Unintentional injury (falls, pedestrian injury, motor vehicle collisions)
- Food insecurity—WIC, SNAP, Child Nutrition & Farm bills
  - Food Safety—multiple foodborne outbreaks currently
- Tobacco control (menthol rule) & vaping
- Growing mental health crisis
- Chronic disease including cancer (screening and case management)
- Health workforce
- Health inequities
- Chronic disease
- Multiple epidemics
  - Opioid
  - Obesity
  - STD
  - Maternal mortality
  - H5N1
  - Mpox
- Building the Next Generation Public Health System

Note. ACA = Affordable Care Act; RSV = respiratory syncytial virus; PEPFAR = US President's Emergency Plan for AIDS Relief; PAHPA = Pandemic and All-Hazards Preparedness Act; WIC = Special Supplemental Nutrition Program for Women, Infants, and Children; SNAP = Supplemental Nutrition Assistance Program; STD = sexually transmitted disease.

So, what is the role of the APHA and the *AJPH* over the next four years? The APHA will take its leadership role as the nation's chief health strategist. We will set our priorities for the nation to drive the national agenda toward optimal health for all. Those priorities include our commitment to diversity, equity, and inclusion and achieving health justice. In doing so, we must speak truth to power. We will lead the fight to prevent regressive policies with every political, advocacy, and legal tool in our toolbox. In addition, the *AJPH* will continue to have a prominent role in ensuring the evidence base for sound public policy, as it has for the past 115 years. As publisher of the *AJPH,* we must ensure the *Journal*'s continued independence as one of the few journals that is still completely owned and managed by a nonprofit association. We must ensure that we continue to provide the resources and the supportive environment to allow the *Journal* to publish the best research to inform, educate, and encourage public health policy and practice for the next 115 years.

Booker T. Washington is credited with having said, "A lie doesn't become truth, wrong doesn't become right, and evil doesn't become good, just because it's accepted by a majority." We in the health sector must not be confused by the degree of disinformation that is being championed by some of our political leaders and policymakers. The APHA and the *AJPH* must collectively speak truth to power and lead the way to building the capacity of the field to make optimal health a top national priority. AJPH

CORRESPONDENCE

Correspondence should be sent to Georges C. Benjamin, 800 I St, NW, Washington, DC 20001 (e-mail: georges.benjamin@apha.org). Reprints can be ordered at https://www.ajph.org by clicking the "Reprints" link.

PUBLICATION INFORMATION

Full Citation: Benjamin GC. Speaking truth to power: making optimal health a top national priority. *Am J Public Health*. 2025;115(3):304–306.

Acceptance Date: December 18, 2024.

DOI: https://doi.org/10.2105/AJPH.2024.307996

ORCID iD:
Georges C. Benjamin https://orcid.org/0000-0003-3453-1654

CONFLICTS OF INTEREST

The author has no conflicts of interest to report.

REFERENCES

1. Gostin LO. Judicial trends in the era of COVID-19: public health in peril. *Am J Public Health*. 2023; 113(3):272–274. https://doi.org/10.2105/AJPH.2022.307211
2. Speer M, McCullough JM, Fielding JE, Faustino E, Teutsch SM. Excess medical care spending: the categories, magnitude, and opportunity costs of wasteful spending in the United States. *Am J Public Health*. 2020;110(12):1743–1748. https://doi.org/10.2105/AJPH.2020.305865
3. McCullough MS, Magnan S, Fielding JE, Kindig D, Teutsch SM. Reduction in US health care spending required to meet the Institute of Medicine's 2030 target. *Am J Public Health*. 2020;110(12):1735–1740. https://doi.org/10.2105/AJPH.2020.305793
4. Fiore JA, Madison AJ, Poisal JA, et al. National health expenditure projections, 2023–32: payer trends diverge as pandemic-related policies fade. *Health Aff (Millwood)*. 2024;43(7):910–921. https://doi.org/10.1377/hlthaff.2024.00469
5. Blumenthal D, Gumas E, Shah A, Gunja M, Williams R. Mirror, mirror 2024: a portrait of the failing US health system—comparing performance in 10 nations. Commonwealth Fund September 2024. https://doi.org/10.26099/ta0g-zp66
6. Woolf SH. Falling behind: the growing gap in life expectancy between the United States and other countries, 1933–2021. *Am J Public Health*. 2023; 113(9):970–980. https://doi.org/10.2105/AJPH.2023.307310
7. Radley D, Williams R, Gunja M, Baumgarther J, Gumas E. Americans, no matter the state they live in, die younger than people in many other countries. To the Point [blog]. Commonwealth Fund, August 11, 2022. https://doi.org/10.26099/8x1n-xg40
8. American Journal of Public Health. Collections page. Available at: https://ajph.aphapublications.org/collections. Accessed January 8, 2025.
9. Colgrove J, Samuel SJ. Freedom, rights, and vaccine refusal: the history of an idea. *Am J Public Health*. 2022;112(2):234–241. https://doi.org/10.2105/AJPH.2021.306504

Threats to Democracy and the Right to Health

Mary T. Bassett, MD, MPH

ABOUT THE AUTHOR

Mary T. Bassett is François-Xavier Bagnoud Professor of the Practice of Health and Human Rights at Havard T. H. Chan School of Public Health, Harvard University, Boston, MA.

See also *AJPH* 115th Anniversary, pp. 301–325.

On November 5, 2024, in a presidential election won by Donald J. Trump, exit polls showed that nearly three quarters of voters believed that democracy was under threat in the United States. Voters also expressed similar views just before the election. That there is a threat to democracy and to well-being seems widely agreed on, but there is disagreement about the source of this threat: Democrats see Republicans who support Trump as the threat; in turn, these Republicans see Democrats as the threat.

The polls did not ask people what the idea of democracy meant to them. In the context of the national elections, one definition might be "one person, one vote." It is worth remembering that this was achieved in the United States only in 1965, 189 years into its nearly 250-year history. Jim Crow laws in the US South effectively barred African Americans from the polls until the passage of the Civil Rights Act (1964) and the Voting Rights Act (1965) a century after the emancipation of their enslaved forebears and following the passage of constitutional amendments that ended enslavement (Thirteenth Amendment), guaranteed the right to citizenship (Fourteenth Amendment), and guaranteed the right to vote (Fifteenth Amendment). The right to vote for Native Americans, whose lands were seized by European settlers, was also secured by the Voting Rights Act. The actual achievement of universal suffrage, typically expected in a democracy, in the United States occurred during the lifetime of many of today's citizens.

But democracy is more than elections. In its most expansive sense, it refers to an inclusive society based on equality, in which residents have substantive input into what it means to have a decent life, have meaningful opportunities to achieve this life, and experience themselves as accountable participants in accomplishing these collective goals. The values underlying these broad goals are enshrined in the United Nations Declaration of Human Rights, agreed to by all member states with no opposing votes in 1948. Article 1 begins, "All human beings are born free and equal in dignity and rights" (https://bit.ly/4glz9nk). The declaration enumerates not only political and civil rights but also social, economic, and cultural rights, including the right to health.

THE RIGHT TO HEALTH IS KEY TO DEMOCRACY

The aspirational goals in the Declaration of Human Rights, some of which the United States has never fully adopted, are a cornerstone of democracy. And public health data suggest these goals are under threat. The COVID-19 pandemic exacted a terrible and unequal toll, but warning signs emerged long before the pandemic. The United States started falling behind its peers in the 1980s. By 2019, the United States had experienced 646 000 excess deaths, compared to the average of the mortality of Canada, Japan, and 16 Western European nations—all democracies. With COVID-19, excess deaths rose to 1.1 million in 2021. One third of all deaths would not have occurred if the United States were just in the "middle of the pack" of its peer nations. Half of deaths to those younger than 65 years would have been averted.[1]

These comparative declines in life expectancy occurred across all racial/ethnic groups, across all ages, among children as well as adults,[2] and across the income distribution except the top 1%.[3] But the magnitude of the life expectancy decline was not equal. The Black–White gap widened to six years, the Latino "advantage" vanished, and for American Indian/Alaska Natives life expectancy declined to 65 years, a life expectancy in our hemisphere experienced by impoverished, unstable Haiti.[4]

It is hard to imagine that any well-functioning democracy would perform so poorly at protecting life.

THE REPUBLICAN TRIFECTA

In 2025, the Republican Party will achieve a federal trifecta, with a Republican president and control of the US House and Senate, along with the most conservative Supreme Court in decades. At the state level, there are now 23 Republican trifectas and 15 Democratic trifectas (down two from before the election). The 47th president

AJPH March 2025, Vol. 115, No. 3

perceives a landslide victory with just below 50% of the popular vote. His opponent and some of his former staff declared that Trump would put the United States on a path to fascism.

We do not yet know what will happen, but in his last term Trump demeaned and vilified opponents, groups, and nations; implemented a Muslim ban; separated immigrant children from their families at the southern border; began withdrawal from the World Health Organization in the midst of a pandemic; mocked climate change and withdrew from the Paris Accords; hollowed out the US Environmental Protection Agency; and, of course, applauded the January 6, 2021, insurrection. The Supreme Court, with three justices appointed by Trump, has undone affirmative action, reversed federal protection of abortion rights, and ended the Chevron doctrine—increasing court oversight of the operational interpretation of legal statutes, previously a task often entrusted to government agency experts. Scholars caution that the path to fascism is not a declaration but a process.

"MAKE AMERICA HEALTHY AGAIN"—OR NOT

Trump has announced Robert F. Kennedy Jr. as his nominee for secretary of Health and Human Services, amid expressions of alarm. With the slogan "Make America Healthy Again," Kennedy will have to overcome the multiple studies that show that Republican, conservative political leadership is associated with poorer population health outcomes.[5,6] Krieger expanded analysis of political determinants by looking at the association between four state-level political metrics (i.e., political ideology based on voting records of US House and Senate members, US state political party control, state policies enacted, and voter political lean) and health outcomes, including infant mortality rates, premature mortality rates, and having health insurance (for adults aged 35–64 years). Each measure of higher state-level political conservatism was associated with worse health outcomes.[7]

Kennedy has identified real problems (e.g., the noncommunicable disease burden, the health risks of ultraprocessed food, and problematic, even lethal actions by Big Pharma) but offered remedies that have scant scientific evidence. He also has not addressed how he will respond to the related corporations, which protect their interests and have politicized the US Federal Drug Administration.[8] Other views of his are misguided and dangerous, including his antivaccine stance, which questions the safety and effectiveness of childhood vaccination, one of the greatest 20th-century public health achievements.[9] Trump's own views have not advanced confidence in vaccination. Despite the success of Operation Warp Speed, which delivered an effective mRNA COVID-19 vaccine in record time, Trump was personally hesitant about receiving it and failed to endorse its widespread use. Undermining confidence in childhood vaccines is especially worrying. The Centers for Disease Control and Prevention and the World Health Organization announced 10.3 million measles cases worldwide in 2023.[10] Unvaccinated children will be increasingly vulnerable.

Trump's budget proposals would reduce the US Department of Health and Human Services budget by $272 billion (18%), cutting the Supplemental Nutrition Assistance Program (food benefits) and Temporary Assistance for Needy Families (financial assistance). A major global health effort, PEPFAR (the President Emergency Plan for AIDS Relief), is set to expire in March 2025. Some recall that the budget cuts made during the Reagan presidency[11] were accompanied by "no harm" promises, which were not kept.

Also at risk is the United States' standing as a preeminent leader in global health and scientific research, which attracts talent from around the world. Plans to redesign the National Institutes of Health may undermine the United States as a producer of scientific knowledge.[12] The plan to treat civil servants, including government scientists, as part of the "deep state" is understandably seen as a threat. During Trump's first term, resistance to public health authorities in regard to handling the COVID-19 pandemic led scores of public health leaders to be fired or quit their jobs.

WINNING PUBLIC TRUST WITH TRUSTWORTHINESS

With so many expectations of dire harm, how has public health, and government more generally, lost the argument? Why is there so little trust?[13] Why do so many invest considerable time in studying material they find on the Internet rather than listening to public health advice from government officials or academics?

Many people are genuinely worried about the safety of vaccines and drugs. They worry about the intentions of Big Pharma and corporations motivated by profit. Kizzmekia Corbett said it clearly: science needs to "move in a direction to be more trustworthy" (https://bit.ly/3Ps6NBN). A first step is to acknowledge that not all concerns are a product of conspiracy theories or quackery. The decline in science education and the insular world of science create a certain inaccessibility. People deserve to be listened to before dismissing their ideas. Next, the mantra to avoid nuance and complexity underestimates the public. So do declarations of certainty, especially when knowledge is limited.

Many promises are being made about regaining the United States' standing and health. Proposed actions include undermining scientific thought and institutions; denigrating groups and individuals; deporting perhaps millions of people who work, pay taxes, and lead lawful lives; and limiting the government's regulatory authority. These do not augur well for either democracy or for health. In his report on a typhus epidemic in Upper Silesia, Rudolf Virchow noted that the solution was "full and unlimited democracy" (https://bit.ly/404F7b4). The job now is to sound the alarm; point to evidence; work with others, especially at the state and local levels; and document harm. Those who believe that the Trump administration will "Make America Healthy Again" should understand that adverse health impacts are anticipated. When we pay the price, they should understand that they were betrayed. AJPH

CORRESPONDENCE

Correspondence should be sent to Mary T. Bassett, M.D, M.P.H, Room 705, 651 Huntington Ave, Boston, MA 02115 (e-mail: mbassett@hsph.harvard.edu). Reprints can be ordered at https://www.ajph.org by clicking the "Reprints" link.

PUBLICATION INFORMATION

Full Citation: Bassett MT. Threats to democracy and the right to health. *Am J Public Health*. 2025;115(3):307–309.

Acceptance Date: December 16, 2024.

DOI: https://doi.org/10.2105/AJPH.2024.307992

ORCID iD:
Mary T. Bassett https://orcid.org/0000-0002-7810-4163

CONFLICTS OF INTEREST

I have no conflicts of interest to declare.

REFERENCES

1. Bor J, Stokes AC, Raifman J, et al. Missing Americans: early death in the United States—1933–2021. *PNAS Nexus*. 2023;2(6):pgad173. https://doi.org/10.1093/pnasnexus/pgad173
2. Woolf SH, Wolf ER, Rivara FP. The new crisis of increasing all-cause mortality in US children and adolescents. *JAMA*. 2023;329(12):975–976. https://doi.org/10.1001/jama.2023.3517
3. Burn-Murdoch J. Why are Americans dying so young? *Financial Times*. Available at: https://www.ft.com/content/653bbb26-8a22-4db3-b43d-c34a0b774303. Accessed November 18, 2024.
4. Andrasfay T, Goldman N. Reductions in 2020 US life expectancy due to COVID-19 and the disproportionate impact on the Black and Latino populations. *Proc Natl Acad Sci U S A*. 2021;118:118(5)e2014746118. https://doi.org/10.1073/pnas.2014746118
5. Lhila A, Algahanem F. Along party lines: examining the gubernatorial party difference in COVID-19 mortality rates in US counties. *Prev Med Rep*. 2023;32:102142. https://doi.org/10.1016/j.pmedr.2023.102142
6. Warraich HJ, Kumar P, Nasir K, Joynt Maddox KE, Wadhera RK. Political environment and mortality rates in the United States, 2001–19: population based cross sectional analysis. *BMJ*. 2022;377:e069308. https://doi.org/10.1136/bmj-2021-069308
7. Krieger N, Moallef S, Chen JT, et al. Politicians, power, and the people's health: US elections and state health outcomes, 2012–2024. *Health Aff Sch*. 2024;2(12):qxae163. https://doi.org/10.1093/haschl/qxae163
8. Wang W, Wertheimer AL. History, status, and politicization of the FDA. *Res Social Adm Pharm*. 2022;18(5):2811–2816. https://doi.org/10.1016/j.sapharm.2021.06.009
9. Centers for Disease Control and Prevention. Ten great public health achievements—United States, 1900–1999. *MMWR Morb Mortal Wkly Rep*. 1999;48(12):241–243.
10. Centers for Disease Control and Prevention. Measles cases surge worldwide, infecting 10.3 million people in 2023. November 14, 2024. Available at: https://www.cdc.gov/media/releases/2024/p1114-measles-cases.html. Accessed November 18, 2024.
11. Campbell O. Here's what happened when Reagan went after healthcare programs. It's not good. Available at: https://medium.com/timeline/reagan-trump-healthcare-cuts-8cf64aa242eb. Accessed January 6, 2025.
12. Kozlov M. Major biomedical funder NIH poised for massive reform under Trump 2.0. *Nature*. 2024;635(8040):792–793. https://doi.org/10.1038/d41586-024-03736-0
13. Pew Research Center. Public trust in government 1958–2024. June 24, 2024. Available at: https://www.pewresearch.org/politics/2024/06/24/public-trust-in-government-1958-2024. Accessed November 18, 2024.

Wide Awake: The Movement for Health Equity Continues

Daniel E. Dawes, JD

ABOUT THE AUTHOR

Daniel E. Dawes is with the School of Global Health, Meharry Medical College, Nashville, TN.

See also *AJPH* 115th Anniversary, pp. 301–325.

In 1860, a movement driven by a keen interest in the most pressing social justice issues of that time was born in the United States to increase political engagement and action. This movement, known as the Wide Awakes, was an unprecedented mobilization of young people who recognized the connection between voting, government, advocacy, and policy to the collective well-being of the nation.[1] They understood that a robust democratic society thrives on the principle that all people, regardless of the characteristics unique to them, factors such as income, education, race, ethnicity, sex, religion, or geographic location, should have the opportunity to lead a healthy life and engage fully in our democracy. As a result of their tireless efforts, Abraham Lincoln was elected president, and the United States realized its first comprehensive, inclusive, and reticulated health policy prioritizing health equity and the social determinants of health among newly freed people and lower socioeconomic people throughout the country—the Freedmen's Bureau Act.[2]

HEALTH EQUITY AND DEMOCRACY INTERCONNECTED

Almost 165 years after the Wide Awakes formed, it is clear that today public health needs a similar movement, a coordinated campaign to increase understanding about public health and underscore how it is a cornerstone of our democracy. Today we need a new movement that can effectively communicate how health equity is the crucial element that enables and empowers public health to benefit the greatest number of people. Health equity ensures that systemic barriers to health are addressed, allowing everyone to achieve their full health potential and well-being. When efforts are made to bypass or prevent the inclusion of health equity in our public health programs, the foundation of our democracy begins to erode. But advancing and actualizing health equity for all populations affirms that democracy remains committed to life, liberty, justice, equality, and shared prosperity. This interconnected relationship underscores the need for continuous investment in public health infrastructure, egalitarian policies, and civic engagement to sustain both a healthy population and a vibrant democracy.

GALVANIZING AND EDUCATING THE NEXT GENERATION

This year presents our country with an inflection point, one that will determine whether people will accept regression toward a system in which health disparities may grow unchecked. More than ever, there will be a need to break down the silos in which we operate and recognize the interconnection between humanity and inhumane outcomes, between groups and issues. There will also be a need to understand how political will shapes public health strategy and how policies are created in the crucible of politics. A cursory knowledge of the political determinants of health will no longer suffice. We need to ensure that our next generation of scholars and leaders comprehensively understand how these determinants—voting, advocacy, government, commercial interests, and policy—have been galvanized throughout history to either hinder or advance health equity.[3]

Equipping public health professionals and health care providers with the knowledge on how to navigate the choppy political waters is essential to moving the needle of health equity forward. And while it is vitally important that we keep in mind the hard-earned teachings of yesteryear, all while still looking toward a brighter tomorrow that we envision, we cannot overlook some of the prescient lessons of recent times. For example, since the COVID-19 pandemic, which has resulted in more than 1.2 million deaths in the United States,[4] there have been more than 1000 legal decisions made at all levels of government regarding public health protections.[5] Many of these legal decisions, coupled with other policy and political decisions at all levels of government, have had profound impacts on the death rates owing to COVID-19 and demonstrated the challenges and threats to our democracy. It is incumbent on public health advocates to avail ourselves of the knowledge of the legal, political, and communications levers that are utilized to advance or hinder health equity moving forward so we can be more effective in our approach.

As we traverse the political actions and inactions that have long deterred previous health equity attempts, it is worth remembering lessons from the past. Forty years ago, the Reagan administration convened a task force to examine population health disparities and concluded that it would take "efforts of monumental proportions" to elevate the health of underresourced and marginalized groups to the level of the rest of the population. Since that time, successive administrations have worked and succeeded in closing some of those health and health care gaps, including child vaccines, and have even secured limited health rights from the judicial branch, including the right to privacy, the right to make reproductive decisions such as the right to use contraception and the right to an abortion, and the right to health care for incarcerated individuals.[3] However, we have rarely been afforded a robust opportunity to engage in the development of comprehensive health equity–focused multilevel policy interventions targeting the root causes of chronic diseases in the United States, interventions that would rise to the level of monumental proportions and significantly improve population health.

POSITIONING AMERICA AMONG THE HEALTHIEST NATIONS

As public health scholars, leaders, students, and professionals, it is paramount that we work to ensure that the movement to advance health equity for all in our nation does not cease because of a single election. We must recognize that to position the United States among the healthiest nations, previous efforts must continue, and new efforts of monumental proportions must be allowed. Our work for a fairer, better, healthier society must continue with resilience and hope. Every step made in this movement, no matter how small, has brought us closer to realizing a tomorrow that is filled with the opportunity to thrive in good health. Consider for example the evidence regarding equity-focused policies such as the 19th Amendment to the US Constitution, which afforded women the right to vote; the Civil Rights Act of 1964, which ended segregated health care; and the Voting Rights Act of 1965, which enabled African Americans to vote in jurisdictions that had limited their right to do so. Research has shown that infant mortality rates improved by up to 15% right after 19th Amendment was ratified,[6] 38 600 Black infant deaths were prevented because of Title VI of the civil rights law,[7] and jurisdictions required to comply with the Voting Rights Act saw reductions of up to 17.5% in infant deaths in their communities.[8]

Since 2016, life expectancy in the United States has fallen from 34th to 60th in ranking among all nations—a trend that is expected to continue unless we take bold steps to reinvest in public health.[9] Additional insights from a study led by Meharry's School of Global Health projects the costs and economic impact owing to disparate and inequitable differences in mental and physical health treatment and outcomes among various populations across the United States at a staggering $1 trillion expenditure in the next 5 years.[10]

TOO CLOSE TO FAIL: PRIORITIZING HEALTH EQUITY

As ominous and undesirable as these facts may be, we need not despair. Instead, let the challenges we face remind us of the urgency of our mission. As I reflect on the election results, and the implications for health equity, I am reminded of those periods in our nation's history when advocates for health equity worked tirelessly to advance this agenda and secured success in realizing egalitarian policies and programs that benefit everyone. I am reminded that they, too, were met with periods of regression and retrenchment but continued to seize opportunities to regroup, educate, activate, and advocate for health equity at all levels. Every setback and challenge also create new opportunities for engagement, for collaboration, and for progress.

As we enter this period of health equity awakening in our country, we must remember that, together, we can continue to make progress. Together, our collective voices can serve as a resounding gong for advancing the health equity needle. Let us remain inspired by the change that we know is possible, and, together, keep pushing forward until health equity becomes a reality for all. Let this moment in time serve as a reminder and call to action that we all must be just as courageous, if not more courageous, in this fight for health equity today, even in what may seem to be the most challenging of times. AJPH

CORRESPONDENCE

Correspondence should be sent to Daniel E. Dawes, JD, Founding Dean, School of Global Health, Meharry Medical College, 1005 Dr DB Todd Jr Blvd, Nashville, TN 37208 (e-mail: ddawes@mmc.edu). Reprints can be ordered at https://www.ajph.org by clicking the "Reprints" link.

PUBLICATION INFORMATION

Full Citation: Dawes DE. Wide awake: the movement for health equity continues. *Am J Public Health*. 2025;115(3):310–312.

Acceptance Date: December 16, 2024.

DOI: https://doi.org/10.2105/AJPH.2024.307991

ORCID iD:
Daniel E. Dawes https://orcid.org/0009-0005-9799-9264

ACKNOWLEDGMENTS

I wish to thank the hardworking team at Meharry Medical College School of Global Health for their support and ongoing efforts to advance health equity.

CONFLICTS OF INTEREST

The author has no financial conflicts of interest to disclose.

REFERENCES

1. Dellinger M. A Civil War political movement reawakens—complete with capes. *New York Times*. September 15, 2020. Available at: https://www.nytimes.com/2020/09/15/style/wide-awakes-civil-war-activists.html. Accessed December 18, 2024.
2. Dawes D. *150 Years of ObamaCare*. Baltimore, MD: Johns Hopkins University Press; 2016. https://doi.org/10.56021/9781421419633
3. Dawes D. *The Political Determinants of Health*. Baltimore, MD: Johns Hopkins University Press; 2020. https://doi.org/10.56021/9781421437903
4. Centers for Disease Control and Prevention. National Center for Health Statistics' National Vital Statistics System provisional COVID-19 mortality surveillance. December 2024. Available at: https://www.cdc.gov/nchs/nvss/vsrr/covid19/index.htm. Accessed December 18, 2024.
5. Parmet WE, Khalik F. Judicial review of public health powers since the start of the COVID-19 pandemic: trends and implications. *Am J Public Health*. 2023;113(3):280–287. https://doi.org/10.2105/AJPH.2022.307181
6. Hesse M. Women's suffrage was a giant leap for democracy. *Washington Post*. August 3, 2020. Available at: https://www.washingtonpost.com/graphics/2020/lifestyle/100-years-of-womens-suffrage-whats-changed. Accessed December 18, 2024.
7. Hahn RA, Truman BI, Williams DR. Civil rights as determinants of public health and racial and ethnic health equity: health care, education, employment, and housing in the United States. *SSM Popul Health*. 2018;4:17–24. https://doi.org/10.1016/j.ssmph.2017.10.006
8. Rushovich T, Nethery RC, White A, Krieger N. 1965 US Voting Rights Act impact on Black and Black versus White infant death rates in Jim Crow states, 1959–1980 and 2017–2021. *Am J Public Health*. 2024;114(3):300–308. https://doi.org/10.2105/AJPH.2023.307518
9. Johnson S. Countries with the longest and shortest life expectancies. *US News and World Report*. March 2024. Available at: https://www.usnews.com/news/best-countries/articles/countries-with-the-longest-and-shortest-life-expectancies. Accessed December 18, 2024.
10. Dawes D, Bhatt J, Dunlap N, et al. *The Projected Cost and Economic Impact of Mental Health Inequities in the United States*. Nashville, TN: Meharry Medical College School of Global Health; 2024.

The Imperative Link Between Civic Engagement and Public Health: Insights From a Former US Surgeon General

Jerome Adams, MD, MPH

ABOUT THE AUTHOR

Jerome Adams is with the Purdue University Center for Health Enhancement and Learning, West Lafayette, IN.

See also *AJPH* 115th Anniversary, pp. 301–325.

At the 2024 American Public Health Association annual meeting, I had the privilege of joining a panel discussion focused on the crucial relationship between democracy and public health. As a former US surgeon general, a state health commissioner in an ultraconservative state, a physician working in an inner-city hospital, and a Black man, I brought a wide range of perspectives to the table. The central question posed to the panelists was whether our democracy is at risk. As we explored challenges such as systemic racism, the January 6 Capitol riots, and voter suppression tactics, it became clear that in a variety of ways, democracy's very foundation is under threat. Although I agreed with my fellow panelists that the aforementioned are critical issues, I also highlighted another equally alarming development: the declining levels of voter participation and civic engagement in the United States, particularly beyond presidential elections.

HISTORICAL CONTEXT: HEALTH BENEFITS OF EXPANDING DEMOCRACY

US history is marked by significant strides toward expanding the electorate, with each extension of the right to vote correlated with improvements in public health outcomes. The women's suffrage movement, culminating in the Nineteenth Amendment in 1920, had profound public health impacts. Studies show that as women gained the right to vote, they became more active in advocating policies that directly affected maternal and child health, leading to substantial improvements in those areas.[1] Similarly, the Voting Rights Act of 1965 not only aimed to eliminate racial discrimination in voting but also had measurable benefits for Black and minority health outcomes, as it expanded political participation and led to policies that addressed social determinants of health.[2]

A more recent study highlights a strong and consistent correlation between voter participation and public health. According to the Health and Democracy Index, which analyzes voter engagement and health outcomes at the state level, states with higher voter turnout tend to have better public health metrics, such as lower infant mortality, higher life expectancy, and improved access to health care services.[3] This is not coincidental: when citizens are active in the democratic process, they are more likely to advocate policies that prioritize health, equity, and well-being. Furthermore, studies show that the act of civic engagement is an independent predictor of health and has even been shown to lower cortisol levels (e.g., https://bit.ly/423BynY).

In recent years, however, voter engagement has been on the decline. In the most recent US presidential election, nearly 40% of eligible voters opted not to participate.[4] This drop-off in participation, which is even more pronounced outside of presidential cycles, is concerning. Local and state elections, in which decisions often have a more direct impact on health policies, suffer from particularly low turnout. This trend undermines the very fabric of democracy and, by extension, public health.

CIVIC DISENGAGEMENT: A PUBLIC HEALTH THREAT

The erosion of civic engagement poses a distinct threat to public health. When large portions of the population, especially those from historically marginalized groups, disengage from the democratic process, their health interests are often sidelined. This is particularly true in states with restrictive policies aimed at suppressing voter turnout among communities of color, low-income individuals, and young people.

AJPH March 2025, Vol. 115, No. 3

Democracy, however, is not limited to presidential elections. One of the more alarming trends I observed during my time as surgeon general and as Indiana health commissioner was the reluctance in the public health community to engage with Republican-led administrations. Although ideological differences are inevitable, it is critical that public health professionals do not retreat into echo chambers or assume that only certain political parties are capable of addressing health issues. On the panel, I highlighted how we were able to expand naloxone availability under the Trump administration and syringe service programs under then Governor Mike Pence. Many minority communities, including Black and Hispanic/Latino populations, reside in states where Republican leaders hold significant power. By refusing to collaborate across party lines, public health advocates risk abandoning the very people who are often most vulnerable and in need of health interventions.

Active participation in local elections, legislative hearings, and even regulatory processes has an outsized impact on public health. As one of my colleagues aptly stated, "Your governor and mayor often have more control over your health than your doctor." Decisions at the local and state levels can shape everything from health care access to environmental regulations to public safety. The failure of individuals, communities, and public health advocates to engage in these processes weakens democracy and directly harms public health outcomes.

REINVIGORATING CIVIC ENGAGEMENT TO IMPROVE PUBLIC HEALTH

To mitigate the risks posed by civic disengagement, public health advocates must lead by example and must take proactive steps to encourage greater participation in the democratic process. Although the challenges are significant, they are not insurmountable. I list several strategies to help restore and amplify civic engagement, particularly in underserved communities.

Community Outreach and Education

Education is a powerful tool in bridging the gap between civic engagement and public health. Public health advocates can launch targeted outreach initiatives to educate marginalized communities about the importance of voting and advocacy. Many people, particularly in communities of color, may not fully understand the direct connection between their vote and their health outcomes. Informational sessions, workshops, and culturally relevant educational materials can help illuminate these connections and encourage active participation in elections and other civic processes.

Collaboration With Community Leaders

To build trust and credibility, public health professionals must collaborate with community leaders—religious leaders, educators, and local activists—who already have strong relationships with their communities. These leaders can serve as conduits for spreading messages about the importance of voting and civic engagement, ultimately amplifying the voice of the community. Working with trusted local influencers can also help address the political and social barriers that prevent some from participating.

Culturally Tailored Messaging

Messaging that resonates with people's cultural and social experiences is essential for fostering engagement. Public health advocates must recognize that different communities face unique challenges, including language barriers, historical mistrust of government institutions, and differing levels of access to information. Tailoring communications to account for these factors—whether through providing multilingual materials or by framing messages in a culturally sensitive manner—can significantly enhance the effectiveness of outreach efforts.

Voter Registration Drives

Making voter registration as simple and accessible as possible is crucial. Public health organizations can organize voter registration campaigns in collaboration with local governments and community groups. This can include helping individuals navigate the registration process and provide necessary documentation and ensuring that those who are eligible are able to participate in local and national elections. Increased voter registration can be the first step toward greater civic engagement and more robust democratic participation.

Advocacy Training

Empowering individuals to become effective advocates for their own health is one of the most significant ways to increase civic participation. Public health organizations should offer advocacy training programs that teach individuals how to engage in legislative processes, communicate with elected officials, and advocate policies that prioritize health equity. Advocacy training fosters a sense of agency and can lead to meaningful, long-term engagement with the democratic process.

CIVIC ENGAGEMENT IS A PUBLIC HEALTH IMPERATIVE

The importance of civic engagement in safeguarding democracy and advancing public health cannot be overstated. Engaged citizens are more likely to advocate policies that promote health equity, improve access to health care, and address the social determinants of health. Conversely, disengaged citizens—especially in marginalized communities—are at risk for having their needs ignored and their voices silenced.

To ensure that civic engagement becomes a cornerstone of public health efforts, we must commit to targeted outreach, collaboration with community leaders, and culturally relevant messaging. As we build these bridges, we can create a more inclusive democracy—one in which every voice is heard and public health outcomes are improved for all. In the end, strengthening democracy strengthens public health, and strengthening public health strengthens democracy. AJPH

CORRESPONDENCE

Correspondence should be sent to Jerome Adams, Executive Director of Health Equity, Purdue University, 610 Purdue Mall, Hovde Hall, Room 140, West Lafayette, IN 47901 (e-mail: adams616@purdue.edu). Reprints can be ordered at https://www.ajph.org by clicking the "Reprints" link.

PUBLICATION INFORMATION

Full Citation: Adams J. The imperative link between civic engagement and public health: insights from a former US surgeon general. *Am J Public Health*. 2025;115(3):313–315.

Acceptance Date: December 18, 2024.

DOI: https://doi.org/10.2105/AJPH.2024.307995

ORCID iD:
Jerome Adams https://orcid.org/0009-0001-3231-937X

CONFLICTS OF INTEREST

The author has no conflicts of interest to disclose.

REFERENCES

1. Miller G. Women's suffrage, political responsiveness, and child survival in American history. *Q J Econ*. 2008;123(3):1287–1327. https://doi.org/10.1162/qjec.2008.123.3.1287
2. Hahn RA, Truman BI, Williams DR. Civil rights as determinants of public health and racial and ethnic health equity: health care, education, employment, and housing in the United States. *SSM Popul Health*. 2018;4:17–24. https://doi.org/10.1016/j.ssmph.2017.10.006
3. Healthy Democracy Healthy People. Health and Democracy Index. 2021. Available at: https://democracyindex.hdhp.us. Accessed November 7, 2024.
4. Foreign Policy. 2024 US presidential election live updates: voter turnout comparison. October 7, 2024. Available at: https://foreignpolicy.com/projects/2024-us-president-election-live-updates-harris-trump/?article_anchor=us-presidential-election-2024-voter-turnout-comparison. Accessed January 7, 2025.

Bearing Witness and Spurring Action for Worker Safety and Health

David Michaels, PhD, MPH, and Gregory R. Wagner, MD

ABOUT THE AUTHORS

David Michaels is with the Milken Institute School of Public Health, George Washington University, Washington, DC. Gregory R. Wagner is with the Harvard T. H. Chan School of Public Health, Boston, MA.

See also *AJPH* 115th Anniversary, pp. 301–325.

More than 40 years ago, soon after the election of Ronald Reagan to US president, Jack Geiger, a pioneering public health and civil rights leader, physician, and activist,[1] spoke with a group of early career worker health and safety and public health trainees. They had expressed frustration and despair about the world they were moving into and uncertainty about what they could do. Drawing from his own experience in Mississippi and nationally, Geiger urged them to "bear witness": to observe, listen, record, analyze, and communicate widely the health conditions of the people they were serving; to work to understand and to help others understand the consequences of changes in policies, practices, and laws.

The mission of *AJPH* is to promote public health research, policy, practice, and education. In fulfilling this mission, it can continue to be a critical vehicle for bearing witness to the consequences of changes in workplace hazards and working conditions, policies, and practices.

AJPH AS A VEHICLE TO IMPROVE WORKER SAFETY AND HEALTH

For decades, *AJPH* has been central to efforts by the public health community to improve working conditions and prevent work-related injuries, illnesses, and fatalities. By publishing original research articles and editorials, the journal has given evidence of the toll of work hazards on worker safety and health and signified that worker safety and health are core components of community health and public health practice, motivating public health practitioners and agencies to apply lessons from this field. As the public health field has become increasingly siloed, *AJPH* has helped to break down barriers and to situate labor issues in the mainstream of the public health arena.

Around the birth of *AJPH*, there was carnage in the nation's workplaces. In 1907, disasters killed 934 coal miners. A 1911 fire in the building housing the Triangle Shirtwaist clothing factory killed 146 garment workers. More than 500 Pittsburgh workers were killed by work each year.[2] Children were commonly employed in dangerous jobs.[3]

These and other outrages spurred reformers to successfully advocate workplace safety regulations. Many states enacted laws limiting child labor and developed workplace inspection programs based in departments of health or labor, along with workers' compensation programs for injured workers. Eventually, propelled by labor activism, Congress passed the Occupational Safety and Health Act of 1970, launching the Occupational Safety and Health Administration (OSHA) and the National Institute for Occupational Safety and Health and, for the first time, requiring employers nationwide to maintain safe workplaces.[4] With new federal agencies charged with investigating hazards and issuing and enforcing workplace standards, many state agencies stepped back, deferring to federal efforts and refocusing resources to address other public health needs.

UNRESOLVED AND NEW THREATS TO WORKER SAFETY AND HEALTH

These reforms brought progress, but the unacceptably high toll of work injuries, illnesses, and deaths continues. Each year in the United States, traumatic workplace injuries kill at least 5000 workers (https://bit.ly/4h4DoZZ), more than three million suffer serious injuries (https://bit.ly/4h29uWe), and an unknown number are sickened and sometimes die from toxic exposures, often long after their exposures have ended.[5] Unfortunately, our surveillance systems for work illnesses and nonfatal work injuries are so poor that we have no accurate figures on the actual toll.[6] Children are again being employed in dangerous jobs. Many injured workers entitled to benefits receive inadequate or no compensation following their injuries.[7]

Recently, the COVID-19 pandemic highlighted disparities in the risk of illness and death from work and, concurrently, weakened public trust in public health. At the pandemic's height, many of the most powerful and highest paid people worked in the comfort and safety of home, while workers in essential industries risked their lives keeping society and the economy running. Thousands died and many more were sickened as a result.[8] At the same time, public health organizations' steps and missteps to limit the spread of COVID-19 were often met with distrust and resistance.

The 2024 presidential election and its aftermath have included threats to public health science, policy, and practice. There is widespread concern among worker health and safety advocates about the abandonment of protective regulations that keep both workers and the general public living healthier and longer. Workers are likely to face greater hurdles to expressing collective voice through unions and other organizations. And the federal government and judiciary are likely to limit efforts to improve worker protections, leaving a void that only some states may attempt to fill. *AJPH* can help those trying to fill the void.

To improve the safety and health of US workers, public health professionals and advocates will need to identify and examine the scientific, social, economic, and political barriers to achieving safe workplaces and tie the knowledge to action. The workplace and workforce are changing. Unions traditionally play an important role in demanding safe working conditions, but only a small proportion of workers are union members. Many workers are employed through online platforms or staffing agencies or work as contractors, so they do not have the same rights as workers in traditional employment relationships. A sizable proportion of workers, especially in high-hazard industries such as agriculture and construction, are unauthorized immigrants, who may accept more hazardous work without protection or complaint. These factors enable the continuation of workplace hazards and impede OSHA's ability to ensure worker safety.[9,10]

HOW *AJPH* CAN MAKE A DIFFERENCE—BEARING WITNESS

AJPH has long published articles that help practitioners understand policies and practices that work and those that do not. *AJPH* should expand its publication of case studies "from the field" that illuminate policies and strategies that drive effective prevention. We need to better understand the complex and sometimes contradictory forces at work in the lives of people who engage in hazardous work. Useful, too, would be reports improving our understanding of what motivates organizational and governmental policy change, including studies examining why some businesses embrace robust safety management and what would encourage those that do not to do so (https://bit.ly/4fKglTh). We should learn through case studies of failures of prevention, for example, the recent outbreak of the ancient disease silicosis among workers who cut, sand, and polish slabs of engineered stone to produce kitchen countertops.

More frequent reports on the results of improved surveillance systems, focusing on both hazards and health outcomes, can inform and stimulate action to reduce risk and mitigate hazards, motivate policy development and implementation, and evaluate intervention effectiveness across locations, industries, and populations. Applications of new tools, such as predictive artificial intelligence, and analyses of new data sets, such as OSHA's Injury Tracking Application, could yield significant advances.[11] Studies employing new technologies and analytic methods, including "wearable" exposure assessment devices, may yield important insights.

Early research on the effects of workplace exposure to substances such as asbestos, benzene, and silica, frequently published in *AJPH*, contributed to preventing many premature deaths. These studies often documented large effects closely tied to specific workplace exposures. Understanding the relationships between hazardous exposures in both workplaces and the general environment can inform and motivate both occupational health and environmental health advocates.[12] More research is clearly needed in traditional areas of study, for example, traumatic injury prevention and the effects of workplace exposure to ergonomic hazards, toxic substances, and airborne pathogens as well as the adequacy of protective equipment. We also need to better understand the causation and prevention of psychosocial hazards[13] and workplace violence (https://bit.ly/3W5rKX1) and the interaction between work-related and non–work-related social determinants of health.[14]

Effective communication is essential to public health practice. Beyond communicating studies on the causes and prevention of illness and injury, *AJPH* could do more to assist practitioners to improve their own communication efforts. It could publish articles that assess innovative methods to communicate research findings and best practices. It should continue to help its audience communicate more effectively, especially in the current context of a profusion of information that is unsupported by science and disinformation that is circulated to advance practices or policies that are antithetical to public health.[15]

AJPH reaches the national public health community and can play a central role in mainstreaming worker health and safety in the larger public health field. Given that work and work-related activities are sources of both adverse and beneficial exposures, the separation of worker protection and mainstream public health activity has worked to the detriment of everyone. It would benefit both workers and the mainstream public health community if these two fields were better integrated.[16]

We hope *AJPH* will expand its publication of transdisciplinary reports of the anticipated or actual consequences of changes in worker exposures and workplace organization. Better understanding the successes and failures of attempts at interventions and the social, economic, legal, and political factors that encouraged or impeded their successes is critically important to communicate broadly as more worker safety and health responsibilities return to the state and local levels.

Worker health and safety, as with all public health concerns, involve the collaborative engagement of many people across disciplines to focus on shared goals. By bearing witness and engaging with and supporting others with a common purpose, *AJPH* will help empower and motivate efforts to help all workers to thrive at work and in their communities. AJPH

CORRESPONDENCE

Correspondence should be sent to David Michaels, Environmental & Occupational Health Department, George Washington University Milken Institute School of Public Health, 950 New Hampshire Ave NW, Washington, DC 20052 (e-mail: drdavidmichaels@gmail.com). Reprints can be ordered at https://www.ajph.org by clicking the "Reprints" link.

PUBLICATION INFORMATION

Full Citation: Michaels D, Wagner GR. Bearing witness and spurring action for worker safety and health. *Am J Public Health*. 2025;115(3):316–318.

Acceptance Date: December 18, 2024.

DOI: https://doi.org/10.2105/AJPH.2024.307997

ORCID iD:
David Michaels https://orcid.org/0000-0001-8558-7733

CONTRIBUTORS

The authors contributed equally to conceptualizing and writing the editorial.

ACKNOWLEDGMENTS

We acknowledge financial support from the McElhattan Foundation. D. Michaels also receives financial support from the Health Action Alliance.

CONFLICTS OF INTEREST

The authors have no conflicts of interest to declare.

REFERENCES

1. Brown TM, Benjamin GC. Dr. H. Jack Geiger, a towering public health leader. *Am J Public Health*. 2021;111(5):792–794. https://doi.org/10.2105/AJPH.2021.306243
2. Rosner D, Markowitz G. A short history of occupational safety and health in the United States. *Am J Public Health*. 2020;110(5):622–628. https://doi.org/10.2105/AJPH.2020.305581
3. Clopper EN. Child labor and public health. *J Am Public Health Assoc*. 1911;1(5):322–328. https://doi.org/10.2105/AJPH.1.5.322
4. Wodka S. OSHA 1971: bringing government to protect the lives of industrial and farm workers. *Am J Public Health*. 2018;108(6):728–729. https://doi.org/10.2105/AJPH.2018.304417
5. Spieler EA, Wagner GR. Counting matters: implications of undercounting in the BLS survey of occupational injuries and illnesses. *Am J Ind Med*. 2014;57(10):1077–1084. https://doi.org/10.1002/ajim.22382
6. Azaroff LS, Levenstein C, Wegman DH. Occupational injury and illness surveillance: conceptual filters explain underreporting. *Am J Public Health*. 2002;92(9):1421–1429. https://doi.org/10.2105/ajph.92.9.1421
7. Boden LI. The Occupational Safety and Health Administration at 50—the failure to improve workers' compensation. *Am J Public Health*. 2020;110(5):638–639. https://doi.org/10.2105/AJPH.2019.305549
8. Michaels D, Spieler EA, Wagner GR. US Workers during the COVID-19 pandemic: uneven risks, inadequate protections, and predictable consequences. *BMJ*. 2024;384:e076623. https://doi.org/10.1136/bmj-2023-076623
9. Michaels D, Barab J. OSHA at 50: protecting workers in a changing economy. *Am J Public Health*. 2020;110(5):631–635. https://doi.org/10.2105/AJPH.2020.305597
10. Weil D. The future of occupational safety and health protection in a fissured economy. *Am J Public Health*. 2020;110(5):640–641. https://doi.org/10.2105/AJPH.2019.305550
11. Michaels D, Wagner GR. OSHA injury data: an opportunity for improving work injury prevention. *Am J Public Health*. In press.
12. Wagner GR. The public health conundrum of coal mining. *Ann Am Thorac Soc*. 2018;15(1):11–13. https://doi.org/10.1513/AnnalsATS.201709-725OI
13. Schulte PA, Sauter SL, Pandalai SP, et al. An urgent call to address work-related psychosocial hazards and improve worker well-being. *Am J Ind Med*. 2024;67(6):499–514. https://doi.org/10.1002/ajim.23583
14. Landsbergis PA, Choi B, Dobson M, et al. The key role of work in population health inequities. *Am J Public Health*. 2018;108(3):296–297. https://doi.org/10.2105/AJPH.2017.304288
15. Michaels D. *The Triumph of Doubt: Dark Money and the Science of Deception*. Oxford, UK: Oxford University Press; 2020.
16. Wagner GR, Michaels D. Work matters: mainstreaming worker health and safety is not limited to pandemic response. *Am J Public Health*. 2024;114(4):372–376. https://doi.org/10.2105/AJPH.2023.307565

Four Distinct Dimensions Through Which Government Actions May Affect Health Insurance Coverage

Sherry Glied, PhD

ABOUT THE AUTHOR

Sherry Glied is with the Robert F. Wagner Graduate School of Public Service, New York University, New York, NY.

See also *AJPH* 115th Anniversary, pp. 301–325.

Health insurance—specifically, an attempt to repeal the Affordable Care Act (ACA), also known as Obamacare—was a centerpiece of President Trump's 2016–2020 first term. Despite Republican majorities in the House (241–194) and Senate (54–46), the 2017 effort was unsuccessful. As Trump prepares to return to the White House, again with Republican majorities in Congress (House, 220–215; Senate, 53–47), coverage advocates fear renewed efforts to erode or eliminate coverage. Beyond ideological differences, because health care spending is the single biggest item in the federal budget, accounting for about 24% of all federal spending,[1] it is an obvious target for Republican efforts to free up budgetary space to renew the tax cuts that would otherwise expire in 2025. Although wholesale repeal of the ACA is unlikely given much slimmer Republican margins in the House and Senate than in 2017, the incoming administration can, and likely will, affect coverage through legislation, regulatory changes, and executive actions.

Government actions that affect coverage will affect people across four distinct dimensions. First, and most obviously, they can change the number of people who are covered by health insurance. A failure by the legislature to renew provisions of the Inflation Reduction Act enhancing the subsidies available to people buying coverage in the marketplaces, which are due to expire at the end of 2025, would directly reduce the number of people participating in this coverage and many[2] would become uninsured. A legislative decision to transform the Medicaid program to a block grant, such as a program with per-capita caps, might not change coverage in the short run, but it could lead to big reductions in insurance in the longer term. Less visible administrative actions could also affect the number of people with insurance. For example, the administration could grant waivers permitting states to restrict Medicaid eligibility to people who are working. Such work requirements would likely prohibit some people and deter many others[3] from participating in the Medicaid program and lead to increases in uninsurance rates.

Second, changes could affect the composition of the insured population. For example, legislative changes to the structure of marketplace subsidies, as were contemplated in the 2017 repeal efforts, would make coverage cheaper[4] for younger, healthier people and increase costs for older, sicker people, shifting the composition of the insured pool. Regulatory changes to the rules governing short-term health insurance plans[5] or changes in the marketplace risk adjustment[6] system, which transfers funds from plans enrolling healthier populations to those enrolling sicker populations, could have similar effects. Although the total number insured might not change much, people with preexisting conditions (including older age) would be worse off (and healthy people would be better off).

Third, changes could affect the financial exposure of people with health insurance. Legislative changes that diminish Medicare's ability to negotiate prescription drug prices,[7] or remove caps on Medicare Part D cost-sharing, could leave beneficiaries with greater financial exposure. Legislators could change ACA rules requiring that marketplace and private employer-sponsored plans cover at least a minimum percentage of expected medical costs (actuarial value), which would leave privately insured people facing greater financial risk. The administration could use its waiver authorities to allow states to impose higher premiums[8] or more cost-sharing for some people (or for some services) in the Medicaid program.

Finally, changes could limit coverage in nonfinancial ways. For example, the administration could relax rules governing formulary and network design,[9] allowing Medicare, Medicaid, and marketplace plans to limit the range of drugs they cover or the number of providers[10] of given types in their networks. Lower payment rates to providers within public programs might also diminish access to care. The administration could also restrict access to preventive services, including contraceptive coverage, by failing to defend a lawsuit against the ACA requirements that these services be offered without cost-sharing.

In 2023 and the first half of 2024 (the most recent data available), less than 8%[11] of the US resident population was uninsured. These historically low[12] rates of uninsurance, with particularly large gains for Black and Hispanic populations, were accompanied by steady declines in the share of people lacking a usual source of care,[13] reporting difficulty in paying medical bills,[14] and having medical debt.[15] Changes in policy could lead to deteriorations across all these fronts—overall coverage, coverage of vulnerable populations, financial protection, and access to care.

It will be important for public health practitioners and scholars to monitor changes across these dimensions. Our ability to track how policy changes—whether legislative, regulatory, or administrative—affect coverage, access, and financial protection depends on a continued commitment to the collection of data measuring these outcomes. Cuts to the budgets or personnel of the data collecting and disseminating agencies won't make program cuts go away—but they will obscure their effects and make it more challenging to address deficiencies in the future. AJPH

CORRESPONDENCE

Correspondence should be sent to Sherry Glied, Robert F. Wagner Graduate School of Public Service, New York University, 105 East 17th St, New York, NY 10012 (e-mail: Sherry.glied@nyu.edu). Reprints can be ordered at https://www.ajph.org by clicking the "Reprints" link.

PUBLICATION INFORMATION

Full Citation: Glied S. Four distinct dimensions through which government actions may affect health insurance coverage. *Am J Public Health*. 2025;115(3):319–320.

Acceptance Date: December 18, 2024.

DOI: https://doi.org/10.2105/AJPH.2024.308002

ORCID iDs:
Sherry Glied https://orcid.org/0000-0001-9432-1662

CONFLICTS OF INTEREST

The author has no conflicts of interest to disclose.

REFERENCES

1. Center on Budget and Policy Priorities. Policy basics: where do our federal tax dollars go? July 18, 2024. Available at: https://www.cbpp.org/research/federal-budget/where-do-our-federal-tax-dollars-go. Accessed January 3, 2025.
2. Lukens G. Health insurance costs will rise steeply if premium tax credit improvements expire. Center on Budget and Policy Priorities. June 4, 2024. Available at: https://www.cbpp.org/research/health/health-insurance-costs-will-rise-steeply-if-premium-tax-credit-improvements-expire. Accessed January 3, 2025.
3. Congressional Budget Office. CBO's estimate of the budgetary effects of Medicaid work requirements under H.R. 2811, the Limit, Save, Grow Act of 2023. April 26, 2023. Available at: https://www.cbo.gov/publication/59109#:~:text=2811%2C%20the%20Limit%2C%20Save%2C%20Grow%20Act%20of%202023.,and%20state%20costs%20would%20increase. Accessed January 3, 2025.
4. Horsley S. The winners and losers in the Republican health care plan. NPR. March 9, 2017. Available at: https://www.npr.org/2017/03/09/519500012/the-winners-and-losers-in-the-republican-health-care-plan. Accessed January 3, 2025.
5. Ding D, Glied S. Tightening the rules around short-term health insurance plans won't lead to more people going without insurance. Commonwealth Fund. October 5, 2023. Available at: https://www.commonwealthfund.org/blog/2023/tightening-rules-around-short-term-health-insurance-plans-wont-lead-more-people-going. Accessed January 3, 2025.
6. American Academy of Actuaries. How changes to health insurance market rules would affect risk adjustment. May 2017. Available at: https://www.actuary.org/content/how-changes-health-insurance-market-rules-would-affect-risk-adjustment. Accessed January 3, 2025.
7. Center for American Progress. Project 2025 Prescription drug plan would increase costs for as many as 18.5 million seniors and others with Medicare. June 13, 2024. Available at: https://www.americanprogress.org/article/project-2025-prescription-drug-plan-would-increase-costs-for-as-many-as-18-5-million-seniors-and-others-with-medicare. Accessed January 3, 2025.
8. Guth M, Ammula M, Hinton E. Understanding the impact of Medicaid premiums & cost-sharing: updated evidence from the literature and section 1115 waivers. KFF. September 9, 2021. Available at: https://www.kff.org/medicaid/issue-brief/understanding-the-impact-of-medicaid-premiums-cost-sharing-updated-evidence-from-the-literature-and-section-1115-waivers. Accessed January 3, 2025.
9. Coleman A, Nuzum R, Ramsay C. What's at stake in the 2024 election for Medicaid. Commonwealth Fund. September 12, 2024. Available at: https://www.commonwealthfund.org/publications/explainer/2024/sep/whats-stake-2024-election-medicaid. Accessed January 3, 2025.
10. Pifer R. CMS proposes stricter network adequacy standards for plans in state-run ACA exchanges. HealthcareDive. November 16, 2023. Available at: https://www.healthcaredive.com/news/cms-proposes-state-aca-provider-adequacy-time-distance-standards/699999. Accessed January 3, 2025.
11. Briones EM, Cohen R. Health insurance coverage: early release of estimates from the National Health Interview Survey, January–June 2024. National Center for Health Statistics. December 2024. Available at: https://www.cdc.gov/nchs/data/nhis/earlyrelease/insur202412.pdf. Accessed January 3, 2025.
12. Assistant Secretary for Planning and Evaluation, Office of Health Policy, US Dept of Health and Human Services. National uninsured rate remains largely unchanged at 7.7 percent in the third quarter of 2023. HP-2024-02. February 2024. Available at: https://aspe.hhs.gov/sites/default/files/documents/e497c623e5a0216b31291cd37063df1d/NHIS-Q3-2023-Data-Point-FINAL.pdf. Accessed January 3, 2025.
13. Peterson-KFF. Usual source of care. Percent of adults who reported not having a usual source of care, 2008–2022. January 3, 2025. Available at: https://www.healthsystemtracker.org/indicator/access-affordability/usual-source-care. Accessed January 3, 2025.
14. Peterson-KFF. Problems paying medical bills. Percent of adults who reported they or a family member had difficulty paying medical bills, 2011–2022. January 3, 2025. Available at: https://www.healthsystemtracker.org/indicator/access-affordability/problems-paying-medical-bills. Accessed January 3, 2025.
15. Kluender R, Mahoney N, Wong F, Yin W. Medical debt in the US, 2009–2020. *JAMA*. 2021;326(3):250–256. https://doi.org/10.1001/jama.2021.8694

AJPH's Coverage of Education in Public Health in the Age of Democracy's Crisis

Laura Magaña, PhD

ABOUT THE AUTHOR

Laura Magaña is president and CEO of the Association of Schools and Programs of Public Health, Washington, DC.

See also *AJPH* 115th Anniversary, pp. 301–325.

As the *American Journal of Public Health* (*AJPH*) marks its 115th anniversary, it is important to reflect on both its storied past and its ongoing role in advancing public health education and workforce development. Over the years, *AJPH* has served as a cornerstone of public health discourse, chronicling the triumphs and challenges within the field. Articles such as "COVID-19 and the Drug Overdose Crisis: Uncovering the Deadliest Months in the United States" and "A Century Later: Rural Public Health's Enduring Challenges and Opportunities" underscore *AJPH*'s commitment to addressing critical public health issues through rigorous scholarship.[1,2]

In an era where democracy faces unprecedented threats, the Journal's influence is more critical than ever. The intersection of democracy and public health is a tangible reality that informs how we educate and equip future professionals. Public health practitioners must not only possess technical expertise but also demonstrate civic engagement to ensure resilience in crises that test both public health systems and democratic principles.[3]

AJPH's role extends beyond documenting these challenges. By sharing stories of transformative programs, *AJPH* can inspire the replication of best practices and provide a platform for institutions and individuals driving meaningful change.

FOSTERING INNOVATION

AJPH must continue to serve as a platform to share cutting-edge approaches to encourage dialogue, adoption, adaptation, and advancement of education on public health. Undergraduate and graduate education, as well as lifelong learning, are critical in ensuring that professionals remain adaptable to evolving challenges and advancements in the field. Higher education has been challenged to integrate student-centered methodologies and increasingly immersive learning technologies, such as simulations, gamification, and augmented and virtual reality, into training programs to provide dynamic, hands-on experiences in outbreak management and community engagement.[4] Technological advancements, such as artificial intelligence (AI), offer additional opportunities. AI-driven predictive analytics and personalized learning pathways can tailor educational experiences to individual career trajectories, enhancing both efficiency and effectiveness. Hybrid learning models are increasing to provide flexibility, enabling professionals to balance academic demands with practical fieldwork. By catering to diverse learning styles, these tools build the practical expertise needed to address real-world health crises while fostering continuous professional growth and resilience.

AJPH can be pivotal in highlighting emerging pedagogical techniques, technological innovations, AI-enhanced decision-making tools, and interdisciplinary and intersectoral training models that bridge public health with technology, social sciences, and other disciplines. Disseminating the scholarship of teaching and learning to an audience seeking evidence-based strategies to enhance the learning experience must be a priority.

EXPANDING PUBLIC HEALTH TRAINING

The global health landscape is marked by crises such as the COVID-19 pandemic, climate change, and persistent health inequities. These challenges, compounded by the erosion of democratic norms—manifesting in disinformation, mistrust of institutions, and rising authoritarianism—demand a multifaceted response.[5,6]

Future public health professionals must be prepared to navigate these complexities through expanded competencies, including sociopolitical literacy, resilience, communication, and leadership. Although disciplines such as epidemiology and biostatistics remain foundational, contemporary public health training must include competencies in combating misinformation and navigating polarized political landscapes. Additionally, integrating policy and advocacy into public health curricula is essential. Professionals need to understand the political determinants of health and advocate for evidence-based policies that strengthen democratic systems.[7] *AJPH* can spotlight interdisciplinary training models that bridge public health with policy, ethics, and communication, providing a road map for the future.

The Framing the Future 2030: Education for Public Health initiative exemplifies this approach. Launched by the Association of Schools and Programs of Public Health in 2020, this initiative seeks to create a resilient and inclusive educational system by integrating antiracism principles and addressing inequities.[8]

By amplifying such efforts, *AJPH* can inspire transformative changes in public health education.

EQUITY AND INCLUSION IN WORKFORCE DEVELOPMENT

Diversity and inclusion are fundamental to the public health workforce. Research consistently demonstrates that diverse teams are better equipped to address complex health issues.[9] We need to ensure that the public health workforce reflects the population it serves. *AJPH* has a strong tradition of championing these values and can build on this foundation by featuring studies that explore strategies to enhance equity in training programs, such as those outlined in the article "Equitable Enforcement of Pandemic-Related Public Health Laws: Strategies for Achieving Racial and Health Justice,"[10] which highlights the importance of addressing racial and health disparities through equitable legal enforcement during public health emergencies.

AJPH must continue to bridge gaps by making resources and knowledge accessible to underserved communities and advancing equity in education and workforce readiness. Highlighting diverse and flexible models such as microcredentials and badges, which offer accessible, bite-sized content, is important to bridge knowledge gaps among underserved populations.[11] This approach aligns with *AJPH*'s mission to promote diverse public health practice models, enhance public understanding of public health challenges, and ensure workforce readiness. Furthermore, disseminating community-based participatory research remains essential, fostering collaboration between public health professionals and the communities they serve.

THE ROLE OF *AJPH* IN LEADERSHIP

It is essential for *AJPH* to continue spotlighting global innovations in public health education. Showcasing scalable models from diverse contexts not only helps to inspire solutions tailored to local needs but also fosters cross-border collaboration. As a leading publication, *AJPH* is uniquely positioned to engage thought leaders from academia, policy, and practice. Beyond traditional publications, the Journal can amplify its impact through its diverse channels such as special issues, podcasts, webinars, and collaborative forums. These platforms allow *AJPH* to address urgent public health challenges and explore their intersection with democratic principles. For example, *AJPH* articles on topics such as the impact of disinformation on vaccination rates (e.g., "Rural–Urban Differences in Vaccination and Hesitancy Rates and Trust: US COVID-19 Trends and Impact Survey on a Social Media Platform"[12]) and the effects of voter suppression on health access (e.g., "Voting Rights as a Key Political Determinant of Health, Then and Now"[13]) can enhance our understanding of how democracy shapes public health outcomes.

PREPARING FOR THE FUTURE

As *AJPH* celebrates its 115th anniversary, it is an exciting opportunity to reaffirm the Journal's commitment to contributing to the future of public health education. Embracing lifelong learning, fostering interdisciplinary approaches, and prioritizing flexible educational models and technological and learning innovations are all key to navigating the contemporary challenges we face. Strengthening the scholarship of teaching and learning will advance evidence-based educational strategies to ensure a competent and future-ready public health workforce.

By continuing to lead discussions on global standards in public health education and encouraging innovation, *AJPH* can ensure that training programs adapt to emerging needs while also addressing ongoing inequities.

The future of public health is intertwined with the future of democracy. Together, we can shape public health training that not only meets today's challenges but also helps to create a healthier, more equitable, and democratic future for all. AJPH

CORRESPONDENCE

Correspondence should be sent to Laura Magaña, President and CEO, Association of Schools and Programs of Public Health, 1615 L St NW, Suite 510, Washington, DC 20036 (e-mail: lmagana@aspph.org). Reprints can be ordered at https://www.ajph.org by clicking the "Reprints" link.

PUBLICATION INFORMATION

Full Citation: Magaña L. *AJPH*'s coverage of education in public health in the age of democracy's crisis. *Am J Public Health.* 2025;115(3):321–323.

Acceptance Date: December 19, 2024.

DOI: https://doi.org/10.2105/AJPH.2024.308001

ORCID iD:

Laura Magaña https://orcid.org/0000-0002-6767-4339

CONFLICTS OF INTEREST

The author declares no potential or actual conflicts of interest related to this editorial.

REFERENCES

1. Friedman J, Akre S. COVID-19 and the drug overdose crisis: uncovering the deadliest months in the United States, January–July 2020. *Am J Public Health.* 2021;111(7):1284–1291. https://doi.org/10.2105/AJPH.2021.306256
2. Ziller E, Milkowski C. A century later: rural public health's enduring challenges and opportunities. *Am J Public Health.* 2020;110(11):1678–1686. https://doi.org/10.2105/AJPH.2020.305868
3. Nelson C, Sloan J, Chandra A. *Examining Civic Engagement Links to Health.* Santa Monica, CA: RAND Corporation; 2019.
4. Marr B. 7 critical education trends that will define learning in 2025. *Forbes.* December 3, 2024. Available at: https://www.forbes.com/sites/bernardmarr/2024/12/03/7-critical-education-trends-that-will-define-learning-in-2025. Accessed January 9, 2025.
5. Scheelbeek PF, Dangour AD, Jarmul S, et al. The effects on public health of climate change adaptation responses: a systematic review of evidence from low- and middle-income countries. *Environ Res Lett.* 2021;16(7):073001. https://doi.org/10.1088/1748-9326/ac092c
6. Ostergard RL Jr. Democracy and health. In: *Handbook on Democracy and Security.* Seltzer NA, Wilson SL, eds. Northampton, MA: Edward Elgar Publishing; 2023:310–328. https://doi.org/10.4337/9781839100208.00027
7. Burkle FM Jr. Declining public health protections within autocratic regimes: impact on global public health security, infectious disease outbreaks, epidemics, and pandemics. *Prehosp Disaster Med.* 2020;35(3):237–246. https://doi.org/10.1017/S1049023X20000424
8. Sullivan LM, Weist EM, Barrington WE, et al. Education for public health 2030: transformation to meet health needs in a changing world. *Front Public Health.* 2023;11:1269272. https://doi.org/10.3389/fpubh.2023.1269272
9. Coggon J, Tahzib F. "The science of social justice": assuring the conditions for ethics and equity at the heart of public health. *J Public Health (Oxf).* 2021;43(4):e629–e631. https://doi.org/10.1093/pubmed/fdaa021
10. Watts MH, Michel KH, Breslin J, Tobin-Tyler E. Equitable enforcement of pandemic-related public health laws: strategies for achieving racial and health justice. *Am J Public Health.* 2021;111(3):395–397. https://doi.org/10.2105/AJPH.2020.306112
11. Omona K, O'dama MK, eds. *Global Perspectives on Micro-Learning and Micro-Credentials in Higher Education.* Hershey, PA: IGI Global; 2024. https://doi.org/10.4018/979-8-3693-0343-6
12. Soorapanth S, Cheung R, Zhang X, Mokdad AH, Mensah GA. Rural–urban differences in vaccination and hesitancy rates and trust: US COVID-19 trends and impact survey on a social media platform, May 2021–April 2022. *Am J Public Health.* 2023;113(6):680–688. https://doi.org/10.2105/AJPH.2023.307274
13. Jones MM. Voting rights as a key political determinant of health, then and now. *Am J Public Health.* 2024;114(3):289–290. https://doi.org/10.2105/AJPH.2024.307579

Buyer's Remorse, Betrayal, and Blame: Who Will Be Held Responsible for the Adverse Health Impacts of the US Elections?

Nancy Krieger, PhD

ABOUT THE AUTHOR

Nancy Krieger is with the Harvard T. H. Chan School of Public Health, Boston, MA.

See also *AJPH* 115th Anniversary, pp. 301–323.

AJPH March 2025, Vol. 115, No. 3

Predictions that US population health and health inequities are likely to grow worse in the wake of the 2024 US elections and that US government support for public health, science, and both global health and climate change initiatives will be curtailed[1,2] have a critical but unspoken counterpart. To wit: who will be blamed?[3]

POLITICAL, ECONOMIC, AND IDEOLOGICAL THREATS TO HEALTH

After all, poorer health and worse health inequities are hallmarks of societies dominated by political ideologies and politicians that prioritize market fundamentalism, individualism, authoritarianism, and so-called "traditional culture" (including religious fundamentalism), as compared with societies where political ideologies and state power uphold social equity and protect collective goods (e.g., keeping healthy the air, soil, water, and relationships on which all life depends).[1,4,5]

Promising a five-alarm fire, *Project 2025*, the right-wing manifesto for the new administration, aims to eviscerate both the "regulatory state" and the "welfare state."[1,2] The agenda includes (1) massive tax cuts for corporations and wealthy individuals, imposition of high tariffs, and mass deportation of both undocumented immigrants and those with temporary protected status; (2) policies curbing health care (e.g., upending the Affordable Care Act, further restricting abortion care), slashing funds for safety net programs, and shredding funding for and authority of public health and environmental agencies; and (3) pulling the United States out of the World Health Organization and the 2015 Paris Climate Agreement, coupled with gutting of US environmental, clean energy, and occupational safety and health regulations.

While not all policies proposed at the time of writing this piece may go into effect, consider the likely myriad impacts of, say, mass deportation of undocumented immigrants in the United States—who work in precarious circumstances with wages driven down precisely because employers wield the threat of deportation. Beyond harms to the health of these immigrants and their communities, costs will rise for food, housing construction, warehouse-dependent commerce, and health aides, and these costs will be exacerbated by intensifying climate change via worse storms, floods, and wildfires. These price hikes will disproportionately impact US adults without a college degree and their families—whose ranks include, among voters, White adults (66% of whom voted for Trump[6]), adults of color (64% of whom did not vote for Trump[6]), and also those who were unable or unwilling to vote.

PUBLIC HEALTH, ACCOUNTABILITY, AND THE POLITICS OF BLAME

Who, however, will be blamed, by whom, when population health profiles tank, health and health care inequities widen, and billionaires reap bonanzas?[3] Will there be "buyer's remorse"?[3] A sense of betrayal?[3] Or, in the time-disgraced playbook of authoritarian governments, will blame be affixed to those deemed to be—in the language of the new administration—internal "enemies of the people" who are demonized as "pests" who "poison the blood" of the nation (echoing the language of eugenicists, Jim Crow supporters, and fascist "racial hygienists" in Europe and the United States in the 1900s to 1940s)?[3,7]

Our job in public health is to prevent scapegoating and to document and make vividly clear, in media and forums of all forms, the causal connections between economic and social inequity, illiberalism, and the people's health. We must ensure that blame for immediate and subsequent health harms is affixed, as warranted, to the new administration's actions, policies, and plutocrat allies. The timeworn excuse so often invoked to explain and explain away past injustice—"they didn't know any better"—is a lie that cannot stand. In keeping with this issue's theme "Threats to democracy are threats to public health," and mindful of the *Journal*'s founding 115 years ago, may the record be clear, 115 years from now, in 2140, that many of us in public health fought back and fought for a better, more equitable future in which all can thrive. AJPH

CORRESPONDENCE

Correspondence should be sent to Nancy Krieger, PhD, Professor of Social Epidemiology, American Cancer Society Clinical Research Professor, Department of Social and Behavioral Sciences (Kresge 717), Harvard T. H. Chan School of Public Health, 677 Huntington Ave, Boston, MA 02115 (e-mail: nkrieger@hsph.harvard.edu). Reprints can be ordered at https://www.ajph.org by clicking the "Reprints" link.

PUBLICATION INFORMATION

Full Citation: Krieger N. Buyer's remorse, betrayal, and blame: who will be held responsible for the adverse health impacts of the US elections? *Am J Public Health*. 2025;115(3):324–325.

Acceptance Date: December 16, 2024.

DOI: https://doi.org/10.2105/AJPH.2024.307985

ORCID iD:
Nancy Krieger https://orcid.org/0000-0002-4815-5947

CONFLICTS OF INTEREST

The author has no conflicts to declare.

REFERENCES

1. Glenza J. Why the Trump administration will be bad for American's health. *The Guardian*. November 12, 2024. Available at: https://www.theguardian.com/us-news/2024/nov/12/trump-adminstration-health-policy. Accessed December 11, 2024.
2. Guarino B, Thompson A, Lewis T, Young LJ. What to know about Project 2025's dangers to science. *Scientific American*. July 19, 2024. Available at: https://www.scientificamerican.com/article/project-2025-plan-for-trump-presidency-has-far-reaching-threats-to-science. Accessed December 11, 2024.
3. Sahar G. *Blame and Political Attitudes: The Psychology of America's Culture War*. Cham, Switzerland: Palgrave MacMillan; 2023. https://doi.org/10.1007/978-3-031-20236-0
4. McGuire JW. *Democracy and Population Health*. Cambridge, UK: Cambridge University Press; 2020. https://doi.org/10.1017/9781108778725
5. Krieger N, Moallef S, Chen JT, et al. Politicians, power, and the people's health: US elections and state health outcomes, 2012–2024. *Health Aff Sch*. 2024;2(12):qxae163, https://doi.org/10.1093/haschl/qxae163
6. NBC News Decision 2024: exit polls. December 2, 2024. Available at: https://www.nbcnews.com/politics/2024-elections/exit-polls. Accessed December 11, 2024.
7. Levine P. *Eugenics: A Very Short Introduction*. New York, NY: Oxford University Press; 2017. https://doi.org/10.1093/actrade/9780199385904.001.0001

Trusted Messengers: Public Health Education and Advocacy in 20th Century Black American Newspapers

Wangui Muigai, PhD

For much of the 20th century, Black readers turned to Black newspapers for health information and advice. The messages reached hundreds of thousands across the United States during a period when the nation's racially separate and unequal health care system limited the ability of Black communities to access vital resources, including public health education. This article, based on an analysis of several hundred health columns published between the 1910s and 1970, traces the origins and evolving role Black newspapers played as trusted messengers of health information. In doing so, it details the strategic ways Black health professionals as well as readers leveraged this form of media to promote health knowledge, address the prevention needs in Black communities, and advocate for better care. (*Am J Public Health*. 2025;115(3):326–332. https://doi.org/10.2105/AJPH.2024.307897)

AJPH March 2025, Vol. 115, No. 3

From 1920 to 1927, Mrs N, a Black middle-aged woman, suffered from irregular bleeding and worried it might be a symptom of "cancer in womb."[1] The doctors she consulted with examined her "very roughly" and insisted she needed an operation, but Mrs N was wary of physicians who seemed "eager" to operate on her. Determined to find a treatment plan she felt comfortable with, she wrote to Albert Wilberforce Williams, MD, editor of a weekly health column in the *Chicago Defender*, the largest Black-run newspaper at the time. "Tell me what you think will help me," she pleaded. "These doctors I have here are white doctors and I want advice from some of my own doctors." In his published reply, Williams condemned the clinicians who treated her poorly and encouraged her to continue searching for a physician with good bedside manner. He went on to explain that her symptom history, indeed, suggested she had uterine cancer and if the condition proved inoperable, advised that radium therapy might "afford you much comfort and may prolong your life." Having responded to her concerns, Williams then used Mrs N's case to emphasize to readers the importance of being proactive and informed about one's health to avoid "an early grave."

Through the early to mid-20th century, Black newspapers were a main channel through which Black medical professionals communicated information about health and disease, and readers across the country sought advice on health issues. The messages reached hundreds of thousands each week at a time when the nation's racially separate and unequal health care system restricted Black Americans' access to public health resources, including educational materials. As one White federal official acknowledged in 1929, "the colored people do not have the same opportunities for knowing . . . literature from Government sources because not so much work has been done by the State and Federal agencies with the negroes as with the white people."[2] For Roscoe Brown, the Black health official who headed the Office of Negro Health Work at the US Public Health Service, the consequences of the government's neglect was dire, as he wrote in 1949, "the Negro people of the nation have suffered greatly from the lack of effective health education."[3] To remedy this situation, Black health leaders and lay people built institutions, nationwide campaigns, and local initiatives that brought health resources directly into their communities.

This article highlights the key role Black newspapers played as a trusted source of health information, drawing on an analysis of several hundred health columns published between the 1910s and 1970, as well as government reports and archival sources. As contemporary studies have shown, collaborating with trusted messengers is an effective strategy for promoting public health.[4] Cancer prevention campaigns, for example, have involved partnerships with Black newspapers, beauty salons, and barbershops to increase disease awareness and early screening, leveraging the longstanding roles these institutions have held as spaces for exchanging information.[5] During the COVID-19 pandemic, public health campaigns that engaged community-based organizations proved essential to improving testing rates, reducing structural barriers to vaccination, and combatting misinformation.[6] This article provides historical context that deepens understanding of these approaches, while also offering a longer perspective on the roles of race and racism, trust, and media in public health. In doing so, it argues for the need to look beyond formal health care settings to recognize the strategies Black Americans have developed to protect their health and advocate for better care in their communities.

THE RISE OF BLACK NEWSPAPERS AND THEIR HEALTH COLUMNS

From their origins in the 1820s, Black newspapers have centered the achievements, concerns, and injustices facing Black Americans, issues that historically have received less attention in White media outlets.[7] The opening decades of the 20th century witnessed the rising influence of Black newspapers as technological innovations in printing and the migration of millions of Black Southerners facilitated the distribution of newspapers into more communities.[8] At its height in the 1920s, the *Chicago Defender* sold 230 000 copies a week. Actual circulation was much higher as copies of the paper were passed along from person to person and read aloud in public areas: waiting rooms, train cars, street corners, and following church services.[9] By the late 1930s, the *Pittsburgh Courier* boasted a readership of a quarter million, relying on similar routes of formal and informal distribution.[10] Through migratory routes and in spaces of communal gathering, Black Americans across geographical regions, class backgrounds, and reading abilities gained regular access to the news.

In 1914, *Chicago Defender*'s editor Robert S. Abbott encouraged readers to turn to the paper not just for news updates but also for health information, writing, "Consult our legal and health editors. Their advice is free. Bring your troubles to us!"[11] Abbott's appeal was more than an effort to boost readership; it anticipated Black newspapers as uniquely positioned to address a growing disparity in public health campaigns. That same year, at the 42nd annual meeting of the American Public Health Association (APHA), a Georgia physician argued that when it came to improving hygiene and health in Black communities, health professionals "might as well try to teach sanitation to mules as to try to teach it to the negroes."[12] Such dehumanizing analogies, rooted in racist cultural stereotypes, served to rationalize and perpetuate health inequities even as some officials recognized that tackling major issues like communicable disease required working across the color line.[13]

With the 1913 debut of "Keep Healthy" in the *Chicago Defender,* Williams aimed to enhance public health awareness in Black communities and disprove claims of Black indifference. He was well-positioned to lead this effort, leveraging his professional reputation and experience treating patients at a municipal tuberculosis sanatorium as well as at Provident Hospital, the first Black-controlled hospital in the United States.[14] A 1887 graduate of Lincoln Institute in Missouri (a historically Black university) Williams earned a medical degree from Northwestern University Medical College in 1894 as well as a certificate in sales from Sheldon Business School in Chicago, Illinois.[15] He drew on his business acumen and medical knowledge to promote his newspaper column as "a weekly talk on preventative measures, first aid remedies, hygienics, sanitation." Emphasizing "no prescriptions given," he sought to dissuade readers from seeking magic bullet solutions to their ailments and placing "too much faith in medicine."[16] Instead he stressed the value of reforming daily habits and home environments to prevent the spread of deadly germs.

By the late 1930s, all of the major Black newspapers debuted health advice columns, following the *Defender*'s lead. Some features ran for only a few editions while others lasted for years and decades including "Keeping Fit" in the *New York Amsterdam News*, "Afro Health Talk," in the *Baltimore Afro-American*, "That Vital Thing Called Health" in the *Philadelphia Tribune*, and others in *Pittsburgh Courier*, *New Journal and Guide*, and *Broad Ax*. With a combined weekly circulation of 1.1 million subscribed readers, Black physicians had built up a significant platform to amplify their health messages.[17] Columnists focused on the leading causes of morbidity and mortality facing their readers: features that ran in the 1910s and 1920s underscored the importance of childhood vaccination and infectious disease control, especially tuberculosis, pneumonia, and venereal diseases. Though they encouraged open discussions on sexual health, medical columnists also adopted a moralizing tone, especially toward unmarried women and Southern migrants, whom they saw as most in need of guidance. Later columns published in the 1930s and 1940s paid growing attention to cancer and chronic conditions.

ESTABLISHING HEALTH COLUMNS AS TRUSTWORTHY SOURCES

Despite the proliferation of health advice columns, Black physicians took on professional risk in communicating to the public through newspapers. Dating back to the 19th century, this form of print media held a reputation as a source of medical misinformation; a platform primarily used by quack doctors to sell patent medicines.[18] During a period when the lack of licensing laws meant anyone could claim to be a doctor, such deceptive marketing tactics, combined with the crowded layout of newspaper pages, made it difficult for even the savviest of readers to differentiate misleading advertisements from messages intended for the public good.[19] But with rising acceptance of the germ theory of disease at the turn of the 20th century, combined with increased federal regulations over drug advertising, many health professionals began to see newspapers in a different light: no longer as platforms for medical quacks to spread misinformation but as tools that modern physicians could use to enlighten the public.

Still, for Black physicians who remained marginalized within the medical profession, dispensing health advice in a newspaper continued to raise questions about their intentions.[20] In an effort to dispel criticism that their columns were just another form of advertising (albeit one that aimed to draw patients to their practice rather than promote a product), Black medical writers emphasized their commitment to public health, that they upheld a professional duty "to sell health and the prevention of disease, instead of sickness or curing disease."[21] The *Philadelphia Tribune* drew a sharp distinction between the health advice provided in its pages from the guidance obtained through face-to-face consultations with a doctor. "It is not the purpose of the articles to take the place of medical examination nor the place of the family physician, but rather to deal with the primary laws of hygiene and right living."[22] Here, too, the editors framed health education and moral instruction as interconnected goals.

To further establish the columnists as trustworthy, newspaper editors highlighted the professional credentials of their medical writers and their experience working to improve health outcomes in Black communities. The 1924 debut of Charles A. Lewis's column in the *Philadelphia Tribune* came with the announcement that the physician "of merit . . . exhibited special interest in the health of his people."[23] A proud graduate of Lincoln University (class of 1905) and the University of Pennsylvania Medical School (1910), Lewis conducted antituberculosis work with Philadelphia, Pennsylvania's Bureau of Public Health and the Henry Phipps Institute, including a detailed survey of the environmental and economic factors that drove higher tuberculosis rates in Black neighborhoods.[24] Other columnists treated patients at Black-serving hospitals, trained and taught at Black universities, held leadership positions in civil rights organizations, and maintained memberships in civic clubs.[25]

Through these community-based and professional ties, Black health writers and their columns contributed to wider social efforts to improve health and living conditions. In health sermons they delivered in Black churches and radio addresses they gave that were broadcast during annual campaigns like National Negro Health Week that ran from 1915 to 1951, health professionals extended the reach of their printed messages to engage audiences across rural and urban locales. In Northern cities, the Urban League and National Association of Colored Women made "a special effort" to get health resources into the hands of newly arriving migrants and new mothers, distributing literature at train stations and community centers, and directing those in need of professional care to Black-serving facilities.[26] The dissemination of health advice in Black newspapers existed within this network of racial uplift work that flourished during the long Jim Crow era.

Across the different modes of outreach, historical survey data indicate that, by the late 1920s, newspapers had become the preferred source of health information in Black households. A national study carried out under the auspices of the 1930 White House Conference on Child Health and Protection, a decennial gathering of child health and welfare leaders, found that for Black parents, newspapers, more so than any other written source (including magazines, pamphlets, and books) served as the primary resource for children's health and infant care. Twenty-seven percent of Black mothers relied exclusively on newspaper advice, compared with 8% of White mothers.[27] The trend was similar for fathers. Writing for the *New York Amsterdam News* in 1928, the Harlem-based physician Lucien Brown observed that through "the medium of the newspaper," Black doctors had found an effective channel to "help thousands."[28] By the time the surgeon Ulysses Dailey launched his "Until the Doctor Comes" column at the *Chicago Defender* in 1940, taking over from Williams, he felt confident to declare that "the medical column as a medium of health education has come to stay, having won the sanction of the medical profession and the interest of the reading public."[29]

FOSTERING READER ENGAGEMENT

Inviting readers to ask questions proved a vital strategy for health columnists seeking to engage and build their readership. This newspaper feature first appeared in the *Chicago Tribune*, the city's daily paper with a largely White audience, where William A. Evans, Chicago's first health commissioner (and future APHA president) briefly responded to readers' questions. Evans saw the question-and-answer format as a valuable strategy for public engagement. Such exchanges, he believed, enabled health professionals to address the concerns of the "average" person, to "know them just as they are and to appeal to them in terms of their daily experiences."[30] Black health writers quickly recognized the potential of this communication strategy, with some, like Algernon Brashear Jackson at the *Baltimore Afro-American*, even listing their home address at the top of their weekly columns to encourage readers to write directly for advice.

Responses published in Black newspapers could be quite detailed, as Black physicians made it a key part of their public engagement to discredit scientific theories about racial susceptibility to disease. When in 1923 Ms. A. L. learned she had a fibroid "the size of a walnut," she wrote to the *Chicago Defender* to learn more about her condition. "Is it true that Negro women are afflicted with fibroid tumors more than women of other races? What causes fibroid tumors?"[31] In answering her questions, Williams first explained that physicians classified fibroids based on their uterine location and that the etiology of the condition "is not known to the medical world." Having established the state of medical knowledge at the time, he turned to address the "speculation and conjecture" that Black women were innately predisposed to fibroids. Such claims, he argued, lacked rigorous data and causal explanation even as they continued to be propagated in medical textbooks and professional articles.

Ms. A. L. was one of hundreds of female and male readers who wrote to Black newspapers with health questions and, in doing so, sent a clear signal that they were not passive recipients of medical advice but actively seeking information that could improve their lives and assessing the merits of such information. At the same time, in replying and publishing many of the letters they received, columnists gave correspondents a degree of agency in shaping public conversations about race and disease that further established health columns as participatory and trustworthy forums.

Some readers also saw value in the columns as a space where they could bare their frustrations over the challenges of accessing quality care. One Cleveland, Ohio, reader recounted the humiliation of traveling to Buffalo, New York, for a surgical procedure only to realize he was admitted to the hospital solely "as an experiment by the young doctors there who had more than a barrel of fun" and discharged him soon after without being fully treated.[32] Another, writing from Mississippi, sought recommendations for treating a painful anal fistula that had swollen in size and was causing "a great deal of trouble."[33] A local physician recommended an operation, but the letter-writer was reluctant to undergo the procedure, explaining, "I am here in the South and the chances are very poor for proper treatment." Many Black women wrote in expressing their reluctance to have reproductive surgeries, fearing the likelihood they would lose the ability to bear children. Their concerns tragically illuminate how Black women understood their vulnerability at a time when eugenic sterilizations were prevalent and how the threat of such harm deterred women from getting care they critically needed. In describing their fears, past medical ordeals, and hopes for "proper treatment," Black readers turned to health columns not just as a repository of expert advice but also a place where they believed they would be listened to and their pain would be taken seriously—not dismissed, ridiculed, or further exploited.

GENDER, RACE, AND PUBLIC HEALTH AUTHORITY

Initially, all of the health columnists who wrote for Black newspapers were men, but by the mid-20th century, some Black women broke through the gendered ranks. Flemmie Pansy Kittrell penned one of the longest-running features, which ran from 1936 to 1944, a column geared specifically to poor and working-class readers of the *New Journal and Guide*, those who "rent houses and work on weekly wages" as she explained.[34] Trained in nutrition science as well as home economics, Kittrell earned her graduate degrees from Cornell University (MA in 1930, PhD in 1936), and over the course of her career taught at leading Black institutions: Bennett College, Hampton Institute, and Howard University.[35] Her columns offered advice that was both scientifically grounded and resourceful, emphasizing the importance of proper nutrition in promoting children's healthy development and including tips on preparing low-cost foods into nutritious meals. As World War II rations made it harder for families to secure basic staples, Kittrell's recommendations became a crucial resource for those confronting food scarcity and insecurity. By 1946, the State Department also sought out Kittrell's expertise, sending her abroad to survey health education and nutritional needs in Liberia.[36]

When Dorothy Boulding Ferebee launched her 1950 column "Women Looking Forward" in the *Afro-American*, she noted with irony that Black women still needed an "invitation" from male news editors to have a space to speak on a national platform.[37] One of the most prominent Black physicians of her generation and president of the National Council of Negro Women, Ferebee recognized the obstacles Black women continued to face to secure positions of leadership despite the fact that Black women carried out the bulk of public health work through their roles as nurses, educators, caregivers, and community organizers. From 1934 to 1942, Ferebee served as medical director of the ακα's annual Mississippi Health Project, guiding her sorority sisters to the Mississippi Delta each summer to provide much-needed preventive services and care to more than 15 000 poor Black families.[38] With her news column, she focused on women's politics, framing the fight for better health care within larger struggles for improving economic and social conditions domestically and globally. One reader found Ferebee's column and its emphasis on Black women's political action, "a source of inspiration."[39] And as the civil rights movement gained momentum in the 1950s and 1960s, more Black health leaders turned to newspapers, alongside magazines and professional journals, to mobilize opposition against health care discrimination and social injustices.

HEALTH ADVOCACY IN BLACK NEWSPAPERS AND IN THE APHA

Within a month of being elected APHA's first Black president in 1969, Paul Bertau Cornely launched the column "Health in Action" that ran in the seven largest Black newspapers based out of Chicago; Philadelphia; Cleveland; Baltimore, Maryland; New York, New York; Pittsburgh, Pennsylvania; and Norfolk, Virginia.[40] The weekly installment had a considerable audience as by the mid-1960s Black newspaper readership approached 10 million.[41] Cornely's editorial carried many of the hallmarks of the earlier generation of health columns. The Guadeloupe, French West Indies–born physician was a widely recognized public health authority having earned three degrees from the University of Michigan (a BA in 1928, MD in 1931, and DrPH in 1934) and spearheaded Howard University's department of preventive medicine and public health. Deeply involved in the civil rights struggle, he co-organized the Imhotep National Conferences on Hospital Integration that brought together physicians working to desegregate health care, and he served as the medical coordinator for the March on Washington for Jobs and Freedom in 1963, among other roles.[42] Cornely's decision to write a news column while holding one of the highest positions of public health leadership signaled that Black health professionals continued to view newspapers as an essential channel for providing health information and promoting community engagement.

Shifting away from previous columns that offered advice on individual health concerns, Cornely announced "Health in Action" would, instead, concentrate on "the ills of the community."[43] He still encouraged readers to write to him, and often referred to questions he received, but kept the focus of his weekly messages on societal-level interventions. For those unsure whether the APHA would advocate for their needs, Cornely emphasized that the association, especially while under his leadership, would be at the forefront on issues that impacted impoverished and disadvantaged communities. Fighting hunger, expanding women's access to abortion services, and regulating environmental hazards like lead exposure marked key policy areas for the organization in the 1960s and 1970s.[44]

As the title of his column underscored, Cornely believed everyone had a responsibility and role to play in advancing the public's health. Laypeople should hold their elected representatives accountable on policy matters, he argued. At the same time, he regularly profiled radical, grassroots efforts to transform health care in underserved areas, including the free medical clinics organized by the Black Panther Party.[45] Cornely brought his call to action to the APHA as well. At the 1970 annual meeting in Houston, Texas, he named racism as a public health "enemy" and urged the organization's 25 000 members to join him in health advocacy, to "come out of their sterile and scientific atmosphere and jump in the polluted waters of the real world where action is the basis for survival."[46] Commitments to advancing health equity, education, and advocacy anchored his leadership vision for the APHA, helping to bring about the creation of the association's Action Board for coordinating grassroots advocacy.

Cornely's column, which ended in 1970, in many ways marked the culmination of Black newspapers as a leading voice on public health in their communities. Subsequent years witnessed declining readership and circulation of Black newspapers because of changes that came with the desegregation of the broader newspaper industry as well as a media landscape that was expanding into television programming. Yet, even as the national prominence of Black newspapers waned, the commitment among Black health professionals to partner with community-based organizations endured. Even today, Black physicians remain more likely than others in their profession to work with local groups and institutions to advocate for the health issues facing the populations they serve.[47]

ADDRESSING HEALTH INEQUITIES AND MISINFORMATION TODAY

Through much of the 20th century, Black newspapers provided a central platform that brought health professionals and everyday people together in their efforts to protect and promote the health of Black communities. The guiding values of education and advocacy resonated deeply with newspaper readers who faced formidable obstacles to accessing health resources. The robust discussions that took place in health education columns, many of them driven by ordinary people's questions, point to the value and continued need to involve and amplify different voices in public health dialogues.

With the 21st-century shift to digital news platforms and social media, public health leaders have sounded alarms that individuals are now exposed to health information that deliberately misleads and undermines public health goals.[48] This situation demands innovative solutions to rebuild trust in public health leadership. Still as this historical case demonstrates, concerns over the harms posed by media are not new. Black communities have long been engaged in combatting false ideas about race and disease and have strategically leveraged media channels to identify, disseminate, and amplify trustworthy information. Ongoing efforts to advance the public's health, especially among those historically underserved, must look to these past efforts as a guide and support institutions that are trusted in their communities. AJPH

ABOUT THE AUTHORS

Wangui Muigai is with the History Department, the African and African American Studies Department, and the Health: Science, Society, and Policy Program, Brandeis University, Waltham, MA.

CORRESPONDENCE

Correspondence should be sent to Wangui Muigai, Brandeis University, 415 South St, Waltham MA, 02453 (e-mail: wmuigai@brandeis.edu). Reprints can be ordered at https://www.ajph.org by clicking the "Reprints" link.

PUBLICATION INFORMATION

Full Citation: Muigai W. Trusted messengers: public health education and advocacy in 20th century Black American newspapers. *Am J Public Health*. 2025;115(3):326–332.

Acceptance Date: October 6, 2024.

DOI: https://doi.org/10.2105/AJPH.2024.307897

ORCID iD:

Wangui Muigai https://orcid.org/0009-0002-3305-1317

ACKNOWLEDGMENTS

This work was supported by the Greenwall Foundation Faculty Scholars Program in Bioethics.

The author is grateful to Vanessa Northington Gamble, Monica Peek, and Theodore M. Brown for their constructive suggestions. The author thanks Sabreen Huq for research assistance.

CONFLICTS OF INTEREST

The author has no conflicts of interest to report.

REFERENCES

1. A. Wilberforce Williams, "The Way to Health: Wants Operation," *Chicago Defender*, December 31, 1927, part 2, page 2.
2. Blanche Haines to Mrs. Walter I. Dolbeare, May 1929, File 0-2-9-1-6, Box 368, Central File (1929–1932), Record Group 102, US Children's Bureau, National Archives, College Park, MD.
3. Roscoe C. Brown, "The Health Education Programs of Government and Voluntary Agencies," *Journal of Negro Education* 18, no. 3 (1949): 377–387.
4. Angela K. Shen et al., "Trusted Messengers and Trusted Messages: The Role for Community-Based Organizations in Promoting COVID-19 and Routine Immunizations," *Vaccine* 41, no. 12 (2023):1994–2002, https://doi.org/10.1016/j.vaccine.2023.02.045
5. Charlene A. Caburnay et al., "Black Newspapers as a Tool for Cancer Education in African American Communities," *Ethnicity and Disease* 18, no. 4 (2008): 488–495; Tracey E. Wilson et al., "Hair Salon Stylists as Breast Cancer Prevention Lay Health Advisors for African American and Afro-Caribbean Women," *Journal of Health Care for the Poor and Underserved* 19, no. 1 (2008): 216–226, https://doi.org/10.1353/hpu.2008.0017; Bill J. Releford et al., "Health Promotion in Barbershops: Balancing Outreach and Research in African American Communities," *Ethnicity and Disease* 20, no. 2 (2010): 185–188.
6. Tiwaladeoluwa B. Adekunle et al., "Continuity of Trust: Health Systems' Role in Advancing Health Equity Beyond the COVID-19 Pandemic," *Community Health Equity Research & Policy* 44, no. 3 (2024): 323–329, https://doi.org/10.1177/2752535X231185221
7. Frankie Hutton, *The Early Black Press in America, 1827–1860* (Westport, CT: Praeger, 1993).
8. Julia Guarneri, *Newsprint Metropolis: City Papers and the Making of Modern Americans* (Chicago, IL: University of Chicago Press, 2017).
9. James R. Grossman, *Land of Hope: Chicago, Black Southerners, and the Great Migration* (Chicago, IL: University of Chicago Press, 1989).
10. Andrew Buni, *Robert L. Vann of the* Pittsburgh Courier (Pittsburgh, PA: University of Pittsburgh Press, 1974).
11. "Leap in Journalism; Eight Pages for the Defender," *Chicago Defender*, September 12, 1914, 2.
12. L. C. Allen, "The Negro Health Problem," *American Journal of Public Health* 5, no. 3 (1915): 194–203, 201.
13. Samuel Kelton Roberts Jr, *Infectious Fear: Politics, Disease, and the Health Effects of Segregation* (Chapel Hill, NC: University of North Carolina Press, 2009).
14. Vanessa Northington Gamble, *Making a Place for Ourselves: The Black Hospital Movement, 1920–1945* (New York, NY: Oxford University Press, 1995), 3.

15. "A. Wilberforce Williams," *Journal of Negro History* 25, no. 2 (1940): 262–263.
16. Williams, "'I Have Heart Trouble, Doctor'," *Chicago Defender*, January 17, 1925, 12.
17. Negro Affairs Division, "Negro Newspapers and Periodicals in the United States" (Washington, DC: US Bureau of Foreign and Domestic Commerce, US Department of Commerce, February 1937), 14.
18. John Parascandola, "Patent Medicines and the Public's Health," *Public Health Reports* 114, no. 4 (1999): 318–321.
19. Richard H. Shryock, *Medical Licensing in America, 1650–1965* (Baltimore, MD: Johns Hopkins University Press, 1967).
20. Robert B. Baker et al., "African American Physicians and Organized Medicine, 1846–1968: Origins of a Racial Divide," *Journal of the American Medical Association* 300, no. 3 (2008): 306–313.
21. Williams, "The Family Physician," *Chicago Defender*, January 27, 1923, 12.
22. "Dr. Charles A. Lewis Agrees to Conduct Health Column," *Philadelphia Tribune*, October 18, 1924, 9.
23. Ibid.
24. David McBride, "The Henry Phipps Institute, 1903–1937: Pioneering Tuberculosis Work With an Urban Minority," *Bulletin of the History of Medicine* 61, no. 1 (1987): 78–97.
25. "Dr. Lucien Brown New Health Writer: Harlem Physician to Continue 'Keeping Fit' Column," *New York Amsterdam News*, October 3, 1928, 2; Cromwell C. Douglas, "Health Is Happiness: The Forward March of Medicine," *New Journal and Guide*, November 28, 1953, 15.
26. Mrs. Mary Waldo Taylor (Chicago Urban League) to Katharine F. Lenroot (Children's Bureau), March 7, 1928, File 0-2-8-1-6, Box 262 (1925–1928), US Children's Bureau; Mary Fitzbutler Waring to US Department of Labor, June 1925, File 0-2-8-1-6, Box 262 (1925–1928), US Children's Bureau.
27. White House Conference on Child Health and Protection, *The Young Child in the Home: A Survey of Three Thousand American Families: Report of the Committee on the Infant and Preschool Child* (New York, NY: D. Appleton-Century Company, 1936), 287–289.
28. Lucien M. Brown, "Keeping Fit: My Impression of Late Dr. Rawlins," *New York Amsterdam News*, October 3, 1928, 16.
29. Ulysses Dailey, "Essay on Medical Columns," Folder 5, Box 3, Manuscripts, Ulysses Grant Dailey Papers, Vivian G. Harsh Research Collection, Carter G. Woodson Regional Library, Chicago, IL.
30. William A. Evans, *How to Keep Well: A Health Book for the Home* (New York, NY: Applewood and Co; 1917), vii, viii.
31. Williams, "Worried About Fibroid Tumors and Ascites," *Chicago Defender* June 23, 1923, 12.
32. Williams, "Worried About Fistula," *Chicago Defender*, August 15, 1925, part 2, page 8.
33. Williams, "The Way to Health: May Be Anal Fistula," *Chicago Defender*, April 30, 1927, part 2, page 2.
34. Flemmie Kittrell, "The Family and National Defense: Child Health Must Be Safeguarded," *New Journal and Guide*, May 23, 1942, 7.
35. Flemmie Pansy Kittrell, "A Study of Negro Infant Feeding Practices in a Selected Community of North Carolina," (PhD dissertation, Cornell University, February 1936).
36. "Dr. Flemmie Kitrell to Make Study of Liberia's Diet Problem," *New Journal and Guide*, December 21 1946, 5.
37. Dorothy Ferebee, "Women Looking Forward," *Afro-American*, January 28, 1950, 1.
38. Susan Smith, *Sick and Tired of Being Sick and Tired: Black Women's Health Activism in America, 1890–1950* (Philadelphia, PA: University of Pennsylvania Press, 2011), 149–167.
39. Elizabeth Williams, "Like Column for Women," *Afro-American*, February 18, 1950, 4.
40. "Top Physician to Pen C & P Column," *Call and Post*, December 20, 1969, 16A; "Dr. Cornely to Write Weekly Column," *Atlanta Daily World*, January 6, 1970, 1.
41. Kimberley Mangun and Earnest L. Perry Jr, "The Negro/National Newspaper Publishers Association and Its Dual Roles as a Trade and Advocacy Organization, 1940–2020," *Journalism & Communication Monographs* 22, no. 4 (2020): 264–336, https://doi.org/10.1177/1522637920965961
42. Theodore M. Brown and Elizabeth Fee, "Paul B. Cornely (1906–2002): Civil Rights Leader and Public Health Pioneer," *American Journal of Public Health* 101, suppl 1 (2011): S164, https://doi.org/10.2105/AJPH.2010.300052
43. "AFRO column by APHA's Cornely," *Afro-American*, December 13, 1969, 21.
44. "Recommended Standards for Abortion Services. Adopted by the Executive Board of the APHA at the 98th Annual Meeting in Houston, Texas, October 29, 1970," *American Journal of Public Health* 61, no. 2 (1971): 396–398.
45. Alondra Nelson, *Body and Soul: The Black Panther Party and the Fight Against Medical Discrimination* (Minneapolis, MN: University of Minnesota Press, 2011); AJPH Special Section: Black Panther Party, *American Journal of Public Health* 106, no. 10 (2016).
46. Paul B. Cornely, "The Hidden Enemies of Health and the American Public Health Association," *American Journal of Public Health* 61, no. 1 (1971), 7–18, 14.
47. Russell L. Gruen, Eric G. Campbell, and David Blumenthal, "Public Roles of US Physicians: Community Participation, Political Involvement, and Collective Advocacy," *Journal of the American Medical Association* 296, no. 20 (2006), 2467–2475, https://doi.org/10.1001/jama.296.20.2467
48. Office of the Surgeon General, *Confronting Health Misinformation: The US Surgeon General's Advisory on Building a Healthy Information Environment* (Washington, DC: US Department of Health and Human Services, 2021).

Racial and Ethnic Representation of the Local Public Health Workforce

Casey P. Balio, PhD, Haleigh Leslie, MPH, MBA, and Michael B. Meit, MA, MPH

See also Masselink, p. 271.

Objectives. To describe racial and ethnic representativeness of the local health department (LHD) workforce compared with the populations served.

Methods. In this study, we used a cross-sectional design of the 2021 Public Health Workforce Interests and Needs Survey, 2019 National Association of County and City Health Officials Profile data, and other sources to estimate the racial and ethnic representativeness of LHD workforce. We calculated representativeness as a binary measure of at least representative of the populations served for each race and ethnicity group. We present bivariate analyses comparing LHD representativeness by region and rurality, and multivariate analyses to estimate the associations between representativeness, agency, and jurisdiction characteristics. This study was conducted in Tennessee in 2023.

Results. Sixty percent of LHDs in the sample were at least representative of the Black, Indigenous, and People of Color populations they serve. For most race and ethnicity groups, urban-serving LHDs were more representative of the populations they serve than rural-serving LHDs.

Conclusions. Racial and ethnic representativeness of the LHD workforce varies by rurality, region, and race or ethnicity. These findings may help inform training, recruitment, and retention efforts in public health. (*Am J Public Health*. 2025;115(3):333–343. https://doi.org/10.2105/AJPH.2024.307903)

AJPH March 2025, Vol. 115, No. 3

Local and state governmental public health is at the forefront of providing a broad array of public health programs and services to the people in their jurisdictions.[1] The demand on public health departments is growing to address evolving and diversifying community needs within a changing political and health context. While the activities and responsibilities of public health agencies across the country have evolved, the 10 Essential Public Health Services remain an important framework for guiding the work of public health, central to which is a focus on health equity.[2] In addition, the Centers for Disease Control and Prevention (CDC) has identified health equity as a priority.[3,4] Inherent to the focus of health equity is a diverse workforce[3] and one that reflects the community served. As the United States becomes more racially and ethnically diverse and works to address health inequities that have been perpetuated for decades, there is a need for attention to the racial and ethnic composition of public servants and the communities they serve, including in governmental public health agencies.[5,6]

Research on bureaucratic representation (the degree to which governmental employees reflect the communities they serve) in other public service sectors has found that when the demographics of the public servants more closely resemble the demographics of the population served—in particular, their race and ethnicity—there is more trust from the community and focus on community needs.[7–10] In more representative bureaucracies, there is more collaboration between the community and public servants on community policies and more accountability of bureaucratic operations.[6] Furthermore, patients who see a health care provider who is the same race as them have better health outcomes.[11–13] The importance of representation may apply to the governmental public health workforce as well, where having a more diverse and representative public health workforce may help to build credibility and trust with communities to address these and future needs.[14]

The most recent iteration of a comprehensive survey of the public health workforce (Public Health Workforce Interests and Needs Survey [PH WINS]) found that the governmental public health workforce is majority White (54%) and female (79%) and has an average age of 46 years.[15] Furthermore, the workforce at the executive level is 66% White,[15] which is not representative of the US population as a whole, and across governmental public health, the intent to leave is higher for staff of color, younger staff, and staff with a graduate degree, all which may influence ongoing objectives of having a representative workforce. However, while the size of most race and ethnicity groups has not significantly changed, the proportion of the public health workforce who are Black, Indigenous, or Persons of Color (BIPOC) is increasing, growing from 41.4% in 2017 to 46.3% in 2021.[15] Among the state-level workforce specifically, there has also been an increase in the number of staff of color and younger staff.[16] While there is greater understanding of the racial and ethnic diversity of the public health workforce at a national level, it is unclear how representative the workforce is of the populations they serve at the local level in which public health operates, and if representation differs by characteristics of agencies or jurisdictions.

The purpose of this study was to describe how racially and ethnically representative the local public health workforce is of the communities they serve. To our knowledge, this analysis is the first of its kind, moving beyond existing evidence not only to look at the overall diversity or representation of individuals working in local health departments (LHDs) but also to consider how representative individual agencies are of their local communities. Findings of this study will be of interest to governmental public health decision-makers at the federal, state, and local levels as a baseline measure of representativeness in the field. Findings may be used in workforce development, to assist schools of public health in their recruitment and placement of students, and to provide insight for additional trainings LHDs may need on cultural humility and diverse and equitable hiring practices. Having a diverse public health workforce throughout skill and education levels may help with addressing health inequities by providing more culturally and linguistically appropriate public health programs and services and a more diverse public health leadership.[17–19]

METHODS

In this cross-sectional study, we used the 2019 National Association of County and City Health Officials (NACCHO) Profile, 2021 PH WINS, 2020 American Community Survey (accessed through IPUMS), and 2022 Agency Health Resources Files to examine the racial and ethnic representation of the local governmental public health workforce compared with the local population served. Each of these data sources has been described in detail elsewhere[15,20–22]; however, for the purposes of the current study, the NACCHO Profile primarily contributed agency-level information, PH WINS contributed individual employee characteristics, and American Community Survey and Agency Health Resources Files provided characteristics of the jurisdiction and population served. Response rates for the NACCHO Profile and PH WINS were 61% and 35%, respectively. Importantly, NACCHO Profile response rates differed by state (from 24% to 100% of invited LHDs within the states responding) and size of the population served (from 53% of agencies serving fewer than 25 000 to 72% of agencies serving 1 million or more).

Study Population

LHDs were included by meeting the following criteria: (1) completed the 2019 NACCHO Profile survey, (2) jurisdiction served as identified in the 2019 NACCHO Profile is defined as serving only county or counties or US Census Bureau Place(s), and (3) the number of respondents in PH WINS was at least 35% of the total number of full-time equivalents reported in NACCHO Profile at the agency level.

Dependent Variables

Dependent variables included several measures of representativeness of the local public health workforce compared with the jurisdiction served. Representation was determined for race and ethnicity categories of Asian, American Indian or Alaska Native, Black or African American, Native Hawaiian or other Pacific Islander, BIPOC, and Hispanic. These race and ethnicity categories were based on survey data collected by PH WINS and matched the categories used in the American Community Survey. BIPOC includes all non-White race and ethnicity groups together. Representation was calculated as the percentage of the workforce of a given race/ethnicity, minus the percentage of the population served that race/ethnicity, divided by the population served that race/ethnicity to scale this measure by the composition of the population served. See Figure A (available as a supplement to the online version of this article at https://ajph.org) for a visual representation of the calculation.

Ultimately, this measure was dichotomized into at least representative or not, indicating that the workforce was either the same or greater representation of a given race/ethnicity as opposed to underrepresentative. A representation calculation of 0% or above was considered at least representative. Not representative was less than 0% representation.

Independent Variables

Independent variables included agency characteristics, geographic characteristics of the jurisdiction, and population served. Agency measures included accreditation status (Public Health Accreditation Board–accredited, in the process, undecided, or not applying), governance structure (state, local, or shared), and binary indicators for characteristics of the agency's top executive (male and with a formal degree in public health). The presence of the agency's top executive with a formal public health degree was included as a covariate as equity is a core principle in public health, as represented in the 10 Essential Public Health Services and included explicitly in public health curricula.[23] Therefore, we expect leaders who have formal public health training to be increasingly cognizant of the potential role of a diverse and representative staff. Geographic characteristics of the jurisdiction included being a rural-serving health department (as defined by NACCHO in the Profile data). Characteristics of the population served included the size of the population served, the percentage of families living in poverty, the percentage of the noninstitutionalized population that is uninsured, the percentage of the population that is unemployed, and the presence of any primary care health professional shortage area (HPSA) in the jurisdiction. The Health Resources and Services Administration defines HPSAs based on having insufficient primary, dental, or mental health care providers for a specific population, geographic area, or a specific organization.[24]

Analyses

We collapsed the data sets to the agency or jurisdiction level to create an agency-level data set. First, we present descriptive and bivariate analyses of the representativeness of included LHDs overall and by rurality. We then present bivariate analyses of representativeness for the highest 3 groups (Black or African American, Hispanic, and BIPOC) by characteristics of the LHDs and communities served. For categorical and binary measures, we conducted bivariate comparisons by rurality with the χ^2 analysis. For continuous measures, we conducted bivariate comparisons by rurality with the *t* test. Next, we present multivariate logistic regression analyses to estimate the association between representativeness and characteristics of the agency and jurisdiction served. We selected these characteristics to reflect the role or need of public health agencies within local communities (including demographic, economic, and health care context), general characteristics of agencies that may reflect the structure of the agency and potential implications for hiring and retention policies and activities (including size, accreditation status, governance), and characteristics of agency leaders that may have implications for culture and inclusivity of the agency. To account for similarities within states, we clustered standard errors at the state level.

RESULTS

A total of 248 LHDs across 32 states met our inclusion criteria and were included in analyses. Most LHDs served small to medium population sizes, were either accredited or in the process, and were decentralized (Table 1). Approximately 91% of agencies served an area with at least 1 primary care HPSA.

Workforce representativeness was highest for the Hispanic population, with 50% of included LHDs being at least representative of the Hispanic population they served (Figure 1). This was followed by Native Hawaiian or other Pacific Islander (29%), Black or African American (29%), Asian (26%), and American Indian or Alaska Native (21%), respectively. When all non-White groups were combined, 60% of included health departments were at least representative of the BIPOC population served.

For all race and ethnicity groups except for Native Hawaiian or other Pacific Islander, urban-serving health departments were significantly more representative than rural-serving health departments. This was most pronounced for Hispanic representation, with 61% of urban LHDs in the sample being at least representative of the Hispanic population they served compared with 35% of rural serving LHDs ($P < .001$). For Native Hawaiian or other Pacific Islanders, rural-serving health departments were significantly more representative than urban-serving health departments (37% vs 22%, respectively; $P = .007$).

Most characteristics of the agency also differed by Black or African American, Hispanic, and BIPOC representativeness in bivariate analyses, including size of the population served, rurality, accreditation status, US Department of

TABLE 1— Characteristics of Local Health Departments and Jurisdictions Served by Rurality: United States, 2019–2021

	Urban (n = 140), No. (%) or Mean ±SD	Rural (n = 108), No. (%) or Mean ±SD	Total (n = 248), No. (%) or Mean ±SD	P
Population served, no.				< .001
< 50 000	16 (11.4)	74 (68.5)	90 (36.3)	
50 000–499 999	94 (67.1)	34 (31.5)	128 (51.6)	
≥ 500 000	30 (21.4)	0 (0.0)	30 (12.1)	
Accreditation status				< .001
PHAB accredited	87 (64.4)	36 (35.6)	123 (52.1)	
In process	21 (15.6)	17 (16.8)	38 (16.1)	
Undecided, do not know	16 (11.9)	25 (24.8)	41 (17.4)	
Not applying for PHAB	11 (8.1)	23 (22.8)	34 (14.4)	
HHS region				.031
1	3 (2.1)	5 (4.6)	8 (3.2)	
2	2 (1.4)	1 (0.9)	3 (1.2)	
3	5 (3.6)	2 (1.9)	7 (2.8)	
4	41 (29.3)	32 (29.6)	73 (29.4)	
5	46 (32.9)	48 (44.4)	94 (37.9)	
6	8 (5.7)	4 (3.7)	12 (4.8)	
7	9 (6.4)	2 (1.9)	11 (4.4)	
8	2 (1.4)	6 (5.6)	8 (3.2)	
9	9 (6.4)	0 (0.0)	9 (3.6)	
10	15 (10.7)	8 (7.4)	23 (9.3)	
2019 LHD governance classification				.1
Centralized	15 (10.7)	22 (20.4)	37 (14.9)	
Decentralized	89 (63.6)	64 (59.3)	153 (61.7)	
Shared	36 (25.7)	22 (20.4)	58 (23.4)	
Top executive male	51 (36.4)	33 (31.1)	84 (34.1)	.39
Top executive with formal public health training	57 (41.6)	28 (26.7)	85 (35.1)	.016
% family poverty	8.5 ±3.5	10.7 ±5.0	9.5 ±4.4	< .001
% uninsured	8.2 ±3.6	9.3 ±4.9	8.7 ±4.3	.039
HPSA 2021	126 (92.6)	97 (89.8)	223 (91.4)	.43
% population with bachelor's degree or above	30.7 ±10.5	19.2 ±7.1	25.7 ±10.8	< .001
% unemployed	5.0 ±1.8	5.5 ±2.6	5.2 ±2.2	.13

Note. HHS = Department of Health and Human Services; HPSA = health professional shortage area; LHD = local health department; PHAB = Public Health Accreditation Board. For categorical measures, bivariate statistical comparisons were conducted with the χ^2 analysis. For continuous measures, bivariate statistical comparisons were conducted with the *t* test. Because of rounding, totals may not sum to 100.

Health and Human Services region, and governance structure (Table 2). For example, representativeness was highest for midsized health departments (serving populations of 50 000–499 999), accredited health departments, and decentralized health departments. Characteristics of the top executive and of the communities served were rarely associated with representativeness with a few exceptions. Agencies that were representative of the Black or African American and BIPOC population they served had higher uninsurance rates than those that were not representative of these populations (Black or African American: 10.4% vs 8.1% [*P* < .001]; BIPOC: 9.6% vs 7.3% [*P* < .001]). Agencies that were representative of the BIPOC population were more likely to be an HPSA than agencies that were not representative (94.5% vs 86.7%, respectively; *P* = .034). Lastly, there were higher rates of the

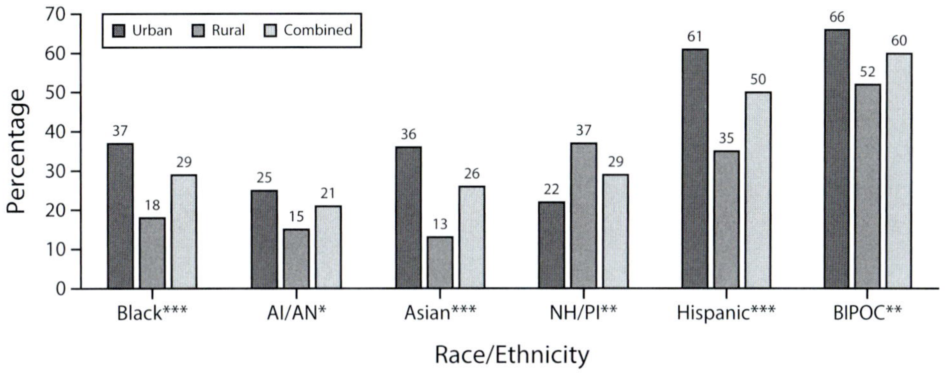

FIGURE 1— Percentage of Local Health Departments That Are at Least Representative of the Populations Served, by Rurality: United States, 2019–2021

Note. AI/AN = American Indian or Alaska Native; BIPOC = Black, Indigenous, or People of Color; NH/PI = Native Hawaiian or other Pacific Islander. Comparisons of the share of local health departments at least representative of each race and ethnicity between rural and urban local health departments were estimated with the *t* test.
$^{*}P < .05$; $^{**}P < .01$; $^{***}P < .001$.

population with at least a bachelor's degree among agencies that were representative of the Black or African American and Hispanic populations they served compared with agencies that were not representative of these populations (Black or African American: 28.4% vs 24.6% [*P* = .012]; Hispanic: 27.6% vs 23.8% [*P* = .006]).

Multivariate regression analyses identified several associations between representativeness and agency and jurisdiction characteristics when controlling for all other characteristics (Table 3). In most instances, LHDs serving larger populations were at greater odds for being at least representative (i.e., the odds of LHDs serving populations of 500 000 or more being at least representative of the Black or African American population served were 6.12 times greater those of LHDs that served fewer than 50 000 people; 95% confidence interval [CI] = 1.15, 32.53). For Hispanic and BIPOC representativeness, shared governance was associated with greater odds of an agency being representative of these populations compared with centralized agencies (Hispanic: odds ratio [OR] = 3.89 [95% CI = 1.04, 14.55]; BIPOC: OR = 4.29 [95% CI = 1.08, 17.01]). The percentage of adults who were uninsured was significantly, positively associated with agencies being at least representative of the population served for Black or African American (OR = 1.16; 95% CI = 1.06, 1.28) and BIPOC (OR = 1.16; 95% CI = 1.04, 1.28). There were also instances where certain characteristics were associated with greater odds of representativeness for certain races or ethnicities while associated with lower odds for other races or ethnicities. For example, having a top executive with formal training in public health was positively associated with American Indian or Alaska Native representativeness (OR = 2.00; 95% CI = 1.09, 3.68) while negatively associated with Asian representativeness (OR = 0.50; 95% CI = 0.28, 0.90). Other characteristics of the agency or jurisdiction were not associated with workforce representativeness for more than 1 race or ethnicity group.

DISCUSSION

As the expectations and responsibilities for public health continue to expand and there is an increased focus on health equity, it is crucial to have a diverse and representative workforce. Previous evidence suggests that the public health workforce is racially and ethnically diverse but is underrepresentative of racial and ethnic minority populations overall.[17–19] This study is the first, to our knowledge, to estimate the racial and ethnic representativeness of the public health workforce on a local level and contributes to a baseline understanding of workforce composition from a different lens. As local public health is highly community-depending, having representation at a local level may be particularly important.

Overall, we estimate that representativeness of LHDs ranges from 21% to 60% of LHDs. Importantly, this varies by race and ethnicity group, rurality, and size of the health department. This suggests some promising levels of

TABLE 2— Characteristics of Local Health Departments and Jurisdictions Served by Black or African American, Hispanic, and BIPOC Representativeness: United States: 2019–2021

	Black or African American			Hispanic			BIPOC		
	Not Rep (n = 177), No. (%) or Mean ±SD	At Least Rep (n = 71), No. (%) or Mean ±SD	P	Not Rep (n = 125), No. (%) or Mean ±SD	At Least Rep (n = 123), No. % or Mean ±SD	P	Not Rep (n = 99), No. (%) or Mean ±SD	At Least Rep (n = 149), No. (%) or Mean ±SD	P
Population served, no.			< .001			< .001			< .001
< 50 000	76 (42.9)	14 (19.7)		60 (48.0)	30 (24.4)		46 (46.5)	44 (29.5)	
50 000–499 999	90 (50.8)	38 (53.5)		58 (46.4)	70 (56.9)		52 (52.5)	76 (51.0)	
≥ 500 000	11 (6.2)	19 (26.8)		7 (5.6)	23 (18.7)		1 (1.0)	29 (19.5)	
Rural	89 (50.3)	19 (26.8)	< .001	70 (56.0)	38 (30.9)	< .001	52 (52.5)	56 (37.6)	.020
Accreditation status			.023			< .001			< .001
PHAB accredited	80 (47.1)	43 (65.2)		46 (39.3)	77 (64.7)		35 (37.2)	88 (62.0)	
In process	29 (17.1)	9 (13.6)		19 (16.2)	19 (16.0)		15 (16.0)	23 (16.2)	
Undecided, do not know	30 (17.6)	11 (16.7)		27 (23.1)	14 (11.8)		21 (22.3)	20 (14.1)	
Not applying for PHAB	31 (18.2)	3 (4.5)		25 (21.4)	9 (7.6)		23 (24.5)	11 (7.7)	
HHS region			< .001			.036			< .001
1	7 (4.0)	1 (1.4)		7 (5.6)	1 (0.8)		6 (6.1)	2 (1.3)	
2	2 (1.1)	1 (1.4)		1 (0.8)	2 (1.6)		2 (2.0)	1 (0.7)	
3	4 (2.3)	3 (4.2)		2 (1.6)	5 (4.1)		2 (2.0)	5 (3.4)	
4	39 (22.0)	34 (47.9)		28 (22.4)	45 (36.6)		14 (14.1)	59 (39.6)	
5	85 (48.0)	9 (12.7)		52 (41.6)	42 (34.1)		53 (53.5)	41 (27.5)	
6	7 (4.0)	5 (7.0)		8 (6.4)	4 (3.3)		5 (5.1)	7 (4.7)	
7	6 (3.4)	5 (7.0)		4 (3.2)	7 (5.7)		3 (3.0)	8 (5.4)	
8	5 (2.8)	3 (4.2)		7 (5.6)	1 (0.8)		6 (6.1)	2 (1.3)	
9	3 (1.7)	6 (8.5)		5 (4.0)	4 (3.3)		0 (0.0)	9 (6.0)	
10	19 (10.7)	4 (5.6)		11 (8.8)	12 (9.8)		8 (8.1)	15 (10.1)	
2019 LHD governance classification			.003			.001			< .001
Centralized	22 (12.4)	15 (21.1)		26 (20.8)	11 (8.9)		20 (20.2)	17 (11.4)	
Decentralized	121 (68.4)	32 (45.1)		80 (64.0)	73 (59.3)		69 (69.7)	84 (56.4)	
Shared	34 (19.2)	24 (33.8)		19 (15.2)	39 (31.7)		10 (10.1)	48 (32.2)	
Top executive male	57 (32.6)	27 (38.0)	.41	36 (29.3)	48 (39.0)	.11	28 (28.9)	56 (37.6)	.16

Continued

TABLE 2— Continued

	Black or African American			Hispanic			BIPOC		
	Not Rep (n = 177), No. (%) or Mean ±SD	At Least Rep (n = 71), No. (%) or Mean ±SD	P	Not Rep (n = 125), No. (%) or Mean ±SD	At Least Rep (n = 123), No. % or Mean ±SD	P	Not Rep (n = 99), No. (%) or Mean ±SD	At Least Rep (n = 149), No. (%) or Mean ±SD	P
Top executive with formal public health training	62 (36.0)	23 (32.9)	.64	36 (29.5)	49 (40.8)	.07	33 (34.4)	52 (35.6)	.84
% family poverty	9.4 ±4.7	9.5 ±3.6	.93	9.7 ±4.7	9.2 ±4.1	.49	9.1 ±4.6	9.7 ±4.2	.25
% uninsured	8.0 ±4.1	10.4 ±4.2	< .001	8.5 ±4.6	8.9 ±3.9	.42	7.3 ±3.8	9.6 ±4.3	< .001
HPSA 2021	159 (90.9)	64 (92.8)	.63	110 (89.4)	113 (93.4)	.27	85 (86.7)	138 (94.5)	.034
% population with bachelor's degree or above	24.6 ±10.7	28.4 ±10.7	.012	23.8 ±9.0	27.6 ±12.1	.006	25.3 ±10.3	25.9 ±11.1	.66
% unemployed	5.1 ±2.2	5.6 ±2.1	.13	5.3 ±2.5	5.2 ±1.7	.77	4.9 ±2.4	5.4 ±2.0	.090

Note. BIPOC = Black, Indigenous, and People of Color; HHS = Department of Health and Human Services; HPSA = health professional shortage area; LHD = local health department; PHAB = Public Health Accreditation Board; Rep = representative. For categorical measures, bivariate statistical comparisons were conducted with the χ^2 analysis. For continuous measures, bivariate statistical comparisons were conducted with the *t* test. Because of rounding, totals may not sum to 100.

representation, but still significant room for improvement. A recent study of the health care workforce across the United States similarly found that the workforce is less than representative of the race or ethnicity of the general population they serve.[25] Similarly, reports of teachers and local election offices also find that the workforce is predominantly non-Hispanic White and female and, therefore, less representative than the children and communities they serve.[26,27] While the methods used for estimating representation differ across studies, together, these findings may suggest that many professions and sectors are lacking in representativeness and that public health is similar to other professions. Furthermore, there is still significant room for improvement, particularly for the field of public health, which is focused on community-level work and health equity, where local representation may be even more important than in other fields.

Workforce diversity and connection to the community have been known to be important characteristics of LHDs to harness trust and facilitate effective public health work in local communities, and representativeness may be another important component that helps to describe these associations. Studies in other areas suggest that greater levels of workforce representation are associated with better outcomes, such as more innovation, improved patient quality, and better financial results in health care settings, and improved mortality rates for Black individuals when they see a Black primary care provider.[28,29] It is not yet understood if these may extend to the public health workforce, but the current study presents a framework for measuring representation of the public health workforce and developing the

TABLE 3— Associations Between Workforce Representativeness, Agency, and Community Characteristics, Multivariate Logistic Regression: United States, 2019–2021

	At Least Rep Black, OR (95% CI)	At Least Rep AI/AN, OR (95% CI)	At Least Rep Asian, OR (95% CI)	At Least Rep NH/PI, OR (95% CI)	At Least Rep Hispanic, OR (95% CI)	At Least Rep BIPOC, OR (95% CI)
Rural	0.95 (0.29, 3.14)	2.22 (0.68, 7.24)	0.62 (0.22, 1.76)	0.84 (0.34, 2.05)	0.89 (0.29, 2.74)	1.00 (0.38, 2.61)
Population served, no.						
< 50 000 (Ref)	1	1	1	1	1	1
50 000–499 000	2.09 (0.47, 9.29)	4.22 (1.85, 9.59)	7.52 (1.75, 32.26)	0.24 (0.11, 0.49)	2.11 (0.92, 4.82)	1.58 (0.42, 5.86)
≥ 500 000	6.12 (1.15, 32.53)	9.49 (2.91, 30.97)	6.42 (1.60, 25.71)	1.17 (0.38, 3.60)	5.49 (1.25, 24.19)	18.96 (1.17, 307.41)
PHAB accreditation process						
Accredited (Ref)	1	1	1	1	1	1
In the process	1.47 (0.51, 4.23)	1.82 (0.61, 5.48)	1.26 (0.56, 2.83)	2.56 (1.11, 5.90)	1.24 (0.47, 3.27)	1.28 (0.54, 3.07)
Undecided or do not know	1.72 (0.42, 6.99)	1.04 (0.26, 4.13)	0.42 (0.09, 1.93)	0.75 (0.24, 2.31)	0.68 (0.20, 2.37)	0.88 (0.27, 2.89)
Not applying for PHAB	0.31 (0.04, 2.15)	0.63 (0.11, 3.65)	0.18 (0.02, 1.31)	1.32 (0.39, 4.42)	0.63 (0.22, 1.85)	0.50 (0.15, 1.7)
Governance						
Centralized (Ref)	1	1	1	1	1	1
Decentralized	0.48 (0.13, 1.73)	0.66 (0.18, 2.35)	0.48 (0.09, 2.71)	0.51 (0.19, 1.38)	1.83 (0.42, 7.92)	2.80 (0.76, 10.37)
Shared	0.72 (0.15, 3.54)	2.15 (0.4, 11.67)	1.77 (0.31, 10.08)	1.13 (0.33, 3.84)	3.89 (1.04, 14.55)	4.29 (1.08, 17.01)
Top executive male	1.04 (0.47, 2.28)	0.92 (0.55, 1.54)	0.83 (0.45, 1.53)	0.66 (0.39, 1.09)	1.53 (0.93, 2.52)	1.67 (0.75, 3.69)
Top executive with formal public health training	0.77 (0.30, 2.00)	2.00 (1.09, 3.68)	0.50 (0.28, 0.90)	0.74 (0.41, 1.37)	1.41 (0.96, 2.09)	0.83 (0.41, 1.66)
% family poverty	0.89 (0.80, 0.98)	1.13 (1.00, 1.28)	0.98 (0.82, 1.18)	0.98 (0.87, 1.1)	1.04 (0.96, 1.14)	0.98 (0.86, 1.12)
% uninsured	1.16 (1.06, 1.28)	0.97 (0.84, 1.11)	0.95 (0.85, 1.07)	1.00 (0.92, 1.09)	1.00 (0.90, 1.12)	1.16 (1.04, 1.28)
Primary care HPSA 2021	0.60 (0.28, 1.29)	4.17 (0.62, 28.09)	1.57 (0.37, 6.76)	0.86 (0.31, 2.43)	1.38 (0.57, 3.32)	1.56 (0.74, 3.30)
% of population with bachelor's degree or above	1.04 (0.99, 1.09)	1.05 (0.99, 1.11)	0.98 (0.95, 1.01)	0.98 (0.94, 1.01)	1.01 (0.97, 1.05)	1.00 (0.95, 1.05)
% unemployed	1.34 (1.13, 1.60)	1.05 (0.84, 1.31)	1.23 (0.94, 1.60)	1.09 (0.88, 1.34)	0.92 (0.75, 1.11)	1.01 (0.79, 1.30)
Constant	0.03 (0.00, 0.38)	< 0.00 (0.00, 0.10)	0.16 (0.01, 2.33)	1.87 (0.27, 13.15)	0.14 (0.01, 1.97)	0.09 (0.00, 2.09)
Pseudo R2	0.20	0.16	0.22	0.15	0.13	0.18
Prob < χ2	< .001	< .001	< .001	< .001	< .001	< .001

Note. AI/AN = American Indian or Alaska Native; BIPOC = Black, Indigenous, and People of Color; CI = confidence interval; HHS = Department of Health and Human Services; HPSA = health professional shortage area; LHD = local health department; NH/PI = Native Hawaiian or other Pacific Islander; OR = odds ratio; PHAB = Public Health Accreditation Board; Rep = representative. ORs greater than 1 represent increased odds of the workforce being at least representative of the race or ethnicity, while ORs less than 1 represent lower odds of the workforce being at least representative of the race or ethnicity. Models included standard errors clustered at the state level.

evidence in this area. Future work should consider the association between representation and agency- or jurisdiction-level outcomes.

Although we are unable to describe why there are differences in the representativeness of the workforce, others have described potential barriers to a diverse public health workforce. First, complete data of the public health workforce is still limited, preventing a comprehensive understanding of the diversity and representativeness of the workforce.[18] Although PH WINS is the most comprehensive data available and is nationally representative, it is not designed to be representative at the local agency level and does not include all public health workers. Furthermore, evidence suggests that most individuals in the public health workforce who identify as BIPOC are in administrative and clerical positions,[18] which may translate to differences in representativeness by type of position. This may be a multifaceted issue arising at least in part from a lack of diversity historically in schools and programs of public health and high educational requirements for certain roles in public health.[18,30] These issues may be further compounded by structural barriers (including hiring practices and policies) and systemic racism. Lastly, variations in the structure of public health by states may also be considered. Differences in hiring practices, if public health is part of an umbrella agency as opposed to a freestanding agency (e.g., public health is within a health and human services agency within the state, including other subagencies and functions such as mental health services, public assistance, and Medicaid),[31] and governance structure may be factors to be considered when identifying potential barriers to a diverse and representative workforce. Larger agencies and those in urban areas may have a larger candidate pool from which to train, recruit, and retain.

Limitations

While this study is the first to consider the representativeness of the workforce at the local level, to our knowledge, it is important to interpret findings within the context of the limitations. First, we used a threshold of 35% of the known full-time equivalents from NACCHO as the required minimum response rate in PH WINS for inclusion in the study, which brings several limitations. PH WINS is not designed to be representative at the agency level. If individuals are differentially likely to respond by race and ethnicity, this may bias our measure of representativeness. Future analyses may use more complete data from agencies, such as those from local or state human resources offices. In addition, future analyses may use a more strict threshold of response rates for inclusion.

Second, our analyses included 248 LHDs, which represents about 10% of health departments invited to participate in the 2019 NACCHO Profile and 17% of health departments that responded to the 2019 NACCHO Profile. As such, findings may not be generalizable to all LHDs and are not intended to reflect the state or federal governmental public health workforce. For example, our sample includes a greater portion of medium and large health departments by population served and higher portion of top executives with a public health degree compared with the full NACCHO sample. However, the response rate for the recently released updated 2022 NACCHO Profile data was significantly lower, at 38%.

Furthermore, our sample was inherently limited by requiring overlapping response rates between NACCHO Profile and PH WINS. Next, this study was cross-sectional in nature and could not estimate causal relationships or identify the potential importance of a representative workforce on population health metrics. Lastly, we only considered representativeness in terms of race and ethnicity. This is only 1 important aspect of representation and diversity. Furthermore, the racial and ethnic composition of the workforce is likely reflective of organizational structures, state and local policies, and structural barriers including systemic racism. Increasing the diversity and representativeness of the workforce will take a multifaceted and comprehensive approach. Future research may also consider the race and ethnicity of agency leadership, which is possible using these data; however, nearly 90% of included agencies had missing data for the top executive's race and ethnicity, and, as such, it was not included in the current analysis.

Conclusions

Solutions for increasing diversity and representativeness of the public health workforce may largely lie with state and local agencies regarding hiring, training, recruitment, and culture in the workforce as well as schools and programs of public health in training the next generation of public health workers. Evidence-based practices to promote diversity, equity, and inclusion and intentional strategies to improve these factors may be adopted by health departments and public health programs. Tracking the diversity of the workforce and identifying structural barriers may serve as a foundation.[18] Furthermore, there is encouraging evidence that the public health workforce is becoming more diverse.[18,32] As public health is experiencing greater attention, increased infrastructure resources, and an influx of workers in response to the pandemic, in parallel with largescale retirements or exiting workers, the workforce composition may change significantly. This study presents a baseline estimate and a method for following these measures in the future to understand public health workforce trends specific to racial and ethnic representation. However, this study is not designed to identify specific factors that may actually improve representativeness of the workforce. Further research is needed to identify evidence-based factors or strategies that improve recruitment efforts and experiences, training, and retention and ultimately strengthen the workforce to support population health improvements and health equity. AJPH

ABOUT THE AUTHORS

Casey P. Balio, Haleigh Leslie, and Michael Meit are with the Center for Rural Health and Research and the Department of Health Services Management and Policy, East Tennessee State University, Johnson City. H. Leslie is a DrPH candidate.

CORRESPONDENCE

Correspondence should be sent to Casey Balio, 2109 W Market St, #116, Johnson City, TN 37604 (e-mail: balioc@etsu.edu). Reprints can be ordered at https://www.ajph.org by clicking the "Reprints" link.

PUBLICATION INFORMATION

Full Citation: Balio CP, Leslie H, Meit MB. Racial and ethnic representation of the local public health workforce. *Am J Public Health*. 2025;115(3):333–343.

Acceptance Date: October 18, 2024.

DOI: https://doi.org/10.2105/AJPH.2024.307903

ORCID iDs:

Casey P. Balio https://orcid.org/0000-0002-2987-4268

Haleigh Leslie https://orcid.org/0009-0005-6069-0722

CONTRIBUTORS

C. P. Balio led the design, data preparation, analysis, interpretation, article development, and article edits. H. Leslie supported the data preparation, analysis, interpretation, article development, and article edits. M. Meit oversaw the overall study design and conduct, interpretation, and article edits.

ACKNOWLEDGMENTS

This project was supported by the Centers for Disease Control and Prevention (CDC) and the Health Resources and Services Administration (HRSA) under awards U81HP47167 and UR2HP47371.

Findings from this work have been previously presented at the 2023 American Public Health Association Annual Meeting (Atlanta, GA), 2023 National Association of County and City Health Officials 360 Conference (Denver, CO), 2024 National Rural Health Association Annual Meeting (New Orleans, LA), and National Network of Public Health Institutes Open Forum Next Generation Meeting (Chicago, IL).

The Public Health Workforce Interests and Needs Survey was developed by the de Beaumont Foundation and the Association of State and Territorial Health Officials to understand the interests and needs of the state and local governmental public health workforce in the United States, and was fielded in 2014, 2017, and 2021. For more information, visit phwins.org. This work was conducted as part of the Consortium for Workforce Research in Public Health, which is led by the University of Minnesota.

Note. This information or content and conclusions are those of the authors and should not be construed as the official position or policy of, nor should any endorsements be inferred by, CDC, HRSA, Department of Health and Human Services, or the US government.

CONFLICTS OF INTEREST

The authors have no conflicts of interest to disclose.

HUMAN PARTICIPANT PROTECTION

This study was deemed non–human participant research by the East Tennessee State University institutional review board.

REFERENCES

1. DeSalvo KB, Wang YC, Harris A, Auerbach J, Koo D, O'Carroll P. Public Health 3.0: A call to action for public health to meet the challenges of the 21st century. *Prev Chronic Dis*. 2017;14:170017. https://doi.org/10.5888/pcd14.170017
2. Public Health Accreditation Board. The 10 essential public health services. September 9, 2020. Available at: https://phaboard.org/center-for-innovation/public-health-frameworks/the-10-essential-public-health-services. Accessed November 8, 2023.
3. Dean HD, Roberts GW, Bouye KE, Green Y, McDonald M. Sustaining a focus on health equity at the Centers for Disease Control and Prevention through organizational structures and functions. *J Public Health Manag Pract*. 2016;22(suppl 1):S60–S67. https://doi.org/10.1097/PHH.0000000000000305
4. Centers for Disease Control and Prevention Office of Health Equity. CDC's CORE commitment to health equity. April 5, 2023. Available at: https://www.cdc.gov/healthequity/index.html. Accessed November 8, 2023.
5. Jensen E, Jones N, Rabe M, et al. The chance that two people chosen at random are of different race or ethnicity groups has increased since 2010. August 12, 2021. Available at: https://www.census.gov/library/stories/2021/08/2020-united-states-population-more-racially-ethnically-diverse-than-2010.html. Accessed January 12, 2023.
6. Riccucci NM, Van Ryzin GG. Representative bureaucracy: a lever to enhance social equity, coproduction, and democracy. *Public Adm Rev*. 2017;77(1):21–30. https://doi.org/10.1111/puar.12649
7. King BA, Barnes A. Descriptive representation in election administration: poll workers and voter confidence. *Elect Law J*. 2019;18(1):16–30. https://doi.org/10.1089/elj.2018.0485
8. Egalite AJ, Kisida B, Winters MA. Representation in the classroom: the effect of own-race teachers on student achievement. *Econ Educ Rev*. 2015;45:44–52. https://doi.org/10.1016/j.econedurev.2015.01.007
9. Monarrez T, Washington K. Racial and ethnic representation in postsecondary education. Urban Institute. 2020. Available at: https://www.urban.org/research/publication/racial-and-ethnic-representation-postsecondary-education. Accessed November 22, 2024.
10. Grissom JA, Kern EC, Rodriguez LA. The "representative bureaucracy" in education: educator workforce diversity, policy outputs, and outcomes for disadvantaged students. *Educ Res*. 2015;44(3):185–192. https://doi.org/10.3102/0013189X15580102
11. Strumpf EC. Racial/ethnic disparities in primary care: the role of physician-patient concordance. *Med Care*. 2011;49(5):496–503. https://doi.org/10.1097/MLR.0b013e31820fbee4
12. Cooper-Patrick L, Gallo JJ, Gonzales JJ, et al. Race, gender, and partnership in the patient–physician relationship. *JAMA*. 1999;282(6):583–589. https://doi.org/10.1001/jama.282.6.583
13. Traylor AH, Schmittdiel JA, Uratsu CS, Mangione CM, Subramanian U. Adherence to cardiovascular disease medications: does patient–provider race/ethnicity and language concordance matter? *J Gen Intern Med*. 2010;25(11):1172–1177. https://doi.org/10.1007/s11606-010-1424-8
14. Lakey D. Providing for the common defense and promoting the general welfare by strengthening the nation's public health system. *J Public Health Manag Pract*. 2023;29(suppl):S4–S6. https://doi.org/10.1097/PHH.0000000000001669
15. de Beaumont Foundation. PH WINS 2021: Key findings and data dashboard. 2022. Available at: https://debeaumont.org/phwins/2021-findings. Accessed January 12, 2023.
16. Bogaert K, Papillon G, Wyche Etheridge K, et al. Seven years, 3 surveys, a changed world: the state public health workforce 2014–2021. *J Public Health Manag Pract*. 2023;29(suppl 1):S14–S21. https://doi.org/10.1097/PHH.0000000000001645

17. Cohen JJ, Gabriel BA, Terrell C. The case for diversity in the health care workforce. *Health Aff (Millwood).* 2002;21(5):90–102. https://doi.org/10.1377/hlthaff.21.5.90
18. Coronado F, Beck AJ, Shah G, Young JL, Sellers K, Leider JP. Understanding the dynamics of diversity in the public health workforce. *J Public Health Manag Pract.* 2020;26(4):389–392. https://doi.org/10.1097/PHH.0000000000001075
19. Jackson CS, Gracia JN. Addressing health and health-care disparities: the role of a diverse workforce and the social determinants of health. *Public Health Rep.* 2014;129(1 suppl 2):57–61. https://doi.org/10.1177/00333549141291S211
20. Health Resources and Services Administration. Area Health Resources Files. Available at: https://data.hrsa.gov/topics/health-workforce/ahrf. Accessed May 30, 2024.
21. IPUMS Center for Data Integration. IPUMS. Available at: https://www.ipums.org. Accessed May 30, 2024.
22. Alford A, Dekker D, Feeser K, et al. 2019 NACCHO Profile of Local Health Departments. 2020. Available at: https://www.naccho.org/uploads/downloadable-resources/Programs/Public-Health-Infrastructure/NACCHO_2019_Profile_final.pdf. Accessed May 30, 2024.
23. Public Health Accreditation Board. The 10 essential public health services. 2020. Available at: https://phaboard.org/wp-content/uploads/EPHS-English.pdf. Accessed July 28, 2024.
24. Health Resources and Services Administration. What is shortage designation? June 2023. Available at: https://bhw.hrsa.gov/workforce-shortage-areas/shortage-designation. Accessed August 20, 2024.
25. Salsberg E, Richwine C, Westergaard S, et al. Estimation and comparison of current and future racial/ethnic representation in the US health care workforce. *JAMA Netw Open.* 2021;4(3):e213789. https://doi.org/10.1001/jamanetworkopen.2021.3789
26. Taie S, Lewis L. Characteristics of 2020–21 public and private K–12 school teachers in the United States: results from the National Teacher and Principal Survey. National Center for Education Statistics. 2022. Available at: https://nces.ed.gov/pubsearch/pubsinfo.asp?pubid=2022113. Accessed August 20, 2024.
27. Manson P, Adona N, Lee J, Gronke P. Staffing the stewards of democracy: gender, race, and representative bureaucracy. Presented at: Midwest Political Science Association. 2021. Available at: https://evic.reed.edu/wp-content/uploads/2022/11/Staffing-the-Stewards_MPSA2021.pdf. Accessed November 22, 2024.
28. Gomez LE, Bernet P. Diversity improves performance and outcomes. *J Natl Med Assoc.* 2019;111(4):383–392. https://doi.org/10.1016/j.jnma.2019.01.006
29. Snyder JE, Upton RD, Hassett TC, Lee H, Nouri Z, Dill M. Black representation in the primary care physician workforce and its association with population life expectancy and mortality rates in the US. *JAMA Netw Open.* 2023;6(4):e236687. https://doi.org/10.1001/jamanetworkopen.2023.6687
30. Barton R. The importance of diversity in public health. Purdue University. December 21, 2021. Available at: https://online.purdue.edu/blog/health-sciences/public-health-diversity. Accessed May 30, 2024.
31. Association of State and Territorial Health Officials. ASTHO profile of state public health. Volume 3: State health agency structure and governance. 2014. Available at: https://legacy.astho.org/Profile/Volume-Three/Issue-Briefs/Structure-and-Governance. Accessed August 20, 2024.
32. Vichare A, Park YH, Plepys CM. Diversity of the US public health workforce pipeline (2016–2020): role of academic institutions. *Am J Public Health.* 2023;113(9):1000–1008. https://doi.org/10.2105/AJPH.2023.307352

Impacts of State COVID-19 Vaccine Mandates for Health Care Workers on Health Sector Employment in the United States

Yin Wang, MA, Kevin Callison, PhD, Julie H. Hernandez, PhD, and Charles Stoecker, PhD

AJPH March 2025, Vol. 115, No. 3

Objectives. To assess the impact of state COVID-19 vaccine mandates for health care workers (HCWs) on health sector employment in the United States.

Methods. Using monthly state-level employment data from the Quarterly Census of Employment and Wages between January and October 2021, we employed a partially pooled synthetic control method that accounted for staggered mandate adoption and heterogeneous treatment effects. We conducted analyses separately for the 4 health care subsectors—ambulatory health care services, hospitals, nursing and residential care, and social assistance—with an additional analysis of 2 industry groups—skilled nursing care and community care for the elderly—under the nursing and residential care subsector. We further explored possible heterogeneous impacts according to the test-out option availability.

Results. Mandate impact estimates were statistically indistinguishable from zero. Results further ruled out a mandate-associated decrease in employment larger than 2.1% of premandate employment levels for the 6 health care domains examined and for states with no test-out option.

Conclusions. State COVID-19 vaccine mandates for HCWs were not found to be associated with significant adverse impacts on health sector employment even in states without a testing alternative to vaccination. The findings support vaccine mandates as a viable preventive measure without material disruption to the health care workforce, including in times of public health emergencies. (*Am J Public Health*. 2025;115(3):344–348. https://doi.org/10.2105/AJPH.2024.307906)

Among the health policies employed during the COVID-19 pandemic, vaccine mandates emerged as particularly contentious because of the potential tradeoff between individual autonomy and public welfare along with their uncertain impact on a weak labor market. This was especially pronounced in the health care sector as 17 states introduced COVID-19 vaccine mandates for health care workers (HCWs) in mid-2021. Concerns were raised given surveys revealing wide variance in mandate acceptance rates (35%–92%) among HCWs[1] and anecdotal evidence of HCWs opting to resign rather than comply with the mandates.[2] On the other hand, supporters maintained that COVID-19 vaccine mandates, like preexisting HCW mandates for other vaccines,[3] would foster a safer workplace and preserve health system capacity.[4]

Despite the polarized debate, there is little empirical evidence for the impact of these state COVID-19 vaccine mandates on health sector employment. To our knowledge, a single study has explored this topic for nursing home facilities and found no significant mandate-associated increase in the proportion of nursing homes reporting staffing shortages.[5] We expand this previous work using highly granular employment data from the Quarterly Census of Employment and Wages (QCEW)[6] to assess the magnitude of employment fluctuations associated with state COVID-19 vaccine mandates for HCWs across the 4 health care subsectors, with an in-depth study of the nursing and residential care subsector. We further stratified vaccine mandate states by test-out option availability (i.e., regular testing in lieu of vaccination) to examine possible heterogeneous impacts.

METHODS

We obtained monthly state-level employment data from the Bureau of Labor Statistics QCEW database.[6] Encompassing more than 95% of jobs in the United States, this near-census program closely monitors labor market fluctuations across each industry sector. The health care sector is classified under North American Industry Classification System (NAICS) 62.

We compiled policies of state COVID-19 vaccine mandates for HCWs from state Web sites and other resources. As mandates may vary in their scopes of applicable health care settings, we conducted separate analyses for the 4 subsectors under NAICS 62—ambulatory health care services (NAICS 621), hospitals (NAICS 622), nursing and residential care (NAICS 623), and social assistance (NAICS 624)—by including states with corresponding mandates in the treated group while maintaining a control group of 29 nonmandate states (details in Section 1 of Appendix, available as a supplement to the online version of this article at http://www.ajph.org). We repeated the analysis for 2 industry groups under the nursing and residential care subsector—skilled nursing care (NAICS 6231) and community care for the elderly (NAICS 6233)—given the acute labor shortages in these settings during the pandemic. Finally, we examined the heterogeneous impacts according to test-out option availability.

To account for state population size, we constructed the outcome variable—the number of HCWs per 10 000 working-age population—using the employment count of each health care domain divided by the state population aged 18 to 64 years in 2021. The study period extended from January 2021, the onset of the COVID-19 vaccination campaign, to October 2021, the month preceding the promulgation of a federal vaccine mandate for HCWs in November 2021. The state vaccine mandates were announced in either July or August 2021, denoting the start of the policy intervention.

To accommodate the fact that states enacted mandates at different points in time, we employed a partially pooled synthetic control method, which allows for multiple treated units with dynamic policy adoption and estimates policy effects by minimizing the preintervention fitting imbalance between treated units and synthetic counterfactuals constructed using units in the control group.[7] We implemented the model using R version 4.3.1 (R Core Team, 2023), which controlled for state-fixed effects and covariates, including state-level percentages of non-Hispanic Black, non-Hispanic White, and Hispanic populations; percentage of population with strong COVID-19 vaccine hesitancy; hospital beds per 10 000 population; percentage of votes for the Republican presidential candidate in the 2020 election; average monthly unemployment rates over the premandate period; and counts of average monthly COVID-19 cases and deaths per 10 000 population over the premandate period (details in Section 2 of online Appendix).

RESULTS

At the time that state vaccine mandates for HCWs were introduced, labor markets for different health care subsectors were experiencing divergent trajectories: employment in ambulatory health care services, hospitals, and social assistance had largely reverted to prepandemic (February 2020) levels (100.51%, 98.85%, and 95.55%, respectively) whereas employment in nursing and residential care facilities remained at 89.97% of the prepandemic level and continued to decline (online Appendix, Figure A). However, despite the disrupted employment trends over the pandemic, a closer examination of 2021 data uncovered no observable differences between mandate and nonmandate states, nor between those with and without a test-out option (online Appendix, Figures B–E).

Results of our analyses corroborated these findings, as none of the estimates indicate that state vaccine mandates were associated with statistically significant changes to health sector employment (Table 1; online Appendix, Figures F–K). The 95% confidence intervals further ruled out mandate-associated decreases in employment larger than 0.88% (ambulatory health care services), 1.44% (hospitals), 1.34% (nursing and residential care), 0.62% (social assistance), 1.56% (skilled nursing care), and 0.69% (community care for the elderly) relative to premandate employment levels. Results from the stratified analyses by test-out option availability remained statistically insignificant and precluded mandate-associated employment decreases larger than 2.09% of premandate levels for states with no test-out option. These findings are supported by similar estimates from models that omit covariates and from a sensitivity test to the synthetic control method pooling parameter[7] (online Appendix, Table C, Figures L–W).

DISCUSSION

Our study did not detect statistically significant adverse impacts of state

TABLE 1— Covariate-Adjusted Impacts of State COVID-19 Vaccine Mandates for Health Care Workers on Employment by 6 Health Care Domains for All Mandate States, States With No Test-Out Option, and States With a Test-Out Option: United States, January–October 2021

	Ambulatory Health Care Services, b (95% CI) or Mean	Hospitals, b (95% CI) or Mean	Nursing and Residential Care, b (95% CI) or Mean	Social Assistance, b (95% CI) or Mean	Skilled Nursing Care, b (95% CI) or Mean	Community Care for the Elderly, b (95% CI) or Mean
All mandate states						
Relative month[a]						
0	−0.45 (−3.00, 1.61)	−0.19 (−4.64, 4.27)	0.36 (−1.11, 1.73)	−0.21 (−3.06, 3.21)	0.18 (−0.80, 1.27)	0.18 (−0.32, 0.71)
1	1.07 (−3.43, 4.14)	0.11 (−3.65, 4.33)	1.75 (−1.58, 4.98)	2.59 (−1.36, 6.66)	1.04 (−1.02, 3.07)	0.57 (−0.27, 1.51)
2	−1.04 (−5.46, 2.53)	−1.60 (−5.16, 2.12)	3.97 (−4.67, 10.02)	2.92 (−2.34, 8.24)	0.98 (−1.50, 3.33)	0.34 (−0.55, 1.28)
Average impact[b]	−0.14 (−3.55, 2.34)	−0.56 (−4.38, 3.41)	2.02 (−2.22, 5.51)	1.77 (−1.71, 5.76)	0.73 (−1.08, 2.54)	0.36 (−0.32, 1.12)
Baseline outcome level[c]	405	303	166	275	69	46
Average impact/baseline[d] (%)	−0.03 (−0.88, 0.58)	−0.18 (−1.44, 1.13)	1.22 (−1.34, 3.32)	0.64 (−0.62, 2.09)	1.06 (−1.56, 3.68)	0.79 (−0.69, 2.44)
States with no test-out option						
Relative month[a]						
0	−0.01 (−3.52, 2.52)	0.24 (−6.46, 6.26)	0.80 (−0.95, 2.42)	0.32 (−3.19, 4.79)	0.05 (−0.91, 1.22)	0.16 (−0.50, 0.94)
1	1.57 (−4.87, 6.01)	0.41 (−5.32, 6.05)	2.51 (−1.22, 6.34)	3.25 (−1.94, 8.73)	0.68 (−1.22, 2.72)	0.59 (−0.39, 1.72)
2	−1.38 (−7.10, 2.96)	−1.34 (−6.55, 3.96)	3.48 (−4.74, 10.12)	1.70 (−2.60, 7.49)	0.35 (−1.81, 2.70)	0.44 (−0.66, 1.76)
Average impact[b]	0.06 (−4.75, 3.33)	−0.23 (−6.04, 5.22)	2.26 (−1.93, 6.26)	1.76 (−2.11, 6.70)	0.36 (−1.16, 2.16)	0.40 (−0.45, 1.44)
Baseline outcome level[c]	408	289	157	305	65	41
Average impact/baseline[d] (%)	0.01 (−1.16, 0.82)	−0.08 (−2.09, 1.81)	1.44 (−1.23, 3.99)	0.58 (−0.69, 2.20)	0.55 (−1.79, 3.32)	0.97 (−1.10, 3.51)
States with a test-out option						
Relative month[a]						
0	−0.55 (−3.39, 2.23)	−0.71 (−4.92, 3.05)	−0.61 (−3.21, 2.14)	−1.21 (−5.03, 2.04)	0.39 (−1.21, 2.27)	0.23 (−0.63, 1.23)
1	0.28 (−1.70, 2.34)	−0.35 (−3.83, 3.09)	−0.04 (−4.77, 4.98)	1.10 (−3.93, 6.67)	1.37 (−2.22, 5.16)	0.86 (−1.16, 3.22)
2	−0.34 (−3.67, 3.36)	−0.91 (−5.46, 3.25)	4.66 (−8.78, 18.21)	5.80 (−9.46, 22.42)	2.03 (−2.87, 7.07)	0.49 (−1.05, 2.38)
Average impact[b]	−0.20 (−2.14, 1.80)	−0.66 (−4.32, 2.88)	1.34 (−4.72, 7.32)	1.90 (−4.59, 8.86)	1.26 (−2.02, 4.78)	0.53 (−0.81, 2.16)
Baseline outcome level[c]	398	331	186	208	78	56
Average impact/baseline[d] (%)	−0.05 (−0.54, 0.45)	−0.20 (−1.30, 0.87)	0.72 (−2.54, 3.94)	0.91 (−2.21, 4.26)	1.62 (−2.58, 6.12)	0.94 (−1.45, 3.85)

Note. CI = confidence interval. Mandate states and jurisdictions include CA, CO, CT, DE, DC, IL, ME, MD, MA, NJ, NM, NY, OR, PA, RI, and WA, of which DE, IL, MD, NJ, and PA were states with a test-out option, defined as those explicitly mentioning a test-out option in the official documents. Nonmandate states include AL, AK, AZ, AR, FL, GA, IN, IA, KS, LA, MI, MO, MT, NE, NH, NC, ND, OH, OK, SC, SD, TN, TX, UT, VT, VA, WV, WI, and WY (details in Section 1 of Appendix, available as a supplement to the online version of this article at http://www.ajph.org).

Source. Authors' analysis by the partially pooled synthetic control method with covariates included.

[a]Period relative to the mandate announcement month.

[b]Average impact over the treatment period.

[c]Mean number of health care workers per 10 000 working-age population across mandate states in the month right before the mandate announcement weighted by state working-age population.

[d]Impact relative to the baseline outcome level.

COVID-19 vaccine mandates on HCW employment. Results further ruled out mandate-associated employment decreases larger than 2.1% of premandate employment levels for the 6 health care domains examined and for the subsample of states with no test-out option. We also found slightly wider confidence intervals in the nursing and residential care subsector and the social assistance subsector. This may reflect lower job attachment in these areas, although we cannot statistically rule out impacts in these subsectors that were the same as in other subsectors.

Concerns about statewide vaccine mandates mainly stem from the severe HCW labor shortages during the pandemic. Indeed, health sector employment was still 481 900 below prepandemic projections as of October 2023.[8] However, we did not find that these mandates materially exacerbated the staffing shortages. Our findings are consistent with previous research on state and federal vaccine mandates for nursing home employees[5,9] and reports from 57 hospitals with employer mandates, where mandate-related resignations were less than 1% of the workforce for 33 hospitals, 1% to 2% for another 15, and 2% to 6% for the remaining 9 hospitals.[10]

Our findings may be partly explained by the relatively high acceptance rate of COVID-19 vaccines among HCWs. Surveys among US nurses in spring 2021 found that 93% of respondents had been, or planned to be, vaccinated.[11] Moreover, statewide mandates, unlike hospital-specific mandates, may have limited the options for HCWs to seek other local employment. News articles also suggest that actual mandate-associated resignations were lower than what was predicted from polls given the cost of actually changing jobs.[12] Furthermore, protection from COVID-19 vaccines likely mitigated infections and severe cases, which may have reduced burnout and thus buttressed the health care workforce.

This work provides important evidence for the magnitude of health sector employment changes associated with statewide COVID-19 vaccine mandates for HCWs. We ruled out a large adverse impact of these mandates on HCW employment and add support for similar practices during future epidemics. AJPH

ABOUT THE AUTHORS

Yin Wang, Kevin Callison, and Charles Stoecker are with the Department of Health Policy and Management and Julie H. Hernandez is with the Department of International Health and Sustainable Development, Celia Scott Weatherhead School of Public Health and Tropical Medicine, Tulane University, New Orleans, LA.

CORRESPONDENCE

Correspondence should be sent to Charles Stoecker, PhD, Suite 1900, 1440 Canal St, New Orleans, LA 70112 (e-mail: cfstoecker@tulane.edu). Reprints can be ordered at https://www.ajph.org by clicking the "Reprints" link.

PUBLICATION INFORMATION

Full Citation: Wang Y, Callison K, Hernandez JH, Stoecker C. Impacts of state COVID-19 vaccine mandates for health care workers on health sector employment in the United States. *Am J Public Health*. 2025;115(3):344–348.

Acceptance Date: October 22, 2024.

DOI: https://doi.org/10.2105/AJPH.2024.307906

ORCID iDs:

Yin Wang https://orcid.org/0000-0002-3554-656X

Kevin Callison https://orcid.org/0000-0003-4181-7407

Julie H. Hernandez https://orcid.org/0000-0002-0868-0958

Charles Stoecker https://orcid.org/0000-0001-5438-9312

CONTRIBUTORS

Y. Wang curated the data and performed the statistical analyses. Y. Wang, K. Callison, and C. Stoecker designed the methodology. Y. Wang and C. Stoecker conceptualized the study. C. Stoecker supervised the study. All authors participated in writing the original draft, reviewed and edited the article, and have read and agreed to the published version of the article.

ACKNOWLEDGMENTS

We thank the participants of the Hunches and Lunches seminar at Celia Scott Weatherhead School of Public Health and Tropical Medicine, Tulane University, for their valuable comments.

CONFLICTS OF INTEREST

The authors have no potential or actual conflicts of interest from funding or affiliation-related activities.

HUMAN PARTICIPANT PROTECTION

The authors received a waiver of institutional review board (IRB) approval from the Tulane University IRB because only publicly available, deidentified data were used.

REFERENCES

1. Politis M, Sotiriou S, Doxani C, Stefanidis I, Zintzaras E, Rachiotis G. Healthcare workers' attitudes towards mandatory COVID-19 vaccination: a systematic review and meta-analysis. *Vaccines (Basel)*. 2023;11(4):880. https://doi.org/10.3390/vaccines11040880
2. Finnerty R. The vaccine mandate for healthcare workers means hospitals are losing staff. Updated September 27, 2021. Available at: https://www.npr.org/2021/09/27/1040983300/the-vaccine-mandate-for-healthcare-workers-means-hospitals-are-losing-staff. Accessed September 11, 2024.
3. Ottenberg AL, Wu JT, Poland GA, Jacobson RM, Koenig BA, Tilburt JC. Vaccinating health care workers against influenza: the ethical and legal rationale for a mandate. *Am J Public Health*. 2011;101(2):212–216. https://doi.org/10.2105/AJPH.2009.190751d
4. Hagan K, Forman R, Mossialos E, Ndebele P, Hyder AA, Nasir K. COVID-19 vaccine mandate for healthcare workers in the United States: a social justice policy. *Expert Rev Vaccines*. 2022;21(1):37–45. https://doi.org/10.1080/14760584.2022.1999811
5. McGarry BE, Gandhi AD, Syme M, Berry SD, White EM, Grabowski DC. Association of state COVID-19 vaccine mandates with staff vaccination coverage and staffing shortages in US nursing homes. *JAMA Health Forum*. 2022;3(7):e222363. https://doi.org/10.1001/jamahealthforum.2022.2363
6. US Bureau of Labor Statistics. Health care and social assistance: NAICS 62. Updated February 9, 2024. Available at: https://www.bls.gov/iag/tgs/iag62.htm. Accessed February 11, 2024.
7. Ben-Michael E, Feller A, Rothstein J. Synthetic controls with staggered adoption. *J R Stat Soc Series B Stat Methodol*. 2022;84(2):351–381. https://doi.org/10.1111/rssb.12448
8. Telesford I, Wager E, Hughes-Cromwick P, Amin K, Cox C. What are the recent trends in health sector employment? Updated December 13, 2023. Available at: https://www.healthsystemtracker.org/chart-collection/what-are-the-recent-trends-health-sector-employment. Accessed February 15, 2024.

9. Plummer E, Wempe WF. Evidence on the effects of the federal COVID-19 vaccine mandate on nursing home staffing levels. *J Am Med Dir Assoc.* 2023;24(4):451-458. https://doi.org/10.1016/j.jamda.2022.12.024

10. Muoio D. How many employees have hospitals lost to vaccine mandates? Here are the numbers so far. Updated February 22, 2022. Available at: https://www.fiercehealthcare.com/hospitals/how-many-employees-have-hospitals-lost-to-vaccine-mandates-numbers-so-far. Accessed June 5, 2023.

11. Rich-Edwards JW, Rocheleau CM, Ding M, et al. COVID-19 vaccine uptake and factors affecting hesitancy among US nurses, March–June 2021. *Am J Public Health.* 2022;112(11):1620–1629. https://doi.org/10.2105/AJPH.2022.307050

12. Barry JJ, Christiano A, Neimand A. Half of unvaccinated workers say they'd rather quit than get a shot—but real-world data suggest few are following through. The Conversation. Updated September 27, 2021. Available at: https://theconversation.com/half-of-unvaccinated-workers-say-theyd-rather-quit-than-get-a-shot-but-real-world-data-suggest-few-are-following-through-168447. Accessed June 5, 2023.

Health Care Facility Characteristics Associated With Providing Telehealth HIV Care Services During the COVID-19 Pandemic

Eduardo E. Valverde, DrPH, Linda Beer, PhD, Dawn Pepin, JD, MPH, Stacy Crim, MPH, and John Weiser, MD, MPH

See also Heckman et al., p. 250.

Objectives. To describe provision of HIV telehealth services during the COVID-19 pandemic using data from the Centers for Disease Control and Prevention (CDC) Medical Monitoring Project Facility Survey for the Ending the HIV Epidemic in the United States initiative, which aims to achieve an at least 90% reduction in new HIV infections by 2030 and highlights telehealth as an important strategy.

Methods. During 2021, we surveyed 1023 facilities providing HIV care to a nationally representative sample of US adults with diagnosed HIV, of which 45% responded. We calculated weighted percentages with 95% confidence intervals comparing the characteristics of facilities providing telehealth services.

Results. Overall, 83.4% of facilities provided HIV care telehealth services by the facility's own providers (82.0%) or by outside providers through remote conferencing (27.0%). Gaps in coverage were identified in smaller facilities and in facilities in rural and primary care health professional shortage areas.

Conclusions. Although most HIV care facilities provided telehealth services during the COVID-19 pandemic, gaps were identified, which must be addressed to meet Ending the HIV Epidemic in the United States goals and better prepare for future health emergencies. (*Am J Public Health*. 2025;115(3):349–353. https://doi.org/10.2105/AJPH.2024.307908)

AJPH March 2025, Vol. 115, No. 3

The Department of Health and Human Services' Ending the HIV Epidemic in the United States (EHE) initiative highlights telehealth as a strategy to achieve an at least 90% reduction in new HIV infections by 2030. Addressing the disproportionate burden of new infections within certain geographic areas and populations is an EHE aim.[1] Telehealth can advance EHE's aims by improving access to and retention in HIV care, particularly for patients with limited transportation options and other barriers to in-person medical visits, and as a tool to expand HIV preexposure prophylaxis for the prevention of new infections.

During the COVID-19 pandemic, use of telehealth increased dramatically.[2] Among directly funded Ryan White HIV/AIDS Program (RWHAP) medical provider grantees (i.e., those funded through Part C or Part D), 99% provided telehealth during August–September 2020, up from 22% before the COVID-19 pandemic.[3] However, information about the availability of HIV care telehealth services at a wide range of types and locations of HIV care facilities nationally during the COVID-19 pandemic has not been available.

We used data from the Centers for Disease Control and Prevention's Medical Monitoring Project (MMP) Facility Survey to describe the availability of telehealth services at facilities where a representative sample of persons with HIV received HIV care.

METHODS

MMP is a 2-stage complex sample survey, including an interview and medical record abstraction, designed to produce nationally representative estimates of US adults with diagnosed HIV.[4] The MMP facility survey was designed to understand the characteristics of facilities providing HIV care to MMP participants, with the survey's methods reported elsewhere.[5] Briefly,

MMP participants reported their most frequent source of HIV care during the previous 24 months to determine the location for medical record abstraction. For the MMP facility survey, we surveyed all HIV care facilities where medical record abstractions were performed for 2019 MMP cycle participants (June 2019–May 2020). Facility data were collected during July–November of 2021; 455 facilities (45%) responded to the survey.

We classified facilities as having provided telehealth services if they provided HIV care by remote conferencing by facility HIV care providers or outside HIV care providers. We used publicly available data to classify facilities by primary care health professional shortage area (HPSA) designation,[6] medically underserved area or population designation,[7] and Rural–Urban Continuum Code.[8]

Data were weighted to reduce nonresponse bias. We calculated weighted percentages with 95% confidence intervals (CIs) to compare characteristics of facilities providing telehealth services and prevalence ratios (PRs) with predicted marginal means to examine associations based on availability of telehealth services. Results with CIs are presented in the tables. The analysis was performed with SAS version 9.4 survey procedures (SAS Institute, Cary, NC) and SAS-callable SUDAAN version 11 (RTI International, Research Triangle Park, NC).

RESULTS

Overall, 83.4% of facilities provided telehealth HIV care services during the COVID-19 pandemic (Table 1). An estimated 82.0% provided telehealth services by the facility's own providers and 27.0% by an outside HIV provider through remote conferencing (Tables A and B, available as supplements to the online version of this article at https://ajph.org).

Facilities located in an HPSA were less likely to offer telehealth HIV care services than facilities not in an HPSA (76.6% vs 89.0%), as were facilities located in nonmetro counties compared with counties with at least 1 million people (68.6% vs 84.8%). Facilities that did not receive RWHAP funding were less likely than those that did to offer telehealth HIV care services (78.9% vs 89.3%). Facilities that did not accept Medicaid compared with those that did were less likely to offer telehealth HIV care services (71.3% vs 85.9%), as were facilities that did not accept AIDS Drug Assistance Program or RWHAP coverage compared with those that did (75.2% vs 89.0%). Compared with facilities with more than 1000 patients, those with fewer than 50 patients (60.4% vs 91.9%) and 50 to 249 patients (76.2% vs 91.9%) were less likely to offer telehealth HIV care services, as were facilities with only primary care physicians (75.6% vs 93.4%) or a combination of infectious disease physicians and primary care physicians (82.9% vs 93.4%), compared with facilities where physicians were only infectious disease specialists. Facilities that did not provide subsistence services were less likely to offer telehealth HIV care services than facilities that did (63.2% vs 87.7%), as were facilities that did not versus did offer preexposure prophylaxis (62.2% vs 87.7%).

DISCUSSION

An estimated 17% of HIV clinical care facilities serving a representative sample of US persons with HIV did not provide telehealth HIV services during a pandemic that required immunocompromised persons to reduce public exposure to severe acute respiratory syndrome coronavirus 2 (SARS-CoV-2) while remaining engaged in HIV care. Patients who received care at facilities caring for fewer than 250 HIV patients, not receiving RWHAP funding, and located in nonmetro counties or HPSAs had particularly low access.

Financial barriers are a potential reason why some HIV care facilities did not provide telehealth services during this critical time. RWHAP-funded facilities received emergency supplemental funding to expand telehealth capacity at the beginning of the pandemic through the Coronavirus Aid, Relief, and Economic Security Act in March of 2020.[9] However, even among directly funded Ryan White providers, a large proportion faced increased operating costs during the pandemic, forcing them to shut down all or most of their HIV prevention services and, to a lesser extent, HIV care services.[3] Non–RWHAP-funded facilities, which account for more than half of HIV care facilities, serving more than one third of HIV patients,[5] might have faced even greater financial challenges.

Staffing resources may also have been a barrier in smaller, nonmetro, and HPSAs, and non–RWHAP-funded facilities. The Extension for Community Healthcare Outcomes project (Project ECHO) may be 1 potential solution to this challenge. Project ECHO is a collaborative model for increasing access to expert specialty care in rural and underserved areas for a variety of conditions, including HIV, by using video conferencing to deliver provider mentoring remotely.[10] HIV care organizations could consider expanding funding for programs like Project ECHO to ensure that smaller, more isolated HIV

TABLE 1— Characteristics of HIV Care Facilities Where Providers Delivered HIV Clinical Care by Remote Conferencing or Patients Received HIV Clinical Care From Outside HIV Providers via Remote Conferencing: Medical Monitoring Project Facility Survey, 2021, United States

	Facilities Utilizing Remote Conferencing for HIV Clinical Care		
	No.[a]	% (95% CI)[b]	PR (95% CI)
Total	374	83.4 (79.6, 87.2)	
Type of facility			
Federally qualified health center (FQHC) or FQHC look-alike			
Yes	88	82.3 (73.9, 90.6)	1 (Ref)
No	283	83.6 (79.3, 87.9)	1.02 (0.91, 1.14)
Hospital-based infectious disease clinic			
Yes	86	88.7 (81.5, 95.8)	1 (Ref)
No	285	81.8 (77.4, 86.3)	0.92 (0.84, 1.02)
Hospital-based primary care clinic			
Yes	34	76.1 (62.1, 90.1)	1 (Ref)
No	337	84.1 (80.1, 88.0)	1.11 (0.91, 1.34)
Private practice			
Yes	114	86.2 (80.2, 92.2)	1 (Ref)
No	257	81.6 (76.7, 86.5)	0.95 (0.86, 1.04)
Primary care health professional shortage area designation			
Yes	166	76.6 (70.2, 82.9)	0.86 (0.78, 0.95)
No	208	89.0 (84.6, 93.4)	1 (Ref)
Medically underserved area/population designation			
Yes	187	85.7 (80.5, 90.8)	1 (Ref)
No	187	81.7 (76.2, 87.1)	0.95 (0.87, 1.04)
Rural-Urban Continuum Code			
Counties in metro areas of > 1 million population	264	84.8 (80.4, 89.1)	1 (Ref)
Counties in metro areas of 250 000–1 million population	62	80.3 (69.9, 90.7)	0.95 (0.82, 1.09)
Nonmetro counties	23	68.6 (50.3, 86.9)[c]	0.81 (0.62, 1.06)
Any Ryan White HIV/AIDS Program funding			
Yes	224	89.3 (85.1, 93.5)	1 (Ref)
No	150	78.9 (73.1, 84.8)	0.88 (0.81, 0.96)
Types of health coverage accepted			
Medicaid			
Yes	328	85.9 (82.1, 89.8)	1 (Ref)
No	43	71.3 (59.8, 82.8)	0.83 (0.70, 0.98)
Medicare			
Yes	349	84.4 (80.6, 88.3)	1 (Ref)
No	22	71.1 (54.3, 87.9)[c]	0.84 (0.66, 1.07)
Private insurance			
Yes	347	84.3 (80.4, 88.2)	1 (Ref)
No	24	73.0 (56.9, 89.1)[c]	0.87 (0.69, 1.08)
AIDS Drug Assistance Program or other Ryan White coverage			
Yes	264	89.0 (85.1, 92.9)	1 (Ref)
No	107	75.2 (67.9, 82.4)	0.84 (0.76, 0.94)
Veterans Administration			
Yes	136	85.8 (79.8, 91.7)	1 (Ref)
No	235	81.9 (77.0, 86.9)	0.96 (0.87, 1.05)

Continued

TABLE 1— Continued

	Facilities Utilizing Remote Conferencing for HIV Clinical Care		
	No.[a]	% (95% CI)[b]	PR (95% CI)
HIV patient load			
< 50	18	60.4 (42.6, 78.1)[c]	0.66 (0.49, 0.89)
50–249	83	76.2 (67.6, 84.8)	0.83 (0.73, 0.95)
250–499	98	89.8 (83.4, 96.2)	0.98 (0.88, 1.08)
500–999	62	85.8 (76.9, 94.7)	0.93 (0.82, 1.06)
≥ 1000	86	91.9 (85.5, 98.3)	1 (Ref)
HIV care provider staffing			
Only full-time HIV care providers	151	88.9 (83.9, 93.9)	1.08 (0.99, 1.19)
A mix of full-time and part-time HIV care providers	166	82.1 (76.1, 88.0)	1 (Ref)
Only part-time HIV care provider	49	74.6 (62.8, 86.5)	0.91 (0.76, 1.08)
Provider types			
Physicians only	74	82.8 (74.7, 90.8)	1 (Ref)
Combined provider types (physicians and nonphysician providers)	280	84.9 (80.6, 89.2)	1.03 (0.92, 1.14)
Physician specialties			
Only infectious disease specialists	77	93.4 (88.3, 98.5)	1 (Ref)
Only primary care specialists	81	75.6 (67.0, 84.2)	0.81 (0.71, 0.92)
Infectious disease and primary care specialists	205	82.9 (77.5, 88.4)	0.89 (0.81, 0.97)
Clinical and supportive services that are currently available onsite or through established outside referral relationships			
Any subsistence services[d]			
Yes	335	87.7 (84.1, 91.4)	1 (Ref)
No	39	63.2 (51.0, 75.5)	0.72 (0.59, 0.88)
HIV preexposure prophylaxis			
Yes	318	87.7 (83.9, 91.4)	1 (Ref)
No	53	62.2 (50.6, 73.8)	0.71 (0.59, 0.86)
HIV postexposure prophylaxis			
Yes	306	84.7 (80.7, 88.8)	1 (Ref)
No	67	76.6 (66.4, 86.8)	0.90 (0.78, 1.04)

Note. CI = confidence interval; PR = prevalence ratio.
[a]Numbers may not add up to the total (374) because of missing data.
[b]Note that these percentages correspond to the percentage of facilities in a given row of the table that utilized remote conferencing.
[c]Estimates have an absolute CI width ≥ 30 or an absolute CI width between 5 and 30 and a relative CI width > 130% and should be interpreted with caution.
[d]Any subsistence services include Supplemental Nutrition Assistance Program or Special Supplemental Nutrition Program for Women, Infants, and Children; transportation assistance; meal or food services; and shelter or housing services.

care facilities can be linked to larger HIV care facilities to strengthen the HIV clinical network.

Limited access to telehealth infrastructure is another barrier to expanding telehealth HIV services. A recent review of successes and unresolved challenges related to telehealth HIV care services identified high-speed Internet access as a challenge particularly affecting poorer, rural, and non-White communities.[11] The review recommended investment in broadband access (particularly in rural regions), equipping health departments with necessary equipment, and training staff to deliver telehealth services.

Limitations

To address the low facility response rate, we minimized potential bias by weighting the data based on information known for all facilities. Also, the survey did not measure use of telehealth services, nor was the quality of those services assessed. A strength of this analysis was the use of data from facilities serving a diverse probability sample of persons with HIV.

Public Health Implications

While most HIV care facilities provided telehealth HIV services during the COVID-19 pandemic, gaps in coverage were identified in smaller facilities and in facilities in rural areas and primary care HPSAs. The reasons for these gaps must be better understood to inform resource allocation to address gaps in the availability of HIV care telehealth services to meet EHE goals and be better prepared for future public health emergencies. AJPH

ABOUT THE AUTHORS

Eduardo E. Valverde and Dawn Pepin are with the Office of the Director, National Center for HIV, Viral Hepatitis, STD, and TB Prevention, Centers for Disease Control and Prevention (CDC), Atlanta, GA. Linda Beer, Stacy Crim, and John Weiser are with the Division of HIV/AIDS Prevention, National Center for HIV/AIDS, Viral Hepatitis, STD, and TB Prevention.

Note. The findings and conclusions in this article are those of the authors and do not necessarily represent the official position of the CDC.

CORRESPONDENCE

Correspondence should be sent to Eduardo E. Valverde, DrPH, Office of the Director, National Center for HIV, Viral Hepatitis, STD, and TB Prevention, Centers for Disease Control and Prevention, 1600 Clifton Rd, NE, Mail Stop MS US8-6, Atlanta, GA 30329 (e-mail: evalverde@cdc.gov). Reprints can be ordered at https://www.ajph.org by clicking the "Reprints" link.

PUBLICATION INFORMATION

Full Citation: Valverde EE, Beer L, Pepin D, Crim S, Weiser J. Health care facility characteristics associated with providing telehealth HIV care services during the COVID-19 pandemic. *Am J Public Health.* 2025;115(3):349–353.

Acceptance Date: October 24, 2024.

DOI: https://doi.org/10.2105/AJPH.2024.307908

ORCID iDs:

Eduardo E. Valverde https://orcid.org/0000-0002-6132-9067

Linda Beer https://orcid.org/0000-0002-5781-8626

Dawn Pepin https://orcid.org/0000-0002-0128-2949

Stacy Crim https://orcid.org/0000-0002-5709-2773

John Weiser https://orcid.org/0000-0003-2310-5641

CONTRIBUTORS

All authors were involved in the analysis and conceptualized, designed, and wrote the research brief.

ACKNOWLEDGMENTS

The authors thank the participating Medical Monitoring Project (MMP) patients, facilities, project areas, and Provider and Community Advisory Board members; the Clinical Outcomes Team; and the Behavioral and Clinical Surveillance Branch at the CDC.

CONFLICTS OF INTEREST

The authors declare no conflicts of interest.

HUMAN PARTICIPANT PROTECTION

In accordance with CDC guidelines for defining public health research (distinguishing public health research and public health nonresearch), CDC determined MMP and the associated MMP surveys were public health surveillance used for disease control, program, or policy purposes. Because no information was collected on individuals, human participants' approvals were not obtained.

REFERENCES

1. Centers for Disease Control and Prevention. Telehealth for HIV prevention and care services. Available at: https://www.cdc.gov/hivpartners/php/effectiveinterventions/pillars.html. Accessed November 23, 2023.
2. Pylypchuk Y, Barker W. Use of telemedicine among office-based physicians, 2021. ONC Data Brief, no. 65. Washington, DC: Office of the National Coordinator for Health Information Technology; 2023.
3. Dawson L, Kates J. Delivering HIV care and prevention in the COVID era: a national survey of Ryan White providers. Kaiser Family Foundation. 2020. Available at: https://www.kff.org/hivaids/issue-brief/delivering-hiv-care-prevention-in-the-covid-era-a-national-survey-of-ryan-white-providers. Accessed November 23, 2023.
4. Beer L, Johnson CH, Fagan JL, et al. A national behavioral and clinical surveillance system of adults with diagnosed HIV (the Medical Monitoring Project): protocol for an annual cross-sectional interview and medical record abstraction survey. *JMIR Res Protoc.* 2019;8(11):e15453. https://doi.org/10.2196/15453
5. Beer L, Williams D, Tie Yunfeng, et al. The capacity of HIV care facilities to implement strategies recommended by the Ending the HIV Epidemic Initiative: the Medical Monitoring Project Facility Survey. *J Acquir Immune Defic Syndr.* 94(4): 290–300. https://doi.org/10.1097/QAI.0000000000003290
6. Health Services and Resources Administration. What is a health professional shortage area (HPSA)? Available at: https://bhw.hrsa.gov/workforce-shortage-areas/shortage-designation#hpsas. Accessed November 20, 2023.
7. Health Services and Resources Administration. What is a medically underserved area/population (MUA/P)? Available at: https://bhw.hrsa.gov/workforce-shortage-areas/shortage-designation#mups. Accessed November 25, 2023.
8. US Department of Agriculture Economic Research Service. Rural-Urban Continuum Codes. Available at: https://www.ers.usda.gov/data-products/rural-urban-continuum-codes.aspx. Accessed November 25, 2023.
9. Kaiser Family Foundation. The Ryan White HIV/AIDS Program: the basics. Available at: https://www.kff.org/hivaids/fact-sheet/the-ryan-white-hivaids-program-the-basics. Accessed November 22, 2023.
10. Arora S, Thornton K, Murata G, et al. Outcomes of treatment for hepatitis C virus infection by primary care providers. *N Engl J Med.* 2011;364(23): 2199–2207. https://doi.org/10.1056/NEJMoa1009370
11. Labisi T, Regan N, Davis P, et al. HIV care meets telehealth: a review of successes, disparities, and unresolved challenges. *Curr HIV/AIDS Rep.* 2022; 19(5):446–453. https://doi.org/10.1007/s11904-022-00623-z

Uptake of Recommended Vaccines During Pregnancy Among Publicly and Privately Insured People in the United States, December 2020–September 2022

Stacey L. Rowe, PhD, MPH, BSc(Hons), Sheena G. Sullivan, PhD, MPH, MSc, BSc(Hons), Flor M. Munoz, MD, MSc, Matthew M. Coates, MPH, Onyebuchi A. Arah, MD, DSc, PhD, MPH, MSc, and Annette K. Regan, PhD, MPH

See also Berenson, p. 247.

AJPH March 2025, Vol. 115, No. 3

Objectives. To estimate maternal COVID-19, influenza, and pertussis vaccine uptake during pregnancy by insurance type and identify factors characterizing those vaccinated and unvaccinated.

Methods. We conducted a US cohort study of pregnant individuals (for pregnancies ending December 11, 2020–September 30, 2022) using insurance claims data. We calculated vaccination probability using Kaplan-Meier methods and identified factors associated with vaccination through binomial regression with inverse probability weights.

Results. Among 695 887 pregnant individuals (median age = 32 years for privately and 27 years for publicly insured), the cumulative probability of COVID-19 vaccination was 43.0% (privately insured) and 11.8% (publicly insured). We observed marked disparities between influenza (33.2% vs 14.2%) and pertussis (70.3% vs 42.8%) vaccination. Only 6.8% (privately insured) and 1.1% (publicly insured) received all 3 vaccines. COVID-19 and influenza vaccination odds were lower among drug and tobacco users. People with high-risk medical conditions, particularly the publicly insured, commonly were vaccinated.

Conclusions. Marked vaccine uptake disparities exist between privately and publicly insured pregnant people. Understanding structural barriers, particularly for Medicaid enrollees, is critical to improving maternal vaccine access. (*Am J Public Health*. 2025;115(3):354–363. https://doi.org/10.2105/AJPH.2024.307899)

Vaccine-preventable diseases, including COVID-19,[1,2] influenza,[3,4] and pertussis,[5] can cause severe illness during pregnancy and infancy. Vaccination against these diseases during pregnancy directly protects the pregnant person and indirectly protects infants via transplacental passage of antibodies. This has led maternal vaccines to be characterized as "two-for-one" strategies.[6]

In the United States, recommendations for influenza vaccines during pregnancy were made in 1960[7] and updated in 2004.[8] Pertussis vaccines were recommended during pregnancy—optimally between 27 and 36 weeks of gestation—in 2012.[9] COVID-19 vaccines were authorized for use in the United States in December 2020 and recommended for those most at risk for severe disease, including health care workers, older people, and those with immune-compromising conditions. At the time, the Advisory Committee on Immunization Practices (ACIP) recommended not withholding COVID-19 vaccines from at-risk pregnant people; however, explicit recommendations for all pregnant people to receive the COVID-19 vaccine were not made until August 2021.[10]

Although the safety and effectiveness of maternal vaccination are well established,[11–14] coverage is chronically suboptimal.[15–20] A survey of pregnant adults reported that 65% received at least 1 dose of COVID-19 vaccine before or during pregnancy.[15] Earlier studies estimating COVID-19 vaccine uptake during pregnancy ranged from 16% in the United States[17] to 37% in Canada.[18] For maternal influenza and pertussis vaccination during pregnancy, coverage has remained relatively stable, with one third of pregnant people receiving an influenza vaccine and just over half receiving a pertussis vaccine.[19] Low uptake of recommended vaccines has been observed among younger people, non-Hispanic Black and Hispanic people, and those experiencing higher socioeconomic disadvantage.[15,17] Few studies have explored differences by insurance type, with some reporting reduced uptake of influenza[15,21] and pertussis[15,22] vaccines among publicly insured individuals.

Monitoring maternal vaccine uptake during pregnancy remains essential to identify gaps in coverage by disease, time, and population. This is particularly important as additional vaccines and therapeutics for pregnant people and infants are introduced.[23] We estimated maternal COVID-19, influenza, and pertussis vaccine uptake during pregnancy by insurance type and identified factors that characterized those vaccinated versus unvaccinated.

METHODS

We followed the REporting of studies Conducted using Observational Routinely collected health Data statement.[24]

Study Design, Setting, and Participants

We conducted a national cohort study of pregnant individuals in the United States using routinely collected administrative health data from insurance claims. Study participants were pregnant people—including women and transgendered people with the ability to become pregnant—aged 18 to 49 years with evidence of at least 1 pregnancy ending between December 11, 2020 (i.e., the COVID-19 vaccine authorization date)[25] and September 30, 2022. We use the term "maternal" to indicate exposures during pregnancy or attributes of a pregnant person and respectfully acknowledge that this may encompass pregnant noncisgendered individuals.

Data Sources

We constructed the study cohort using 2 data sources. First, we assembled a claims-based cohort of commercially insured (herein referred to as "privately insured") pregnant people from the Merative Marketscan Commercial Database (the "Commercial data set"). This database captures nationwide de-identified patient-level data from privately insured employees and their dependents. Second, we assembled a cohort of publicly insured pregnant people from the Merative Marketscan Multistate Medicaid claims database, capturing de-identified patient-level data for more than 47 million Medicaid enrollees. Collectively, these databases capture inpatient and outpatient medical encounters—including pregnancy-related procedures and tests, laboratory work and drug prescriptions, and vaccinations—recorded by physicians, employers, insurance companies, mail order prescriptions, and specialty pharmacies (supplementary material, available as a supplement to the online version of this article at http://www.ajph.org). Data on geographical area of residence were available in the Commercial data set, and data on race/ethnicity (i.e., White, Black, Hispanic, other, missing) were available in the Multistate Medicaid data set.

Data Preparation

We used a previously validated algorithm to identify pregnancy outcomes, pregnancy start date, and gestational age at pregnancy end.[26] We excluded pregnant people without prescription benefits or continuous enrollment in their insurance plan (supplementary material). We additionally restricted pertussis vaccine analyses to pregnancies ending at 27 weeks or later of gestation to align with recommendations.[9] The assembled cohort represented pregnancies, not unique people. We included all pregnancy outcomes, including spontaneous or medical abortions, trophoblastic pregnancies, whether live or stillbirth, and other unknown outcomes of pregnancy.

Outcomes

We assessed uptake of all vaccines routinely recommended to pregnant people. For COVID-19, a person was considered vaccinated if they (1) received at least 1 COVID-19 vaccine during pregnancy, or (2) completed their primary COVID-19 vaccine course before pregnancy. We did not consider individuals vaccinated if only 1 dose of a 2-dose primary vaccine series was received before pregnancy.[15,20] In sensitivity analyses, we explored more sensitive and specific case definitions (supplementary material). For influenza, we considered a person vaccinated if at least 1 influenza vaccine was administered during pregnancy, irrespective of influenza season timing. For pertussis, we considered a person vaccinated if at least 1 pertussis vaccine was administered during pregnancy. We considered a vaccine administered during pregnancy if it was given between the estimated date of the last menstrual period and 1 day before the infant's date of birth, inclusive.

Descriptive Factors

We explored several sociodemographic and maternal factors that characterized vaccinated versus unvaccinated people. These were insurance type; maternal and gestational age at pregnancy end; US region of residence (privately insured people only); race (publicly insured people only); tobacco, drug, or alcohol use complicating pregnancy, childbirth, or the puerperium; singleton or multiple pregnancy; whether the pregnancy was the outcome of assisted reproductive technology; history of preterm birth; and administration of other recommended maternal vaccines. Other factors included the presence of a high-risk medical condition in the 12 months before pregnancy (supplementary material).

Statistical Analyses

We used statistics (counts; medians; and minimum, maximum, and interquartile ranges) to describe study participants and their characteristics. For each vaccine, we calculated crude vaccine uptake as the number of pregnant people vaccinated as a proportion of all pregnancies ending during the period of interest. We used the Kaplan-Meier survival analysis to calculate the cumulative probability of vaccination for each vaccine over time and by insurance type. For COVID-19 vaccines, we estimated cumulative coverage in weeks since COVID-19 vaccine availability in the United States (December 11, 2020). Additionally, for all vaccines, we estimated the cumulative probability of vaccination by gestational week of vaccination. We censored unvaccinated persons at the week of pregnancy end. We estimated the cumulative probability of vaccination at time (t) as 1 minus the survival probability (S): $1 - S(t)$.

We used binomial regression models with robust (sandwich) variance estimation to quantify variations in vaccine uptake across each descriptive factor of interest to characterize vaccinated versus unvaccinated participants. We used inverse probability weights (IPW) to standardize each estimate to the distribution of all other covariates when quantifying the marginal vaccine uptake per factor. We used logistic regression models to generate the probability (propensity) of each factor of interest. We calculated unstabilized IPWs as the inverse of the probability of having a factor of interest, given all other factors. In total, we considered 22 covariates (described in Descriptive Factors) when building these models and in the calculation of the IPWs.

We assessed covariate balance after weighting using standardized mean differences (SMD), with an SMD less than 0.10 considered adequate. We calculated crude and adjusted odds ratios (AORs) and 95% confidence intervals (CIs) to quantify the multivariable standardized vaccine uptake by factor, accounting for all other factors. We incorporated insurance type into the model as a product term to derive separate estimates for each insurance type and to evaluate heterogeneity between the groups. We performed data preparation and analyses in Stata version 14.0 (StataCorp, College Station, TX).

RESULTS

We identified 695 887 pregnancies ending between December 11, 2020, and September 30, 2022. After applying exclusion criteria, we included 568 071 and 555 656 pregnancies in the analyses of COVID-19 and influenza vaccines, respectively; and we included 477 734 pregnancies in the pertussis vaccine analyses (Figure A, available as a supplement to the online version of this article at http://www.ajph.org). Characteristics of the cohort are shown in Table A (available as a supplement to the online version of this article at http://www.ajph.org). The median maternal age was 32 years (range = 18–49 years) among privately insured people and 27 years (range = 18–49 years) among publicly insured people.

Among pregnant individuals who were publicly insured, just under half were White, one third were Black, and 8.4% were Hispanic. Among privately insured people, the geographical distribution roughly followed the US population, with approximately half of pregnancies identified in the South (45.3%) and one fifth in the West (56 493; 18.1%).[27] The median gestational age at pregnancy end was 38 weeks for both insurance types. Proportionally, more publicly insured people had medical records indicating tobacco or drug use that complicated pregnancy, obesity, or a history of preterm birth. Proportionally more privately insured pregnancies were a result of assisted reproductive technology. The presence of specific high-risk medical conditions varied by insurance type (Table A, available as a supplement to the online version of this article at http://www.ajph.org). After we applied the IPWs for our adjusted models (data not shown), the SMDs indicated good balance across covariates.

The uptake of maternal vaccines during pregnancy varied considerably by insurance type. Overall, 21.4% (95% CI = 21.3, 21.5) of privately insured people were vaccinated against COVID-19 during pregnancy compared with 4.9% (95% CI = 4.8, 5.0) of publicly insured people. We observed a similar pattern of disparity for influenza (24.8%; 95% CI = 24.6, 25.0 vs 12.4%; 95% CI = 12.2, 12.5) and pertussis (68.1%; 95% CI = 67.9, 68.3 vs 40.9%; 95% CI = 40.6, 41.1) vaccines. On average, uptake of these vaccines was nearly 56% lower ($P < .001$) for publicly compared with privately insured pregnant people. Very few people were vaccinated with all 3 recommended maternal vaccines (6.8%; 95% CI = 6.7, 6.9 for privately insured and 1.1%; 95% CI = 1.0, 1.1 for publicly insured; Table B, available as a supplement to the online version of this article at http://www.ajph.org).

Vaccine uptake also varied over time. Maternal COVID-19 vaccine uptake peaked at 36.6% in February 2022 for privately insured people and 10.6% in January 2022 for publicly insured people (data not shown). Using sensitivity analyses assessing COVID-19 vaccine uptake and a more sensitive case definition, we identified a 52.5% vaccination rate among privately insured people by September 2022 compared with only 17.8% among publicly insured people (supplementary material). We observed notable increases in the cumulative probability of COVID-19 vaccination near key pandemic milestones, including when the Centers for Disease Control and Prevention and the American College of Obstetricians and Gynecologists recommended that all pregnant people be vaccinated (August 2021) and following their recommendations for booster doses to be administered to the general population (November 2021).[25]

These increases were more pronounced among privately insured people. The cumulative probability of COVID-19 vaccination reached 43.0% among privately insured and 11.8% among publicly insured people by September 30, 2022 (Figure 1). We also observed lags in the time of vaccination relative to gestational age by insurance type. Compared with the publicly insured, privately insured people had a higher probability of COVID-19 vaccination at each week of pregnancy (Figure 1).

Influenza vaccine uptake varied by seasonal vaccine availability, peaking at 39.5% in December 2020 for the

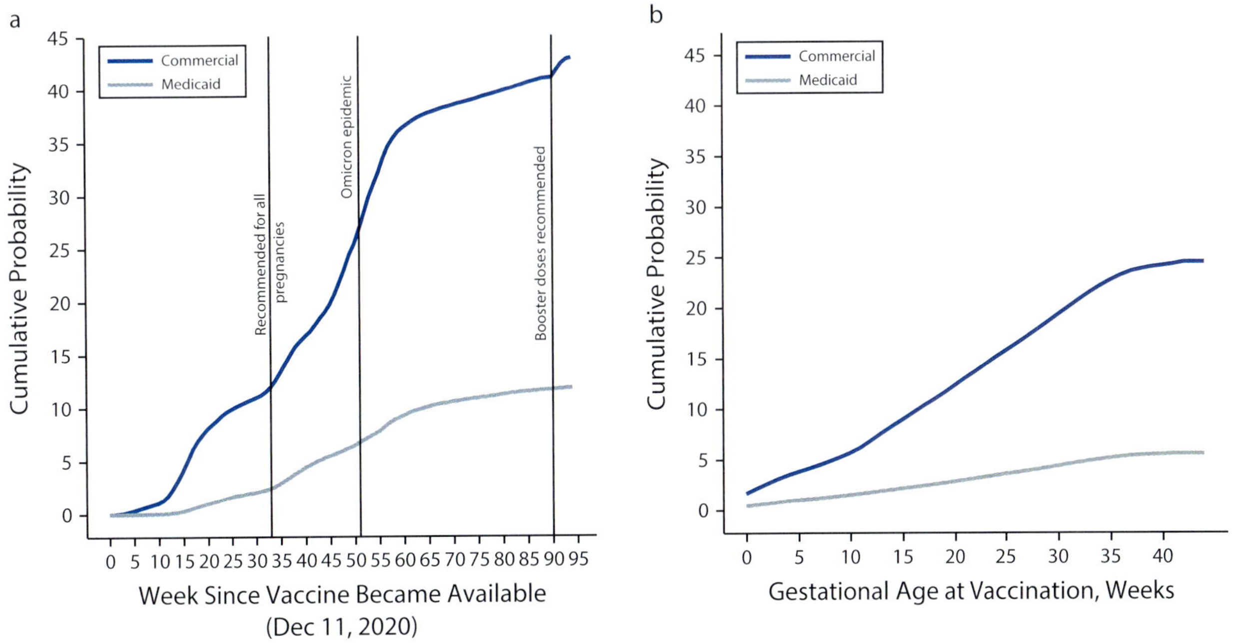

FIGURE 1— Cumulative Probability of COVID-19 Vaccination During Pregnancy by Insurance Type and (a) Week Since Vaccine Availability (December 11, 2010) and (b) Gestational Age in Weeks at Vaccine Administration: United States, December 2020–September 2022

AJPH March 2025, Vol. 115, No. 3

privately insured and 22.5% for the publicly insured (Figure 2). Privately insured people also had a higher probability of influenza vaccination throughout each week of pregnancy, with the gap between privately and publicly insured people widening over time relative to gestational age. After 40 weeks gestation, 33.2% of privately insured people were vaccinated against influenza during their pregnancy compared with 14.2% of publicly insured people (Figure 3).

Pertussis vaccine uptake remained relatively stable over the study period, peaking at 70.4% in October 2021 for privately insured people and 45.3% in December 2021 for publicly insured people (Figure 2). Consistent with COVID-19 and influenza vaccination rates, we observed disparities between privately and publicly insured people throughout pregnancy in pertussis vaccination rates: the cumulative probability of vaccination after 40 weeks of gestation was 70.3% among privately insured compared with 42.8% among publicly insured people (Figure 3).

In our adjusted models, we identified several factors more likely to describe vaccinated versus unvaccinated people, with some notable differences between insurance types. For both insurance types, people with a record of tobacco or drug use complicating pregnancy had a reduced odds of COVID-19 and influenza vaccination. This finding was also reflected among privately insured people regarding pertussis vaccination. Similarly, for both insurance types, COVID-19 vaccination was higher among older people. This was also observed among privately insured people with regard to influenza and pertussis vaccination. Among publicly insured people, Hispanic people had higher odds of COVID-19 (AOR = 1.50; 95% CI = 1.38, 1.62) and influenza (AOR = 1.95; 95% CI = 1.85, 2.05) vaccination compared with the referent group (White). Among privately insured pregnant people, compared with those living in the Northeastern United States, people in all other US regions had lower odds of COVID-19 vaccination, most notably in the South (AOR = 0.74; 95% CI = 0.70, 0.78; Figure 4; Figure B, Figure C, available as a supplement to the online version of this article at http://www.ajph.org).

We observed variations in the odds of vaccination among people with high-risk medical conditions. Publicly insured people with immunocompromising conditions had higher odds of influenza vaccination than did people without these conditions (AOR = 1.41; 95% CI = 1.22, 1.60); by contrast, privately insured people with these conditions

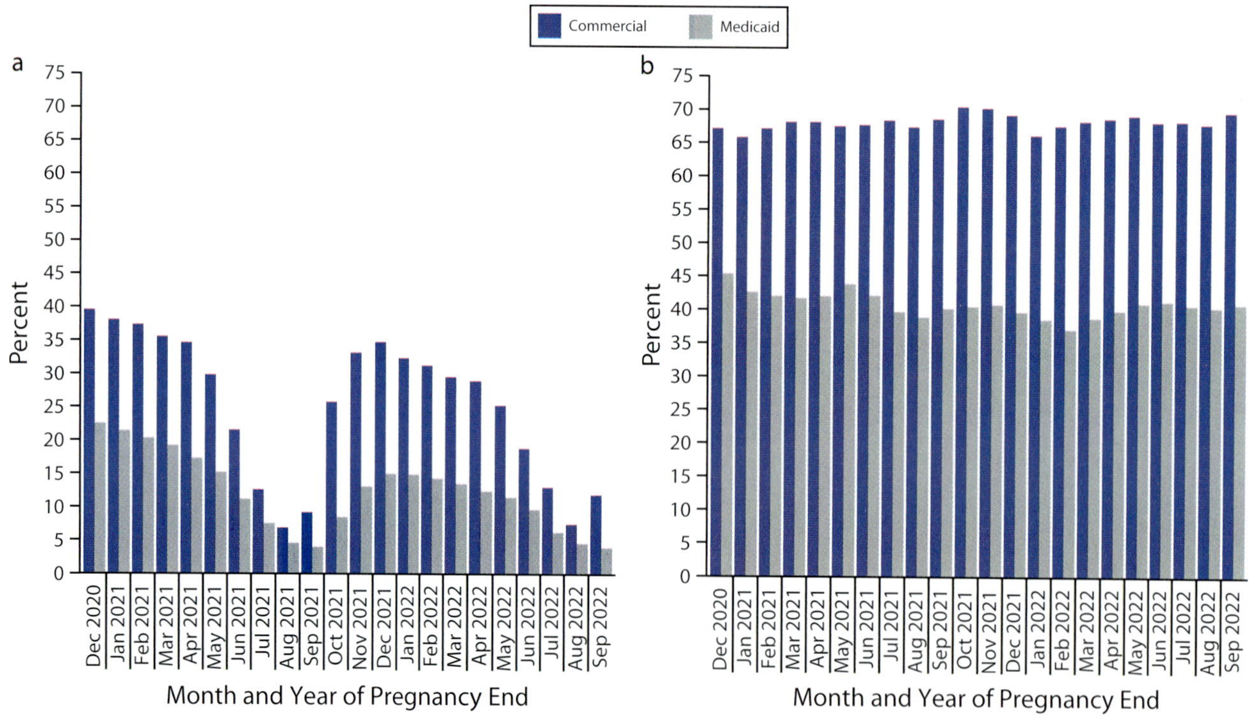

FIGURE 2— Percentage of People Vaccinated During Pregnancy, by Insurance Type and Month and Year of Pregnancy End, Against (a) Influenza or (b) Pertussis: United States, December 2020–September 2022

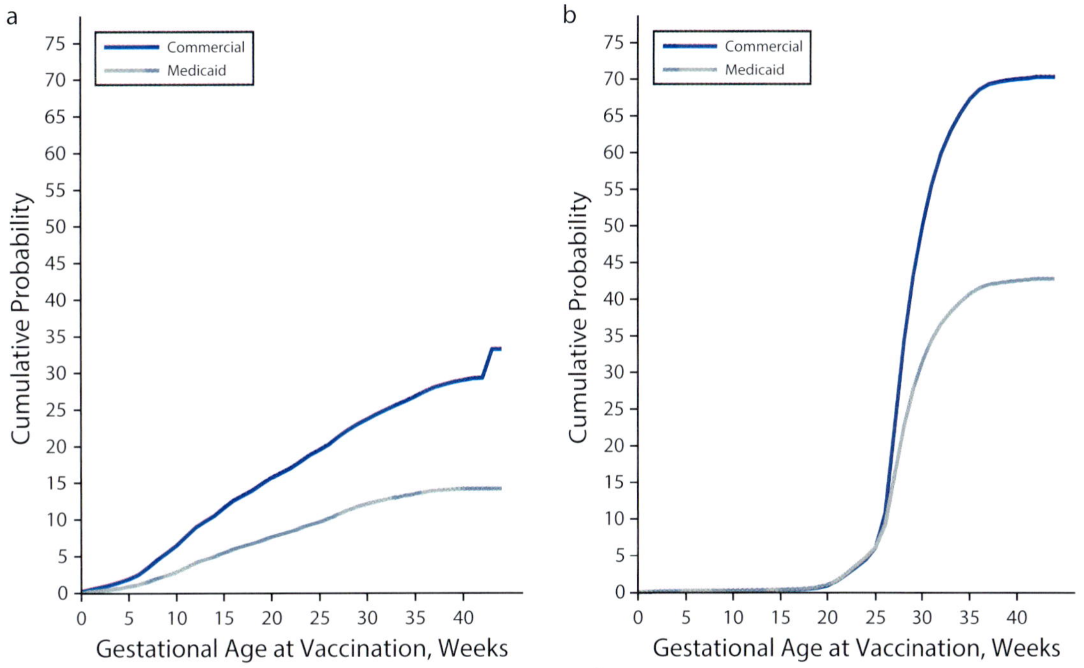

FIGURE 3— Cumulative Probability of Vaccination During Pregnancy, by Gestational Age in Weeks at Administration, of (a) Influenza and (b) Pertussis: United States, December 2020–September 2022

had reduced odds of influenza vaccination (AOR = 0.85; 95% CI = 0.76, 0.95). Differences in the estimates between these 2 groups were statistically significant ($P < .001$). We observed similar results for other high-risk medical conditions, such as liver disease and obesity (Figure 4; Figures B and C, available as a supplement to the online version of this article at http://www.ajph.org).

We also observed differences in vaccine uptake between insurance types among people with a history of preterm birth. Publicly insured people with a history of preterm birth had slightly higher odds of COVID-19 (AOR = 1.15; 95% CI = 1.07, 1.24) and pertussis (AOR = 1.16; 95% CI = 1.12, 1.20) vaccination; by contrast, privately insured people with a history of preterm birth had reduced odds of being vaccinated against these diseases (COVID-19: AOR = 0.89; 95% CI = 0.84, 0.94; pertussis: AOR = 0.82; 95% CI = 0.78, 0.86). Among both insurance types and across all vaccines examined, individuals vaccinated with any 1 maternal vaccine had higher odds of receiving other maternal vaccines (Figure 4; Figures B and C).

DISCUSSION

In this large cohort study, we found considerable variations in the uptake of COVID-19, influenza, and pertussis vaccines among pregnant people. Very few people received all 3. There were marked disparities in uptake of these vaccines between privately and publicly insured people, with exceptionally low uptake among Medicaid enrollees. This was most apparent for COVID-19 vaccination: uptake reached only 11.8% among publicly insured people compared with 43.0% among privately insured people. We identified several factors that characterized the vaccinated versus unvaccinated people and noted the differences by insurance type.

In the United States—as in other parts of the world—the COVID-19 vaccine rollout was staged, initially focusing on those at highest risk for severe disease. Pregnancy was not a contraindication to vaccination for people who met eligibility criteria. In our study, most pregnant people vaccinated in the first 8 months of rollout were privately insured; this likely reflects the eligibility of pregnant health care workers for early vaccination because of their employment status. However, when COVID-19 vaccines were recommended for all pregnant people, observed coverage gaps between privately and publicly insured people persisted. This was despite national policy enabling the provision of COVID-19 vaccines for all, including Medicaid enrollees with limited benefit packages, who generally did not have access to the full range of ACIP-recommended vaccines.[28] Observed disparities in vaccine coverage between privately and publicly insured

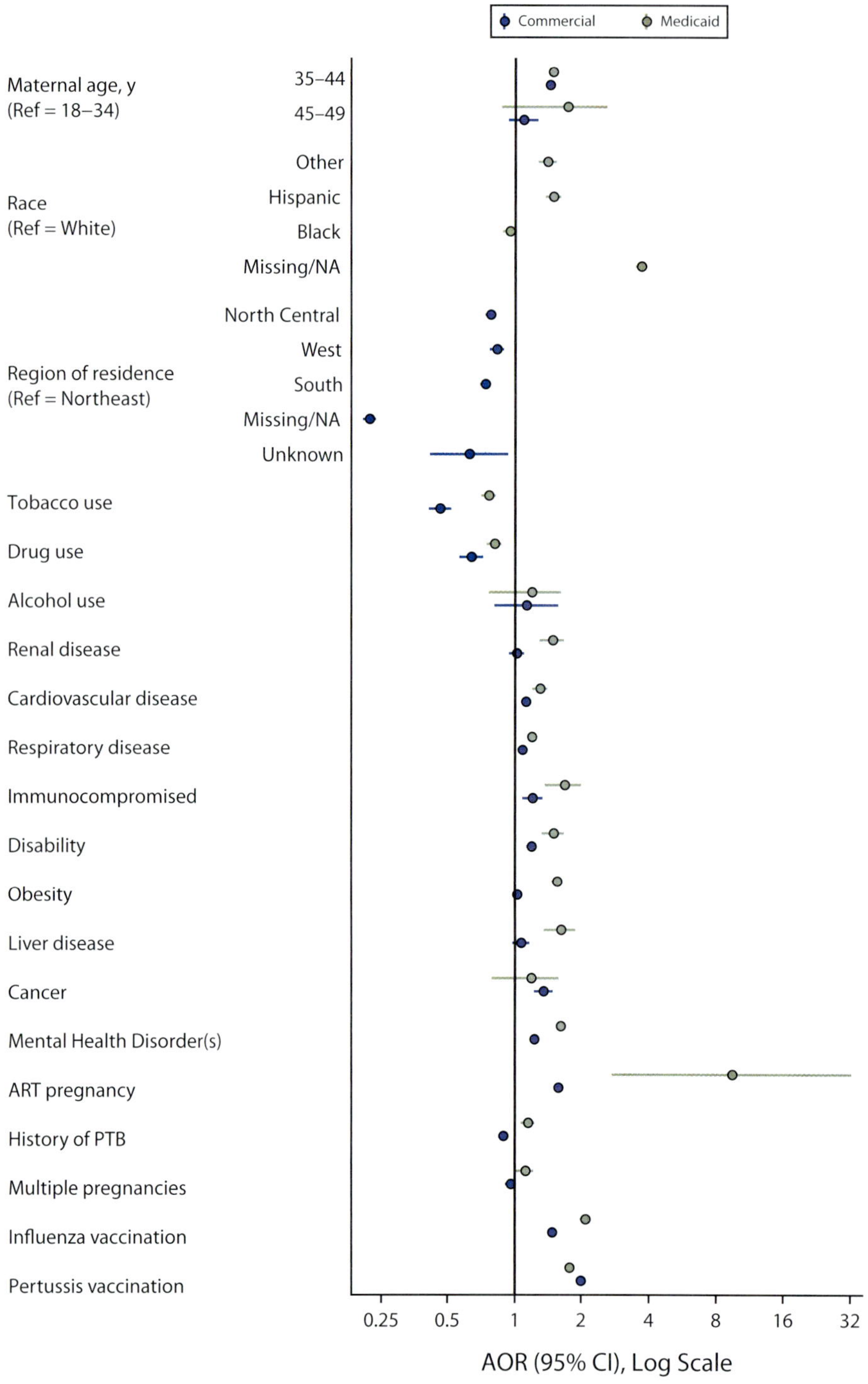

FIGURE 4— Characteristics of People Vaccinated During Pregnancy Against COVID-19 by Insurance Type: United States, December 2020–September 2022

Note. AOR = adjusted odds ratio; ART = assisted reproductive technology; CI = confidence interval; PTB = preterm birth. All factors listed without a reference group are binary 1 = yes; 0 = no outcomes, and the reference group is 0 = no. For race, the category listed as "other" is commonly used in Medicaid claims data to represent people of Asian descent. Missing/NA represents data from the Commercial data set for which data on race was not available. For region, missing/NA represents data from the Medicaid data set for which region was not available. Unknown represents data from the Commercial data set for which the region was recorded as "unknown."

people were not unique to COVID-19; they were also evident with influenza and pertussis vaccines, both of which have long-established programs supported by robust evidence of safety and effectiveness[11,12] and—particularly for maternal pertussis vaccination—high levels of acceptability among patients and providers.[29]

Our findings point to a systematic lack of access to vaccines among publicly insured people. Barriers to uptake of ACIP-recommended vaccines among adult Medicaid enrollees include variations or restrictions in vaccine coverage policies by state; limited provider support, access, and availability; and inadequate support and education for beneficiaries.[28] Although restrictions were lifted for Medicaid enrollees during the COVID-19 pandemic[28]—theoretically removing barriers to vaccine availability—our results suggest that other barriers to accessing vaccines may have affected COVID-19 vaccine uptake in this population.

In pandemic and nonpandemic settings, governments and health care providers may need to tailor vaccine delivery approaches to meet the specific needs of Medicaid beneficiaries and other underserved populations. This could involve addressing logistical barriers to accessing care, implementing financial policies or incentives to remove cost barriers, and developing culturally and linguistically sensitive support and communication material.[30] The proposed Vaccines for Adults program currently under consideration as part of the federal budget would increase the availability of ACIP-recommended vaccines to all Medicaid beneficiaries and uninsured individuals. Nonetheless, broader access barriers need to be addressed as part of local implementation.

Consistent with other studies,[15,21] we found that maternal influenza vaccine coverage was low among both publicly and privately insured pregnant people. Coverage estimates for pertussis vaccination were moderately high among privately insured pregnant people (reaching 70.3% at > 40 weeks gestation). Although uptake of pertussis vaccine among publicly insured people was lower (42.8% at > 40 weeks gestation), it was high relative to the uptake of COVID-19 and influenza vaccines among this group. These results demonstrate that moderate to high levels of vaccine uptake during pregnancy can be achieved irrespective of insurance type. Variations in uptake by vaccine may reflect differences in attitudes toward the diseases against which they are designed to protect, rather than a hesitancy to be vaccinated during pregnancy.[31] Further work is required to understand the factors driving the relative success of the maternal pertussis vaccination program in the United States and to characterize structural or attitudinal factors driving vaccine-specific differences. Emerging insights could strengthen existing maternal vaccination programs and support the delivery of new maternal and neonatal therapeutics against other vaccine-preventable diseases, such as respiratory syncytial virus.[23]

We also described maternal and sociodemographic characteristics of vaccinated versus unvaccinated participants. Although some characteristics are shared between privately and publicly insured unvaccinated people (e.g., tobacco use, younger maternal age), several other characteristics were more dominant in the publicly insured. For example, vaccination was generally higher among those with high-risk medical conditions, likely reflecting increased contact with health care providers during pregnancy and in line with recommendations for people with preexisting medical conditions to be vaccinated. Reasons for the observed differences between privately and publicly insured individuals are unclear but may be attributable to attitudinal differences toward vaccination among providers and patients in the 2 insurance types. These coverage gaps warrant further investigation, as do our contrasting findings related to vaccine coverage among people with a history of preterm birth. Observed differences in vaccine uptake by insurance type may be explained by increases in vaccine hesitancy in populations of higher socioeconomic position.[32]

Regardless of insurance type, provider hesitancy to recommend vaccines during pregnancy has been implicated in low vaccine coverage, particularly for COVID-19[10,32] and influenza.[33] Patient-level vaccine hesitancy also plays a role, with more hesitancy against influenza and pertussis vaccines during the COVID-19 pandemic period.[15] Vaccine hesitancy can be overcome, but it requires a multimodal approach that addresses both provider- and patient-level barriers. Provider recommendations are the most important predictors of vaccination during pregnancy,[29] even when patients previously refused vaccine.[34] Other provider-level strategies include ensuring adequate vaccine stock in obstetric practices, implementing standing orders, and strengthening provider to patient discussions that focus on safety and benefits to the infant.[34]

Limitations

Our use of national data that captured comprehensive medical information from a large cohort of publicly and privately insured pregnancies provided a robust platform to assess maternal vaccine uptake, contrasting with single-site studies or those drawing on cross-sectional or panel survey data. Nonetheless, several limitations exist.

First, misclassification of vaccination status is likely in claims data, with 1 study demonstrating that claims data may underestimate COVID-19 vaccination status by up to 15 percentage points.[35] Additionally, the timing of vaccine exposures relative to pregnancy may be misclassified because of the algorithm used to estimate gestational age at pregnancy end. Conversely, misclassification of pregnancy start and end dates is likely to be low, with 1 study demonstrating high agreement between claims-based algorithms and physician adjudication of electronic medical records.[26] Misclassification may have influenced the magnitude of our estimates (in either direction); however, it is unlikely to explain all disparities observed. Underascertainment of COVID-19 vaccination may have occurred because of the rapid rollout, but our coverage estimates (including results from our sensitivity analyses) are not unlike other studies.[15,17,20] Our influenza and pertussis vaccine coverage estimates also align with previously reported national estimates,[19,22] providing reassurance about external validity.

Second, our results may be affected by selection bias, as we did not exclude pregnancies ending early (e.g., owing to early termination). People whose pregnancies end early have reduced opportunity for vaccination and may systematically differ from people whose pregnancies end at later stages of gestation. Nonetheless, inclusion of early losses reflects the general pregnant population and offsets sampling bias introduced by including only healthy pregnancies ending in live birth or closer to term.

Third, in our analyses describing characteristics of those vaccinated, we were unable to include factors not captured in claims data, limiting our ability to draw inferences about the role of race and region. Nonetheless, Medicaid data are considered a surrogate for socioeconomic status, as they correlate with several socioeconomic measures. Further, we included several factors commonly unreported in other studies, such as maternal medical history and tobacco and drug use.

Fourth, our data sources precluded the assessment of vaccine uptake among uninsured pregnant people. It is likely that coverage in this group is lower than in the Medicaid sample.

Public Health Implications

We examined uptake of 3 vaccines recommended during pregnancy in a pandemic setting and identified considerable disparities in uptake by vaccine and insurance type. Very few people were vaccinated with all 3 recommended vaccines. Structural and attitudinal barriers to the accessibility, availability, and uptake of maternal vaccines—particularly among publicly insured people—should be explored. The complexity of structural barriers facing socioeconomically disadvantaged pregnant people likely requires multimodal solutions, including reform in the way public health interventions are delivered to this population. Enhanced vaccine promotion and delivery efforts will be needed to ensure maternal vaccination equity. AJPH

ABOUT THE AUTHORS

Stacey L. Rowe is with the School of Nursing and Health Professions, University of San Francisco, San Francisco, CA. Sheena G. Sullivan is with the School of Clinical Sciences, Monash University, Melbourne, Australia. Flor M. Munoz is with the Department of Pediatrics, Baylor College of Medicine, Houston, TX. Matthew M. Coates and Onyebuchi A. Arah are with the Department of Epidemiology, Fielding School of Public Health, University of California, Los Angeles. Annette K. Regan is with the Department of Research and Evaluation, Kaiser Permanente Research, Pasadena, CA.

CORRESPONDENCE

Correspondence should be sent to Stacey L. Rowe, University of San Francisco, 2130 Fulton St, San Francisco, CA 94117 (e-mail: srowe3@usfca.edu; stacey.rowe@monash.edu). Reprints can be ordered at https://www.ajph.org by clicking the "Reprints" link.

PUBLICATION INFORMATION

Full Citation: Rowe SL, Sullivan SG, Munoz FM, Coates MM, Arah OA, Regan AK. Uptake of recommended vaccines during pregnancy among publicly and privately insured people in the United States, December 2020–September 2022. *Am J Public Health*. 2025;115(3):354–363.

Acceptance Date: October 7, 2024.

DOI: https://doi.org/10.2105/AJPH.2024.307899

ORCID iDs:

Stacey L. Rowe https://orcid.org/0000-0002-9226-1376

Sheena G. Sullivan https://orcid.org/0000-0002-0856-0294

Matthew M. Coates https://orcid.org/0000-0002-8474-4992

Onyebuchi A. Arah https://orcid.org/0000-0002-9067-1697

Annette K. Regan https://orcid.org/0000-0002-3879-6193

CONTRIBUTORS

S. L. Rowe designed the study, analyzed the data, interpreted the results, and wrote the article. S. G. Sullivan supported figure preparation. S. G. Sullivan, F. M. Munoz, M. M. Coates, and O. A. Arah provided critical feedback on study design and article content. O. A. Arah provided direction for statistical analyses. A. K. Regan conceptualized the study, secured funding for the research, extracted the data to define the study cohort, and provided critical input during study design and execution. All authors reviewed and approved the final version of the article.

ACKNOWLEDGMENTS

This study received funding from the National Institute of Allergy and Infectious Diseases, National Institutes of Health (NIH; grant R01AI169239).

Note. The NIH had no role in the conduct of the study or in the decision to publish study findings.

CONFLICTS OF INTEREST

S. G. Sullivan reports paid consulting of or advisory board participation in CSL Seqirus, Evo Health, Moderna, Novavax, and Pfizer but declares no nonfinancial competing interests. All other authors declare no financial or nonfinancial competing interests.

HUMAN PARTICIPANT PROTECTION

This research was conducted using previously collected de-identified data and was deemed by the National Institutes of Health to be an activity that did not involve human participants. The University of San Francisco Institutional Review Board (IRB) for the Protection of Human Subjects Institutional determined that no IRB approval was necessary.

REFERENCES

1. Allotey J, Fernandez S, Bonet M, et al. Clinical manifestations, risk factors, and maternal and perinatal outcomes of coronavirus disease 2019 in pregnancy: living systematic review and meta-analysis. *BMJ*. 2020;370:m3320. https://doi.org/10.1136/bmj.m3320
2. Smith ER, Oakley E, Grandner GW, et al. Adverse maternal, fetal, and newborn outcomes among pregnant women with SARS-CoV-2 infection: an individual participant data meta-analysis. *BMJ Glob Health*. 2023;8(1):e009495. https://doi.org/10.1136/bmjgh-2022-009495
3. Mertz D, Geraci J, Winkup J, Ortiz J, Loeb M. Pregnancy as a risk factor for severe outcomes from influenza virus infection: a systematic review and meta-analysis of observational studies. *Open Forum Infect Dis*. 2015;2(suppl 1):1153. https://doi.org/10.1093/ofid/ofv133.865
4. Wang R, Yan W, Du M, Tao L, Liu J. The effect of influenza virus infection on pregnancy outcomes: a systematic review and meta-analysis of cohort studies. *Int J Infect Dis*. 2021;105:567–578. https://doi.org/10.1016/j.ijid.2021.02.095
5. Decker MD, Edwards KM. Pertussis (whooping cough). *J Infect Dis*. 2021;224(12 suppl 2): S310–S320. https://doi.org/10.1093/infdis/jiaa469
6. Rasmussen SA, Jamieson DJ. COVID-19 vaccination during pregnancy—two for the price of one. *N Engl J Med*. 2022;387(2):178–179. https://doi.org/10.1056/NEJMe2206730
7. Burney LE. Influenza immunization: statement. *Public Health Rep (1896)*. 1960;75(10):944.
8. Centers for Disease Control and Prevention. Prevention and control of influenza: recommendations of the Advisory Committee on Immunization Practices (ACIP). *MMWR Recomm Rep*. 20048;53(RR-6):1–40. [Update in: *MMWR Recomm Rep*. 2005;54(RR-8):1–40; Erratum in: *MMWR Recomm Rep*. 2004;53(32):743.]
9. Centers for Disease Control and Prevention. Updated recommendations for use of tetanus toxoid, reduced diphtheria toxoid, and acellular pertussis vaccine (Tdap) in pregnant women—Advisory Committee on Immunization Practices (ACIP), 2012. *MMWR Morb Mortal Wkly Rep*. 2013;62(7):131–135.
10. Grunebaum A, Chervenak FA. Physician hesitancy to recommend COVID-19 vaccination in pregnancy as a cause of maternal deaths—Robert Brent was prescient. *Birth Defects Res*. 2023;115(14): 1255–1260. https://doi.org/10.1002/bdr2.2136
11. Nunes MC, Madhi SA. Influenza vaccination during pregnancy for prevention of influenza confirmed illness in the infants: a systematic review and meta-analysis. *Hum Vaccin Immunother*. 2018;14(3):758–766. https://doi.org/10.1080/21645515.2017.1345385
12. Vygen-Bonnet S, Hellenbrand W, Garbe E, et al. Safety and effectiveness of acellular pertussis vaccination during pregnancy: a systematic review. *BMC Infect Dis*. 2020;20(1):136. https://doi.org/10.1186/s12879-020-4824-3
13. Rowe SL, Leder K, Perrett KP, et al. Maternal vaccination and infant influenza and pertussis. *Pediatrics*. 2021;148(3):e2021051076. https://doi.org/10.1542/peds.2021-051076
14. Prasad S, Kalafat E, Blakeway H, et al. Systematic review and meta-analysis of the effectiveness and perinatal outcomes of COVID-19 vaccination in pregnancy. *Nat Commun*. 2022;13(1):2414. https://doi.org/10.1038/s41467-022-30052-w
15. Centers for Disease Control and Prevention. Influenza, Tdap, and COVID-19 vaccination coverage and hesitancy among pregnant women—United States, April 2023. *MMWR Morb Mortal Wkly Rep*. 2023;72(39):1065–1071. https://doi.org/10.15585/mmwr.mm7239a4
16. Rowe SL, Perrett KP, Morey R, et al. Influenza and pertussis vaccination of women during pregnancy in Victoria, 2015–2017. *Med J Aust*. 2019; 210(10):454–462. https://doi.org/10.5694/mja2.50125
17. Centers for Disease Control and Prevention. COVID-19 vaccination coverage among pregnant women during pregnancy—eight integrated health care organizations, United States, December 14, 2020–May 8, 2021. *MMWR Morb Mortal Wkly Rep*. 2021;70(24):895–899. https://doi.org/10.15585/mmwr.mm7024e2
18. Fell DB, Török E, Sprague AE, et al. Temporal trends and determinants of COVID-19 vaccine coverage and series initiation during pregnancy in Ontario, Canada, December 2020 to December 2021: a population-based retrospective cohort study. *Vaccine*. 2023;41(10):1716–1725. https://doi.org/10.1016/j.vaccine.2023.01.073
19. Law AW, Judy J, Atwell JE, Willis S, Shea KM. Maternal Tdap and influenza vaccination uptake 2017–2021 in the United States: implications for maternal RSV vaccine uptake in the future. *Vaccine*. 2023;41(51):7632–7640. https://doi.org/10.1016/j.vaccine.2023.11.009
20. Zerbo O, Ray GT, Fireman B, et al. Individual and neighborhood factors associated with being unvaccinated against COVID-19 among pregnant persons. *Hum Vaccin Immunother*. 2023;19(2): 2256042. https://doi.org/10.1080/21645515.2023.2256042
21. Cambou MC, Copeland TP, Nielsen-Saines K, Macinko J. Insurance status predicts self-reported influenza vaccine coverage among pregnant women in the United States: a cross-sectional analysis of the National Health Interview Study data from 2012 to 2018. *Vaccine*. 2021;39(15):2068–2073. https://doi.org/10.1016/j.vaccine.2021.03.026
22. Isenhour CJ, Skoff TH, Lindley MC, Zhou F, Hariri S. Tetanus, diphtheria, and acellular pertussis vaccination coverage among publicly insured pregnant women, US, 2016–2019. *AJPM Focus*. 2022;2(1):100060. https://doi.org/10.1016/j.focus.2022.100060
23. Yonts AB, Gaviria-Agudelo C, Kimberlin DW, O'Leary ST, Paulsen GC. Fall 2023 ACIP update on meningococcal, RSV, COVID-19, and other pediatric vaccines. *Pediatrics*. 2024;153(3): e2023064990. https://doi.org/10.1542/peds.2023-064990
24. Benchimol EI, Smeeth L, Guttmann A, et al. The REporting of studies Conducted using Observational Routinely-collected health Data (RECORD) statement. *PLoS Med*. 2015;12(10):e1001885. https://doi.org/10.1371/journal.pmed.1001885
25. Centers for Disease Control and Prevention. CDC Museum COVID-19 timeline. Available at: https://www.cdc.gov/museum/timeline/covid19.html. Accessed April 18, 2024.
26. Moll K, Wong HL, Fingar K, et al. Validating claims-based algorithms determining pregnancy outcomes and gestational age using a linked claims-electronic medical record database. *Drug Saf*. 2021;44(11):1151–1164. https://doi.org/10.1007/s40264-021-01113-8
27. US Census Bureau. State population totals and components of change: 2020–2024. December 2024. Available at: https://www.census.gov/data/tables/time-series/demo/popest/2020s-state-total.html. Accessed December 28, 2024.
28. Medicaid and CHIP Payment and Access Commission. June 2022 report to Congress on Medicaid and CHIP. June 2022. Available at: https://www.macpac.gov/publication/june-2022-report-to-congress-on-medicaid-and-chip. Accessed December 28, 2024.
29. Myers KL. Predictors of maternal vaccination in the United States: an integrative review of the literature. *Vaccine*. 2016;34(34):3942–3949. https://doi.org/10.1016/j.vaccine.2016.06.042
30. Hutchins SS, Fiscella K, Levine RS, Ompad DC, McDonald M. Protection of racial/ethnic minority populations during an influenza pandemic. *Am J Public Health*. 2009;99(suppl 2):S261–S270. https://doi.org/10.2105/AJPH.2009.161505
31. Zimmerman M, Zapata LP, Bachiller K, et al. Comparison of attitudes toward routine maternal vaccines and COVID-19 vaccines among pregnant patients in an urban safety-net setting. *J Natl Med Assoc*. 2023;115(4):362–376. https://doi.org/10.1016/j.jnma.2023.04.003
32. Bhattacharya O, Siddiquea BN, Shetty A, Afroz A, Billah B. COVID-19 vaccine hesitancy among pregnant women: a systematic review and meta-analysis. *BMJ Open*. 2022;12(8):e061477. https://doi.org/10.1136/bmjopen-2022-061477
33. Morales KF, Menning L, Lambach P. The faces of influenza vaccine recommendation: a literature review of the determinants and barriers to health providers' recommendation of influenza vaccine in pregnancy. *Vaccine*. 2020;38(31): 4805–4815. https://doi.org/10.1016/j.vaccine.2020.04.033
34. Rand CM, Olson-Chen C. Maternal vaccination and vaccine hesitancy. *Pediatr Clin North Am*. 2023;70(2):259–269. https://doi.org/10.1016/j.pcl.2022.11.004
35. Schneider KL, Bell EJ, Zhou CK, et al. Use of immunization information systems in ascertainment of COVID-19 vaccinations for claims-based vaccine safety and effectiveness studies. *JAMA Netw Open*. 2023;6(5):e2313512. https://doi.org/10.1001/jamanetworkopen.2023.13512

Direct Estimation of Alcohol-Attributable Fractions for Suicide in the United States, 2021

Julien Robitaille, MPH, Jürgen Rehm, PhD, Mark S. Kaplan, DrPH, Carolin Kilian, PhD, Laura Llamosas-Falcón, MD, and Shannon Lange, PhD

Objectives. To estimate the alcohol-attributable fraction (AAF) for suicide in the United States.

Methods. Using restricted-access data from the National Violent Death Reporting System for 2021, we estimated the sex-specific AAF for suicide, among those 15 years of age and older, by sociodemographic characteristics and suicide means. An alcohol-attributable suicide was defined as that for which the decedent had a blood alcohol concentration of 0.10 grams per deciliter or higher.

Results. In 2021, the AAF for suicide for males (20.2%) was significantly higher than that for females (17.8%; $P < .001$). The AAF for suicide was higher for both males and females who used a firearm as the means of suicide (23.4% and 22.8%, respectively) compared with their counterparts who used other means (16.5% and 15.9%, respectively).

Conclusions. Despite some variation, AAFs for suicide were consistently high, with about 1 in 5 suicides being attributable to alcohol use. Therefore, suicide prevention initiatives in the United States should also target excessive alcohol use. (*Am J Public Health*. 2025;115(3):364–368. https://doi.org/10.2105/AJPH.2024.307910)

AJPH March 2025, Vol. 115, No. 3

Alcohol use is an established risk factor for suicide.[1] Up-to-date, sex-specific estimates of the proportion of suicides attributable to alcohol use for the United States are absent. The aims of the current study were to (1) estimate the proportion of suicides attributable to alcohol—that is, the alcohol-attributable fraction (AAF), and (2) determine whether there are sociodemographic differences and means-specific differences in the AAF for suicide.

METHODS

We used restricted access data from the National Violent Death Reporting System (NVDRS) for 2021. In 2021, data were available for 48 states, the District of Columbia, and Puerto Rico. (The NVDRS excluded data from Florida and Hawaii because of incomplete case reporting.)

Measures

We restricted all analyses to solitary suicides (i.e., incidents involving only 1 suicide decedent). In line with previous estimates,[2] we defined alcohol-attributable suicides as those suicides where the decedent had a blood alcohol concentration (BAC) of 0.10 grams per deciliter (g/dL) or higher. BAC is available only for decedents for whom a toxicology examination was performed and the presence of alcohol was ascertained. The percentage of decedents with BAC available varies across states (Table A, available as a supplement to the online version of this article at http://www.ajph.org), which likely reflects the medicolegal death investigation system in each state. We used a continuous measure of BAC (weight by volume) to create a categorical variable (i.e., 0 = BAC < 0.10 g/dL and 1 = BAC ≥ 0.10 g/dL). We restricted analyses to those 15 years of age or older and stratified by sex.

Statistical Analysis

We performed sex-specific univariate and multivariate logistic regression analyses. We excluded sociodemographic variables from the multivariate models if there was no statistically significant association in the univariate model. We tested interactions between sex and the other sociodemographic variables to determine if sex-stratified models were appropriate (Table B, available as a supplement to the online version of this article at http://www.ajph.org).

Sensitivity Analyses

We calculated sex-specific AAFs for suicide, excluding data from California and Texas, where only a portion of violent deaths were reported to the NVDRS, and compared them with the AAFs calculated using the full sample to get a sense of whether their inclusion affected the estimates obtained. Additionally, to explore whether the varying state-specific percentage of decedents with BAC available had an impact on the estimated AAFs for suicide, we calculated sex-specific AAFs for (1) those states with 50% or more of suicide decedents with BAC available and (2) those states with fewer than 50% of suicide decedents with BAC available.

RESULTS

Data for a total of 21 993 suicide decedents (78.0% male and 22.0% female) were available for 2021 (Figure A, available as a supplement to the online version of this article at http://www.ajph.org). The percentage of suicide decedents with BAC available was not correlated with the percentage of decedents with a positive BAC (r = 0.013; 95% confidence interval [CI] = −0.263, 0.288; P = 0.928; Figure B, available as a supplement to the online version of this article at http://www.ajph.org). Overall, the AAF for suicide was 19.7% (males: 20.2%; females: 17.8%; $\chi^2 = 13.42$; df = 1; $P < .001$).

Decedents of an alcohol-attributable suicide had a mean BAC of 0.200 g/dL (SD = 0.076; range = 0.100–0.580; median = 0.186); BAC was 0.200 g/dL for both males (SD = 0.076; range = 0.100–0.580; median = 0.186) and females (SD = 0.076; range = 0.100–0.578; median = 0.188).

For those younger than 64 years of age, the AAF for suicide was higher among both males (15–34 years: 22.3%; 35–64 years: 23.8%) and females (15–34 years: 18.8%; 35–64 years: 19.9%) compared with those aged 65 years and older (males: 6.4%; females: 7.8%; Table 1). Among male suicide decedents, having an education level below that of a bachelor's degree was associated with higher odds of an alcohol-attributable suicide (for high school diploma or less, adjusted odds ratio [AOR] = 1.26; 95% CI = 1.12, 1.41; for some college but not a bachelor's degree, AOR = 1.27; 95% CI = 1.12, 1.44). Among female suicide decedents, an education level of some college but not a bachelor's degree was associated with higher odds of an alcohol-attributable suicide (AOR = 1.36; 95% CI = 1.11, 1.68). The odds of an alcohol-attributable suicide were lower among males who were never or not currently married (single or never married: AOR = 0.70; 95% CI = 0.63, 0.77; separated, widowed, or divorced: AOR = 0.84; 95% CI = 0.75, 0.93); among females, however, marital status was not significantly associated with dying from an alcohol-attributable suicide. Whereas males showed some differences in the odds of an alcohol-attributable suicide between race/ethnicity categories, females did not.

The AAF for suicide was higher for both males and females who used a firearm as the means of suicide (23.4% and 22.8%, respectively) compared with their counterparts who used other means (16.5% and 15.9%, respectively).

In contrast with the AAF for suicide when we included all states with available data, the AAF for suicide when we excluded California and Texas was 20.1% (males: 20.6%; females: 18.3%), a difference of 0.4 percentage points (males: 0.4 percentage points; females: 0.5 percentage points). The AAF for those states where 50% or more of suicide decedents had BAC data available was not statistically significantly different from the AAF for those states where fewer than 50% of suicide decedents had BAC data available (overall: $\chi^2 = 1.03$; df = 1; $P = .310$; males: $\chi^2 = 0.92$; df = 1; $P = .336$; females: $\chi^2 = 0.02$; df = 1; $P = .900$; Table C, available as a supplement to the online version of this article at http://www.ajph.org).

DISCUSSION

The AAF for suicide among males in 2021 was statistically significantly higher than among females, albeit only by about 2 percentage points. Interestingly, although males on average tend to consume alcohol more heavily than females,[3] the mean BAC among male and female decedents of an alcohol-attributable suicide was found to be equivalent. Overall, the directionality in the odds of dying from alcohol-attributable suicide within sociodemographic categories was largely consistent across the sexes, with the exception of marital status and race/ethnicity. Concerning firearm-involved suicides, there was near parity in the AAF across the sexes.

This study has limitations. First, although the NVDRS has greatly expanded its coverage since its inception in 2003, it does not include all suicide decedents in the United States.

TABLE 1— Alcohol-Attributable Fractions for Suicide and the Odds Ratio of Dying From an Alcohol-Attributable Suicide, by Sex: United States, 2021

	No.	AAF[a] (%)	OR[b] (95% CI)	AOR[c] (95% CI)
Males				
No.	17 156[d]	20.2		
Age, y				
15–34	6 260	22.3	4.10 (3.51, 4.80)	6.02 (5.04, 7.19)
35–64	7 629	23.8	4.40 (3.77, 5.13)	5.57 (4.74, 6.55)
≥ 65	2 861	6.4	1 (Ref)	1 (Ref)
Education level				
High school diploma or less	9 594	20.8	1.33 (1.20, 1.49)	1.26 (1.12, 1.41)
Some college, but no bachelor's degree	4 117	21.8	1.42 (1.26, 1.60)	1.27 (1.12, 1.44)
Bachelor's degree or higher	3 039	16.5	1 (Ref)	1 (Ref)
Race/ethnicity				
Non-Hispanic White	12 610	21.0	1 (Ref)	1 (Ref)
Non-Hispanic Black or African American	1 342	14.5	0.63 (0.55, 0.75)	0.54 (0.46, 0.64)
Hispanic	1 788	20.5	0.97 (0.86, 1.09)	0.91 (0.80, 1.04)
Non-Hispanic other races	1 010	18.2	0.84 (0.71, 0.99)	0.84 (0.71, 0.99)
Marital status				
Single/never married	7 727	20.1	0.87 (0.80, 0.95)	0.70 (0.63, 0.77)
Separated/widowed/divorced	3 758	18.1	0.77 (0.69, 0.84)	0.84 (0.75, 0.93)
Married/civil union/domestic partnership	5 265	22.4	1 (Ref)	1 (Ref)
Firearm involvement				
Yes	9 194	23.4	1.56 (1.45, 1.69)	1.76 (1.62, 1.90)
No	7 556	16.5	1 (Ref)	1 (Ref)
Females				
No.	4 837[e]	17.8		
Age, y				
15–34	1 590	18.8	2.80 (2.05, 3.82)	2.70 (1.97, 3.71)
35–64	2 487	19.9	2.95 (2.18, 3.99)	2.89 (2.13, 3.93)
≥ 65	640	7.8	1 (Ref)	1 (Ref)
Education level				
High school diploma or less	2 218	17.1	1.13 (0.93, 1.37)	1.09 (0.90, 1.33)
Some college, but no bachelor's degree	1 322	21.2	1.45 (1.18, 1.77)	1.36 (1.11, 1.68)
Bachelor's degree or higher	1 177	15.6	1 (Ref)	1 (Ref)
Race/ethnicity				
Non-Hispanic White	3 549	18.1	1 (Ref)	. . .
Non-Hispanic Black or African American	335	15.2	0.82 (0.61, 1.11)	. . .
Hispanic	428	20.3	1.12 (0.87, 1.43)	. . .
Non-Hispanic other races	405	15.6	0.82 (0.62, 1.08)	. . .
Marital status				
Single/never married	1 784	16.2	0.86 (0.71, 1.03)	. . .
Separated/widowed/divorced	1 492	19.1	1.05 (0.87, 1.26)	. . .
Married/civil union/domestic partnership	1 441	18.4	1 (Ref)	. . .

Continued

TABLE 1— Continued

	No.	AAF[a] (%)	OR[b] (95% CI)	AOR[c] (95% CI)
Firearm involvement				
Yes	1 342	22.8	1.58 (1.35, 1.85)	1.53 (1.31, 1.80)
No	3 375	15.9	1 (Ref)	1 (Ref)

Note. AAF = alcohol-attributable fraction; AOR = adjusted odds ratio; OR = odds ratio.
[a]Cases where the blood alcohol concentration was > 0.60 g/dL were excluded per the recommendation of the National Violent Death Reporting System.
[b]Produced using univariate logistic regression.
[c]Produced using multivariate logistic regression.
[d]A total of 16 750 male suicide decedents older than 15 years with data on blood alcohol concentration had complete sociodemographic data.
[e]A total of 4 717 female suicide decedents older than 15 years with data on blood alcohol concentration had complete sociodemographic data.

Second, as specified in the Methods section, BAC is available only for those suicide decedents who underwent a toxicology examination, and the rates vary across states as testing is dependent on local resources. Although the percentage of decedents with BAC available was not correlated with the percentage of decedents with a positive BAC—nor did the varying levels of BAC ascertainment appear to affect the AAFs calculated here—there are BAC measurement limitations to note. The different medicolegal death investigation systems across states result in variations in expertise and a lack of standardization not only across jurisdictions but also across coroners and medical examiners.[4] As discussed in detail elsewhere,[4] particularly noteworthy limitations of the NVDRS data are the lack of standardization for ascertaining substance use information, including alcohol use, and possible selection bias in that toxicological data are collected only from decedents for whom this information is important for the determination of the cause of death.

It should also be noted that, although the proportion of suicides for which excessive alcohol consumption occurred prior to the incident is referred to as "alcohol-attributable," it cannot be concluded that alcohol was the only causal factor. Suicide is a phenomenon that results from many multifaceted social and cultural factors, and its prevention requires multisectoral collaboration targeting health and social well-being in society.

Further, this study represents 1 method of estimating the AAF for injuries—the direct method. In contrast, the indirect method involves integrating the prevalence of alcohol use and the relative risk associated with it. Each method is not without its limitations. However, it has been previously reported that when the 2 methods are compared, the indirect method produced AAFs for injuries that were notably higher than those produced via the direct method.[5]

PUBLIC HEALTH SIGNIFICANCE

The need for a comprehensive suicide prevention strategy to include alcohol—an often overlooked risk factor[6]—is supported by the current finding that about 1 in every 5 suicides in the United States in 2021 was alcohol-attributable. AJPH

ABOUT THE AUTHORS

Julien Robitaille, Jürgen Rehm, Carolin Kilian, Laura Llamosas-Falcón, and Shannon Lange are with the Institute for Mental Health Policy Research, Centre for Addiction and Mental Health, Toronto, Ontario, Canada. Mark S. Kaplan is with the Luskin School of Public Affairs, University of California, Los Angeles.

CORRESPONDENCE

Correspondence should be sent to Shannon Lange, Centre for Addiction and Mental Health, 250 College St, Room 938, Toronto, Ontario, Canada M5T 1R8 (e-mail: Shannon.lange@camh.ca). Reprints can be ordered at https://www.ajph.org by clicking the "Reprints" link.

PUBLICATION INFORMATION

Full Citation: Robitaille J, Rehm J, Kaplan MS, Kilian C, Llamosas-Falcón L, Lange S. Direct estimation of alcohol-attributable fractions for suicide in the United States, 2021. *Am J Public Health*. 2025;115(3):364–368.

Acceptance Date: October 28, 2024.

DOI: https://doi.org/10.2105/AJPH.2024.307910

ORCID iDs:

Julien Robitaille https://orcid.org/0009-0009-2659-3864

Jürgen Rehm https://orcid.org/0000-0001-5665-0385

Laura Llamosas-Falcón https://orcid.org/0000-0003-4718-9376

Shannon Lange https://orcid.org/0000-0002-8067-8932

CONTRIBUTORS

J. Robitaille analyzed the data and contributed to drafting the manuscript. J. Rehm and M. S. Kaplan critically reviewed and commented on the article. C. Kilian and L. Llamosas-Falcón contributed to the methodology and revising the article. S. Lange led the conceptualization and design of the study, and contributed to the statistical analysis, interpretation of the data, and writing of the article. All authors read and approved the final manuscript.

CONFLICTS OF INTEREST

The authors have no conflicts of interest to disclose.

HUMAN PARTICIPANT PROTECTION

Approval for the current study was obtained from the Centre for Addiction and Mental Health, Research Ethics Board (REB#2024/004).

REFERENCES

1. GBD 2016 Alcohol Collaborators. Alcohol use and burden for 195 countries and territories, 1990–2016: a systematic analysis for the Global Burden of Disease Study 2016. *Lancet.* 2018; 392(10152):1015–1035. https://doi.org/10.1016/S0140-6736(18)31310-2
2. Centers for Disease Control and Prevention. Alcohol-related disease impact (ARDI) application. 2022. Available at: www.cdc.gov/ARDI. Accessed November 1, 2023.
3. White AM. Gender differences in the epidemiology of alcohol use and related harms in the United States. *Alcohol Res.* 2020;40(2):01. https://doi.org/10.35946/arcr.v40.2.01
4. Kaplan MS, Caetano R, Giesbrecht N, et al. The National Violent Death Reporting System: use of the restricted access database and recommendations for the system's improvement. *Am J Prev Med.* 2017;53(1):130–133. https://doi.org/10.1016/j.amepre.2017.01.043
5. Ye Y, Shield K, Cherpitel CJ, Manthey J, Korcha R, Rehm J. Estimating alcohol-attributable fractions for injuries based on data from emergency department and observational studies: a comparison of two methods. *Addiction.* 2019;114(3):462–470. https://doi.org/10.1111/add.14477
6. Marcotte DE, Hansen B. *The Re-Emerging Suicide Crisis in the US: Patterns, Causes and Solutions.* Cambridge, MA: National Bureau of Economic Research; 2023. NBER Working Paper No. 31242. https://doi.org/10.3386/w31242

Parental Factors Associated With Measles–Mumps–Rubella Vaccination in US Children Younger Than 5 Years

Eric Geng Zhou, PhD, Jonathan Cantor, PhD, Autumn Gertz, MS, Brian Elbel, PhD, MPH, John S. Brownstein, PhD, and Benjamin Rader, PhD, MPH

Objectives. To determine the association between parental characteristics and MMR (measles–mumps–rubella) vaccination status of children in the United States.

Methods. We conducted a cross-sectional study from July 2023 to April 2024 using a digital health survey via OutbreaksNearMe, weighted to target national population characteristics. We analyzed the responses of 19 892 parents of children younger than 5 years to examine the association between self-reported parental characteristics (i.e., sociodemographics, politics, COVID-19 vaccination status) and children's MMR vaccination rates using logistic regression.

Results. Children of parents who received at least 1 dose of the COVID-19 vaccine had higher MMR vaccination rates (80.8%) than did children of unvaccinated parents (60.9%; odds ratio [OR] = 1.84; 95% confidence interval [CI] = 1.68, 2.00). We observed lower MMR vaccination rates among children of parents who identified as Republican versus Democratic (OR = 0.73; 95% CI = 0.64, 0.82), parents on Medicaid or Medicare versus private insurance (OR = 0.85; 95% CI = 0.76, 0.95), and minority (OR = 0.44) versus White (OR = 0.71) parents. We found higher MMR vaccination rates in the Northeast and Midwest United States.

Conclusions. Early data indicate that parental sociodemographic characteristics and COVID-19 vaccine status are associated with children's MMR vaccine uptake, emphasizing the need for further investigations into multipronged public health interventions. (*Am J Public Health*. 2025;115(3):369–373. https://doi.org/10.2105/AJPH.2024.307912)

AJPH March 2025, Vol. 115, No. 3

Measles is a highly contagious disease that poses severe risks to pediatric health.[1] Despite the well-established safety and efficacy of the measles–mumps–rubella (MMR) vaccine,[2] long-standing vaccine hesitancy—exacerbated by the COVID-19 pandemic[3]—has led to a concerning decrease in overall immunization rates and notable recent increases in measles outbreaks,[4,5] which are linked to social clustering and international travel.[6]

Recent measles outbreaks disproportionately affected children, a population with significant sociodemographic disparities in pediatric vaccination rates.[7] However, data on MMR vaccine uptake for US children younger than 5 years—the first birth cohort influenced by the COVID-19 pandemic—remain limited. Understanding vaccine uptake in this age group is crucial for informing public health strategies and outbreak prevention, as pandemic-related hesitancy may extend to other pediatric vaccines. Given that MMR vaccination is required for children aged 5 years and older to attend school, variability in US MMR vaccination rates is likely concentrated in children younger than 5 years, subject to various state exemption rules. Current US MMR vaccine surveillance relies primarily on administrative data collected at kindergarten entry and the National Immunization Survey,[8] which uses nonanonymous telephone collection procedures that may leave gaps in measuring early childhood MMR vaccine rates.

In this study, we used a nationwide anonymous participatory surveillance system with minimal data collection delay to present data on MMR vaccine uptake among US children younger than 5 years. This study complements existing surveillance measures with a digital survey to assess the association between MMR vaccine uptake and parental characteristics. We aimed to identify factors associated with low MMR vaccination rates in children younger than 5 years to inform targeted interventions.

METHODS

We used OutbreaksNearMe, a large-scale digital health surveillance survey, to query the MMR vaccination status of children in the contiguous United States. OutbreaksNearMe uses nonprobability river sampling, drawing from SurveyMonkey's diverse multimillion-person daily user base. Between July 2023 and April 2024, randomly selected adult participants anonymously answered questions about demographics, politics, health, and whether they had children younger than 5 years (questionnaire appears in Appendix A, available as a supplement to the online version of this article at http://www.ajph.org). Participation required no incentives or accounts. Our analytic sample included all respondents with children younger than 5 years, and we weighted the sample using census demographic data to approximate the US population, a method validated by the Centers for Diseases Control and Prevention for measuring sensitive outcomes such as COVID-19 testing.[9,10]

The primary outcome was children's MMR vaccination (at least 1 dose vs none) as reported by their parents. Exposures included parent's self-reported age, sex, race/ethnicity, educational attainment, household income, geographical region, political party affiliation, health insurance source, COVID-19 vaccine status (≥ 1 dose vs none), and chronic health conditions (further details are provided in Appendix A).

We analyzed the relationship between parental characteristics and children's MMR vaccine uptake using summary statistics and multivariable logistic regression. We adjusted overall summary statistic MMR vaccine rates to reflect the proportion of children (older than 6 months) eligible for the vaccine. We conducted all analyses in R version 4.3.2 (RStudio, Boston, MA).

RESULTS

In this analysis of parent responses (n = 19 892), 71.8% (95% confidence interval [CI] = 70.4%, 73.2%) reported that their children received at least 1 dose of MMR vaccine. Children of COVID-19–vaccinated parents were more likely to be MMR vaccinated (80.8% vs 60.9%; Appendix B, Table A, available as a supplement to the online version of this article at http://www.ajph.org). Child MMR vaccine rates differed by respondent sex (75.0% vs 67.4%; female vs male parents) and race (81.2% vs 57.4%; White vs Black parents). Uninsured parents (58.3%) or those with Medicare or Medicaid (65.7%) reported lower uptake than did those with private or employer-provided insurance (80.3%). Parents identifying as Democrats reported higher vaccination rates (77.6%) than did those identifying as Independents (68%) or Republicans (72.1%). Vaccine uptake differed by US census divisions: New England, East North Central, and East South Central reported higher uptake than did other divisions (Appendix B, Figure A). Stark differences in demographic and geographic MMR vaccine uptake emerged when stratified by parental COVID-19 vaccination status.

Using multivariable logistic regression, we identified several factors associated with MMR vaccination (Figure 1). Compared with female respondents, males had lower odds (odds ratio [OR] = 0.69; 95% CI = 0.63, 0.75) of having a child younger than 5 years vaccinated for MMR. Racial/ethnic minority parents showed lower uptake than did White parents: Asian (OR = 0.63; 95% CI = 0.52, 0.78), Black (OR = 0.44; 95% CI = 0.39, 0.49), and Hispanic (OR = 0.50; 95% CI = 0.44, 0.57).

Higher education levels and yearly household income were associated with increased uptake: college degree (OR = 1.54; 95% CI = 1.40, 1.70) compared with high school or less and more than $100 000 versus less than $50 000 (OR = 1.21; 95% CI = 1.04, 1.40). Higher uptake was associated with parents vaccinated against COVID-19 (OR = 1.84; 95% CI = 1.68, 2.00) and without chronic conditions (OR = 1.18; 95% CI = 1.08, 1.29).

Parents with private or employer-provided insurance had higher uptake than did those with Medicare or Medicaid (OR = 0.84; 95% CI = 0.76, 0.94) or no insurance (OR = 0.78; 95% CI = 0.67, 0.90). Lastly, self-identifying Republicans (OR = 0.72; 95% CI = 0.64, 0.82) and Independents (OR = 0.79; 95% CI = 0.71, 0.88) had lower uptake than did self-identifying Democrats. By contrast, living in a county where the majority voted for Trump (vs Biden) in the 2020 presidential election did not influence uptake (OR = 0.92; 95% CI = 0.84, 1.01).

DISCUSSION

We present survey data on MMR vaccine uptake among the first birth

Variable		OR (95% CI)
Sex	Female	1 (Ref)
	Male	0.69 (0.63, 0.75)
Race/Ethnicity	White	1 (Ref)
	Asian	0.63 (0.52, 0.78)
	Black or African American	0.44 (0.39, 0.49)
	Hispanic	0.50 (0.44, 0.57)
	Other	0.71 (0.60, 0.85)
Education	High school or less	1 (Ref)
	Some college education	1.54 (1.40, 1.70)
	College degree	1.60 (1.40, 1.83)
	Postgraduate degree	1.82 (1.53, 2.16)
Household Income, $	< 50 000	1 (Ref)
	50 000–100 000	1.11 (0.99, 1.24)
	> 100 000	1.21 (1.04, 1.40)
Political Identification	Democrat	1 (Ref)
	Republican	0.72 (0.64, 0.82)
	Independent	0.79 (0.71, 0.88)
County-Level Presidential Vote in 2020	Democrat	1 (Ref)
	Republican	0.92 (0.84, 1.01)
COVID-19 Vaccine Status	Not vaccinated	1 (Ref)
	Vaccinated	1.84 (1.68, 2.00)
Chronic Conditions	Has chronic condition(s)	1 (Ref)
	None	1.18 (1.08, 1.29)
Type of Health Insurance	Private or employer-provided	1 (Ref)
	Medicaid or Medicare	0.84 (0.76, 0.94)
	Uninsured	0.78 (0.67, 0.90)
Region	Midwest	1 (Ref)
	Northeast	0.98 (0.85, 1.14)
	South	0.88 (0.79, 0.98)
	West	0.90 (0.79, 1.03)

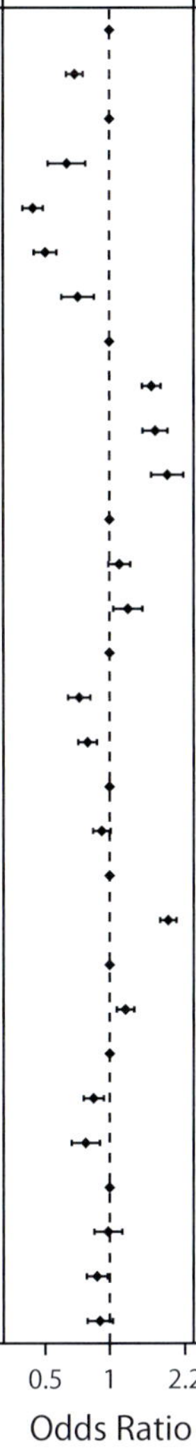

FIGURE 1— Multivariable Logistic Regression Analysis of Parental Characteristics on Reported Uptake of at Least 1 Dose of the MMR Vaccine for Children Younger Than 5 Years: United States, July 2023–April 2024

Note. CI = confidence interval; MMR = measles–mumps–rubella; OR = odds ratio. The sample comprised all respondents with children younger than 5 years who completed the OutbreaksNearMe survey between July 2023 and April 2024, excluding those in Alaska, where election outcomes were not reported at the county level. We adjusted our analysis by using survey weights to ensure that it represents the larger population. The results are shown as ORs, with error estimates that account for differences in data variability.

cohort of children since the onset of the COVID-19 pandemic. Our findings indicate that parental sociodemographics, political beliefs, and COVID-19 vaccination are associated with differences in reported MMR vaccine uptake, highlighting potential disparities in measles risk in the sampled population.

Nonvaccination is a complex issue shaped by personal beliefs, health care access, and pandemic-related delays.[11] Although misinformation[2] has historically driven MMR nonvaccination, we did not examine nonvaccination reasoning. However, our findings indicate that factors associated with health disparities[12] and pediatric nonvaccination[9,13] (e.g., socioeconomic disadvantages) remain influential. Additionally, the strong association between parental COVID-19 vaccination and MMR vaccination introduces further complexity into vaccination efforts, as COVID-19–related factors may affect the uptake of routine childhood vaccines.

Self-reported political beliefs were associated with children's MMR vaccination, whereas county-level preferences were not, underscoring the importance of individual-level data. Future research should focus on geographically detailed data to better identify areas at higher risk for outbreaks owing to clusters of unvaccinated children.[14] The overall reported MMR vaccination rates for children aged 6 months through 5 years are lower than are those reported for kindergarteners,[8] which may reflect immunization delay rather than refusal.

Limitations

Although overall vaccination rates fell below the 95% threshold for herd immunity,[15] these results should be interpreted cautiously because of the data limitations and because MMR vaccination is not indicated for most children until aged 12 months. Self-reported responses may be prone to recall and social desirability bias, and the generalizability of the results depends on the validity of the weighting procedures. These limitations may also explain differences in reported rates[16] by respondent sex. Additionally, because we did not collect the exact ages of the children and because parents might report a single vaccination status for all children younger than 5 years, the overall uptake may be underestimated if the youngest child's status was reported. However, the potential bias is unlikely to vary across demographic groups, so the relative differences in MMR vaccine rates should hold.

Public Health Implications

Decreases in MMR vaccine uptake are a growing public health challenge. Our data suggest that socioeconomic disparities are associated with MMR vaccination and that the influence of COVID-19 vaccine hesitancy may present an additional challenge. Tailored interventions, such as community outreach in areas with lower vaccine uptake, guided by further research, remain actionable and effective ways to promote uptake and reduce delays.[17,18] Recognizing the influence of COVID-19 on pediatric MMR vaccine uptake is crucial for assessing and managing risks of measles outbreak in the postpandemic era. AJPH

ABOUT THE AUTHORS

Eric Geng Zhou is with the Center for Child Health Services Research, Icahn School of Medicine at Mount Sinai, New York, NY. Jonathan Cantor is with RAND, Santa Monica, CA. Autumn Gertz, John S. Brownstein, and Benjamin Rader are with Innovation and Digital Health Accelerator, Boston Children's Hospital, Boston, MA. Brian Elbel is with the Department of Population Health, Grossman School of Medicine, New York University, New York.

CORRESPONDENCE

Correspondence should be sent to Benjamin Rader, PhD, MPH, 401 Park Dr, 7th Floor West, Boston, MA 02215 (e-mail: benjamin.rader@childrens.harvard.edu). Reprints can be ordered at https://www.ajph.org by clicking the "Reprints" link.

PUBLICATION INFORMATION

Full Citation: Zhou EG, Cantor J, Gertz A, Elbel B, Brownstein JS, Rader B. Parental factors associated with measles-mumps-rubella vaccination in US children younger than 5 years. *Am J Public Health*. 2025;115(3):369–373.

Acceptance Date: October 28, 2024.

DOI: https://doi.org/10.2105/AJPH.2024.307912

ORCID iDs:

Eric Geng Zhou https://orcid.org/0000-0003-2423-2204

Jonathan Cantor https://orcid.org/0000-0003-4468-833X

Autumn Gertz https://orcid.org/0000-0002-1642-8912

Benjamin Rader https://orcid.org/0000-0002-6095-0193

CONTRIBUTORS

E. G. Zhou performed the statistical analyses. E. G. Zhou, A. Gertz, J. S. Brownstein, and B. Rader acquired, analyzed, and interpreted the data. E. G. Zhou and B. Rader drafted the article; they had full access to the study data and take responsibility for the data integrity and the accuracy of the data analysis. A. Gertz provided administrative, technical, and material support. J. S. Brownstein and B. Rader supervised the study. All authors conceptualized and designed the study and critically revised the article for important intellectual content.

ACKNOWLEDGMENTS

B. Rader received funding from the Thrasher Research Fund (Boston Children's Hospital grant FP00000397). E. Geng Zhou and B. Elbel received funding from the National Institute of Nursing Research of the National Institutes of Health (U01NR020443).

The authors thank Juliana Sopko (Boston Children's Hospital) for her assistance.

Note. The funders had no role in the design and conduct of the study; collection, management, analysis, and interpretation of the data; preparation, review, or approval of the article; or decision to submit the article for publication.

CONFLICTS OF INTEREST

The authors have no conflicts of interest to report.

HUMAN PARTICIPANT PROTECTION

This study was approved by the Boston Children's Hospital institutional review board (IRB-P00023700) and received a waiver of informed consent.

REFERENCES

1. Moss WJ. Measles. *Lancet*. 2017;390(10111):2490–2502. https://doi.org/10.1016/S0140-6736(17)31463-0
2. DeStefano F, Shimabukuro TT. The MMR vaccine and autism. *Annu Rev Virol*. 2019;6:585–600. https://doi.org/10.1146/annurev-virology-092818-015515
3. DeSilva MB, Haapala J, Vazquez-Benitez G, et al. Association of the COVID-19 pandemic with routine childhood vaccination rates and proportion up to date with vaccinations across 8 US health systems in the vaccine safety datalink. *JAMA Pediatr*. 2022;176(1):68–77. https://doi.org/10.1001/jamapediatrics.2021.4251
4. Phadke VK, Bednarczyk RA, Omer SB. Vaccine refusal and measles outbreaks in the US. *JAMA*. 2020;324(13):1344–1345. https://doi.org/10.1001/jama.2020.14828
5. Centers for Disease Control and Prevention. Measles—United States, January 1, 2020–March 28, 2024. *MMWR Morb Mortal Wkly Rep*. 2024;73(14):295–300. https://doi.org/10.15585/mmwr.mm7314a1
6. Sarkar S, Zlojutro A, Khan K, Gardner L. Measles resurgence in the USA: how international travel compounds vaccine resistance. *Lancet Infect Dis*. 2019;19(7):684–686. https://doi.org/10.1016/S1473-3099(19)30231-2
7. Kempe A, Saville AW, Albertin C, et al. Parental hesitancy about routine childhood and influenza vaccinations: a national survey. *Pediatrics*. 2020;146(1):e20193852. https://doi.org/10.1542/peds.2019-3852
8. Centers for Disease Control and Prevention. Coverage with selected vaccines and exemption from school vaccine requirements among children in kindergarten—United States, 2022–23 school year. *MMWR Morb Mortal Wkly Rep*. 2023;72(45):1217–1224. https://doi.org/10.15585/mmwr.mm7245a2

9. Rader B, Chiang ME, Kriner DL, Weintraub RL, Brownstein JS. Persistent drop in confidence following US recommended pause of Ad26.COV$_2$.S vaccine administration. *Vaccine*. 2023;41(1):5–9. https://doi.org/10.1016/j.vaccine.2022.11.035
10. Centers for Disease Control and Prevention. Use of at-home COVID-19 tests—United States, August 23, 2021–March 12, 2022. *MMWR Morb Mortal Wkly Rep*. 2022;71(13):489–494. https://doi.org/10.15585/mmwr.mm7113e1
11. Health Resources and Services Administration. Impacts of the COVID-19 pandemic, 2021. October 2022. Available at: https://www.ncbi.nlm.nih.gov/books/NBK603013. Accessed October 1, 2022.
12. Braveman PA, Cubbin C, Egerter S, Williams DR, Pamuk E. Socioeconomic disparities in health in the United States: what the patterns tell us. *Am J Public Health*. 2010;100(suppl 1):S186–S196. https://doi.org/10.2105/AJPH.2009.166082
13. Sehgal NKR, Rader B, Gertz A, Astley CM, Brownstein JS. Parental compliance and reasons for COVID-19 vaccination among American children. *PLOS Digit Health*. 2023;2(4):e0000147. https://doi.org/10.1371/journal.pdig.0000147
14. Gastañaduy PA, Funk S, Lopman BA, et al. Factors associated with measles transmission in the United States during the postelimination era. *JAMA Pediatr*. 2020;174(1):56–62. https://doi.org/10.1001/jamapediatrics.2019.4357
15. Centers for Disease Control and Prevention. Measles cases and outbreaks. Available at: https://www.cdc.gov/measles/data-research/index.html. Accessed June 1, 2024.
16. Waters E, Doyle J, Wolfe R, Wright M, Wake M, Salmon L. Influence of parental gender and self-reported health and illness on parent-reported child health. *Pediatrics*. 2000;106(6):1422–1428. https://doi.org/10.1542/peds.106.6.1422
17. Sadaf A, Richards JL, Glanz J, Salmon DA, Omer SB. A systematic review of interventions for reducing parental vaccine refusal and vaccine hesitancy. *Vaccine*. 2013;31(40):4293–4304. https://doi.org/10.1016/j.vaccine.2013.07.013
18. Hendrix KS, Finnell SME, Zimet GD, Sturm LA, Lane KA, Downs SM. Vaccine message framing and parents' intent to immunize their infants for MMR. *Pediatrics*. 2014;134(3):e675–e683. https://doi.org/10.1542/peds.2013-4077

Research Funded by National Institutes of Health Concerning Sexual and Gender Minoritized Populations: A Tracking Update for 2012 to 2022

Ben C. D. Weideman, MS, Alexandra M. Ecklund, MPH, Rhea Alley, MPH, B. R. Simon Rosser, PhD, MPH, and G. Nic Rider, PhD

See also Friedman, p. 255.

Objectives. To investigate trends in awards funded by the National Institutes of Health (NIH) focusing on sexual and gender minoritized (SGM) populations from 2012 to 2022 in the United States.

Methods. Replicating the method of Coulter et al., we identified NIH-funded awards for SGM research from 2012 to 2022 using the NIH RePORTER (Research Portfolio Online Reporting Tools Expenditures and Results) system. We coded for SGM subpopulations, demographics, and health content areas. We also inflation adjusted awards to 2022 dollar values.

Results. NIH funded 1093 unique awards concerning SGM health, which totaled $491.7 million in first-year funding and made up 0.8% of the NIH portfolio. Frequency of awards nearly tripled over our study period. Most awards focused on HIV/AIDS (65.5%), mental health (29.5%), illicit drug use (19.9%), or sexual health issues (17.0%). We found funding differences across subpopulations: sexually minoritized men (67.8%; $357.9 million), transgender women (18.1%; $77.6 million), sexually minoritized women (13.9%; $57.6 million), transgender men (8.2%; $37.6 million), and nonbinary people (4.4%; $17.6 million). Only 42.2% of awards explicitly examined racial/ethnic identities of participants.

Conclusions. Although NIH funding for SGM-related research has increased, persistent inequities indicate the need for systemic changes to advance health equity. (*Am J Public Health*. 2025;115(3):374–386. https://doi.org/10.2105/AJPH.2024.307913)

AJPH March 2025, Vol. 115, No. 3

Over the past decade, the National Institutes of Health (NIH) strengthened its research infrastructure to advance the health of sexual and gender minoritized (SGM) communities. In 2011, an Institute of Medicine (now National Academy of Medicine) report, commissioned by NIH, brought to national attention evidence of stark SGM health disparities (e.g., suicidality, violence, barriers to care) and the need for more research.[1] In 2015, NIH established the Sexual and Gender Minority Research Office.[2] In 2016, NIH formally designated SGM individuals as a health disparity population.[2] In 2019, NIH contracted the National Academies of Sciences, Engineering, and Medicine to provide an update on the state of SGM research.[3] The report highlighted how scientific advancements have increased our knowledge and awareness of health inequities across SGM subgroups and emphasized the need for more work and funding to achieve health equity. NIH afterward put forth a strategic plan to advance SGM health research for 2021 through 2025 that included a commitment to increase grant support.[4] The plan also raised key considerations: priority for underresearched SGM subgroups, focus on aging, and need for intersectionality in study design.

SGM communities are diverse, and sociostructural power dynamics significantly affect their lives and well-being, particularly in regard to resource allocations. Consequently, taking intersectionality into account is crucial for research on SGM populations and public health more broadly.[5,6] Intersectionality is a critical framework rooted in Black feminism that interrogates how systems of power and interlocking structural inequalities affect the lives of people based on their multiple social positions.[6–10] Thus, to achieve SGM health equity, we must contend with the confluence of oppressive systems (e.g., cisheterosexism, racism, sexism, classism) that direct resources to advantaged groups and produce disparate health outcomes among marginalized groups. Both NIH-commissioned reports and the NIH strategic plan promote intersectionality as foundational to SGM research.[1,3,4]

NIH is the largest medical and public health research funder in the world.[11] NIH wields immense power in its mission to enhance health and reduce illness across all populations in the United States, including SGM people. Our objective was to use an intersectionality lens to investigate trends in NIH funding for SGM population research.

More than a decade ago, Coulter et al. collected LGBT (lesbian, gay, bisexual, or transgender)-related abstracts from the NIH Research Portfolio Online Reporting Tools Expenditures and Results (RePORTER) system. Their key finding was that only 0.5% of all NIH funding awards from 1989 to 2011 focused on SGM populations.[12] Most of those awards were for research on cisgender, sexually minoritized men (86.1%), with much less research involving cisgender, sexually minoritized women (13.5%) or transgender people (6.8%). HIV/AIDS was the most commonly funded area (79.1%), followed by illicit drug use (30.9%) and mental health (23.2%). Relatively few abstracts mentioned race or ethnicity (31.4%) or people younger than 18 years (9.7%) or 50 years or older (0.3%). Coulter et al. argued that the lack of SGM research funding before 2011 perpetuated health inequities, including funding that would support sufficient research at the intersections of race/ethnicity and age. Since 2011, the proportion of US adults who report SGM identities has more than doubled (3.2% in 2012 to 7.6% in 2024), largely driven by increases in bisexual women and transgender or nonbinary people in the youngest generations.[13–15]

Altogether, the size and rapid growth of SGM communities, the persistence of SGM health inequities and research gaps, and the improvements in SGM research infrastructure since 2011 indicate a need for updated estimates of NIH funding for SGM-focused studies. Therefore, we replicated the evaluation of Coulter et al. of NIH awards for SGM research from 2012 to 2022. We also have made novel additions: we included transgender and gender-diverse subgroups (i.e., transgender men, transgender women, and nonbinary people), report explicit mentions of racialized identities (e.g., Asian, Black), describe new health content areas (e.g., intersectionality), and analyzed inflation-adjusted funding for all awards.

METHODS

We replicated the method of Coulter et al.[12] using NIH RePORTER[16] to collect abstracts of research that received an NIH award. We collected 4 award types (research project grants, research career awards, fellowships, and training grants) with a project start date between January 1, 2012, and December 31, 2022. By limiting the search to project numbers ending in -01 and new awards, we identified 142 280 unique awards. We then conducted an advanced text search using the same keywords as Coulter et al. with the following additions[12]: "agender," "asexual," "cisgender," "genderqueer," "intersex," "nonbinary," "same gender loving," "transfeminine," "transmasculine," "transphobia," "Two-Spirit," and "queer." This yielded 1653 abstracts potentially related to SGM health.

Data Coding

We classified an award as related to SGM health if the research abstract in NIH RePORTER explicitly indicated that the research examined outcomes by sexual orientation or gender modality (i.e., relation between gender identity and sex assigned at birth)[17] or if the abstract explicitly mentioned at least 1 SGM subpopulation. We coded abstracts by the specific SGM population or populations mentioned. We excluded awards without an SGM focus from subsequent coding and analyses. We coded abstracts that stated outcomes were also examined by race or ethnicity, following Coulter et al.,[12] and we noted specific racial/ethnic subgroups that were explicitly mentioned in the abstract. We coded abstracts that explicitly included people aged 50 years or older or younger than 18 years, as well as those examining populations outside the United States.

Next, we classified the health focus or foci for each abstract and whether the award was for an intervention, directed by the categories used by Coulter et al.[12] We added codes for transphobia, racism, COVID-19, gender-affirming care, and neurologic disorders. We also coded research that explicitly mentioned applying an intersectionality lens or structural systems of oppression. A codebook with definitions is included as Appendix A (available as a supplement to the online version of this article at http://www.ajph.org).

Each of the 1653 abstracts was coded by 1 of 4 authors (B. C. D. W., A. M. E., R. A., G. N. R.), with any coding uncertainties addressed collaboratively. To assess interrater reliability, this group randomly selected 80 (4.8%) abstracts, and an author who did not code it initially recoded each abstract. Coders agreed on 96.9% of codes and reached consensus on all disagreements.

We validated our intersectionality findings as we advanced the method of Coulter et al. First, we randomly sampled half of 2014 SGM-related awards and evaluated the proportion of NIH RePORTER-linked articles published within 7 years meeting our intersectionality criteria. Second, we searched NIH RePORTER to determine the proportion of non-SGM awards during the study period that mentioned intersectionality in the abstract.

Data Analysis

We assessed the proportion of NIH awards related to SGM health and funding across various sample characteristics (Table 1). Funding represented total cost in the first year of the award, inflation adjusted to 2022 values using the Biomedical Research and Development Price Index.[18] We also explored changes in NIH awards for SGM health research over time (Figure 1); content areas, including HIV/AIDS studies by SGM subpopulations (Table 2); and content areas, excluding HIV/AIDS studies by subpopulations (Table 3).

RESULTS

From 2012 to 2022, NIH issued 142 280 unique awards totaling $60.1 billion. Of these, 1093 (~0.8%) awards were for research focused on SGM health, at a cost of $491.7 million (~0.8% of awarded dollars). The 1093 awards were composed of multiple grant mechanisms: research grants (76.9%), career awards (14.0%), fellowships (8.7%), and training grants (0.3%). Based on the NIH RePORTER abstracts, the SGM studies receiving most of the awards focused on HIV/AIDS (716 awards; 65.5%; $339.8 million), and many were interventions (436 awards; 39.9%; $219.2 million). Excluding HIV/AIDS awards, 377 abstracts focused on SGM health (0.3% of all NIH awards for research in the period), with funding totaling $151.9 million. Of these awards, 75 (19.9%) were interventions, with funding totaling $36.2 million.

Subpopulations

Of the 1093 SGM-related awards (including those involving HIV/AIDS), 741 (67.8%; $357.9 million) abstracts indicated the research focused on sexually minoritized men, and 152 (13.9%; $57.6 million) focused on sexually minoritized women. Among all awards for SGM research, 606 (55.4%) abstracts explicitly indicated that the studies included men who have sex with men, 151 (13.8%) included gay men, 142 (13.0%) included bisexual men, 93 (8.5%) included lesbian women, 86 (7.9%) included bisexual women, 5 (0.5%) included women who have sex with women, 1 included asexual women, and none included asexual men. Awards for SGM research including transgender gender modality numbered 298 (27.3%; $124.2 million). A total of 198 (18.1%; $77.6 million) awards explicitly mentioned transgender women, 90 (8.2%; $37.6 million) mentioned transgender men, and 48 (4.4%; $17.6 million) mentioned nonbinary people in their NIH RePORTER abstracts. Only 9 (0.8%; $4.5 million) awards mentioned intersex people, and zero explicitly mentioned including Two-Spirit people.

Among the 377 non-HIV/AIDS–related awards, 149 (39.5%; $62.7 million) abstracts of awards for SGM research focused on sexually minoritized men and 130 (34.5%; $43.7 million) focused on sexually minoritized women. Awards for SGM research that included transgender gender modality numbered 144 (38.2%; $58.6 million); 69 (18.3%; $25.2 million) abstracts explicitly mentioned transgender women, 66 (17.5%; $25.3 million) mentioned transgender men, and 42 (11.1%; $16.1 million) mentioned nonbinary people. Awards for SGM research often involved more than 1 SGM subgroup in their NIH RePORTER abstract, which is undifferentiated in Table 1, so we provide additional detail in Appendix B (available as a supplement to the online version of this article at http://www.ajph.org).

Racial/ethnic identity was explicitly noted in 461 (42.2%; $228.9 million) of the 1093 NIH awards for SGM health research, including those related to HIV/AIDS. Racialized subgroups were explicitly mentioned in abstracts at the following frequencies: Black (223; 20.4%; $107.9 million), Hispanic or Latino/a/x/e (108; 9.9%; $60.8 million), White (25; 2.3%; $11.5 million), Asian (14; 1.3%; $5.4 million), American Indian/Alaska Native (3; 0.3%; $8.3 million), and

TABLE 1— NIH-Funded Awards for Research on the Health of SGM Populations: United States, 2012–2022

Content Area/Subpopulation	NIH-Funded SGM Health-Related Awards, No. (%), $ in Millions	
	Total Awards for Studies Including HIV/AIDS (n = 1093, $ = 491.7 million)	Awards for Studies Excluding HIV/AIDS (n = 377, $ = 151.9 million)
SGM health-related studies		
Total	1093 (100), 491.7	377 (100), 151.9
Studies focusing on HIV/AIDS	716 (65.5), 339.8	. . .
Studies focusing on topics other than HIV/AIDS	377 (34.5), 151.9	. . .
SGM health-related intervention studies		
Total	436 (39.9), 219.2	75 (19.9), 36.2
Studies focusing on HIV/AIDS	361 (33.0), 182.8	. . .
Studies focusing on topics other than HIV/AIDS	75 (6.9), 36.4	. . .
Studies involving sexually minoritized women[a]		
Total	152 (13.9), 57.6	130 (34.5), 43.7
Involving lesbian women	93 (8.5), 35.2	86 (22.8), 28.7
Involving bisexual women	86 (7.9), 31.9	79 (21.0), 25.4
Involving women who have sex with women	5 (0.5), 1.4	4 (1.1), 0.7
Involving asexual women	1 (0.1), 0.1	1 (0.3), 0.1
Studies involving sexually minoritized men[a]		
Total	741 (67.8), 357.9	149 (39.5), 62.7
Involving gay men	151 (13.8), 65.7	77 (20.4), 27.8
Involving bisexual men	142 (13.0), 62.3	68 (18.0), 25.5
Involving men who have sex with men	606 (55.4), 302.3	49 (13.0), 25.9
Involving asexual men	0 (0), 0	0 (0), 0
Studies involving transgender people[b]		
Total	298 (27.3), 124.2	144 (38.2), 58.6
Involving transgender women	198 (18.1), 77.6	69 (18.3), 25.2
Involving transgender men	90 (8.2), 37.6	66 (17.5), 25.3
Involving nonbinary people	48 (4.4), 17.6	42 (11.1), 16.1
Studies involving Two-Spirit people, total	0 (0), 0	0 (0), 0
Studies involving intersex people, total	9 (0.8), 4.5	9 (2.4), 4.5
Studies involving children or older adults		
Involving people aged < 18 y	207 (18.9), 110.5	94 (24.9), 35.9
Involving people aged ≥ 50 y	36 (3.3), 17.5	22 (5.8), 11.0
Studies examining racial/ethnic identity		
Total	461 (42.2), 228.9	154 (40.8), 63.9
Involving American Indian/Alaska Native people	3 (0.3), 8.3	1 (0.3), 0.7
Involving Asian people	14 (1.3), 5.4	7 (1.9), 2.1
Involving Black people	223 (20.4), 107.9	37 (9.8), 15.7
Involving Hispanic or Latino/a/x/e people	108 (9.9), 60.8	24 (6.4), 8.1
Involving Native Hawaiian/Pacific Islander people	3 (0.3), 2.6	0 (0), 0
Involving White people	25 (2.3), 11.5	8 (2.1), 1.8
Studies involving populations outside the United States, total	157 (14.4), 54.9	16 (4.2), 6.7

Note. NIH = National Institutes of Health; SGM = sexual and gender minoritized. Some awards involved ≥ 1 subpopulations so numbers may not sum to 100%. All dollar amounts are inflation adjusted using the Biomedical Research and Development Price Index to represent purchasing power in 2022.
[a]Awards involving sexually minoritized people did not necessarily specify gender modality.
[b]Awards involving gender minoritized people included diverse sexual orientations.

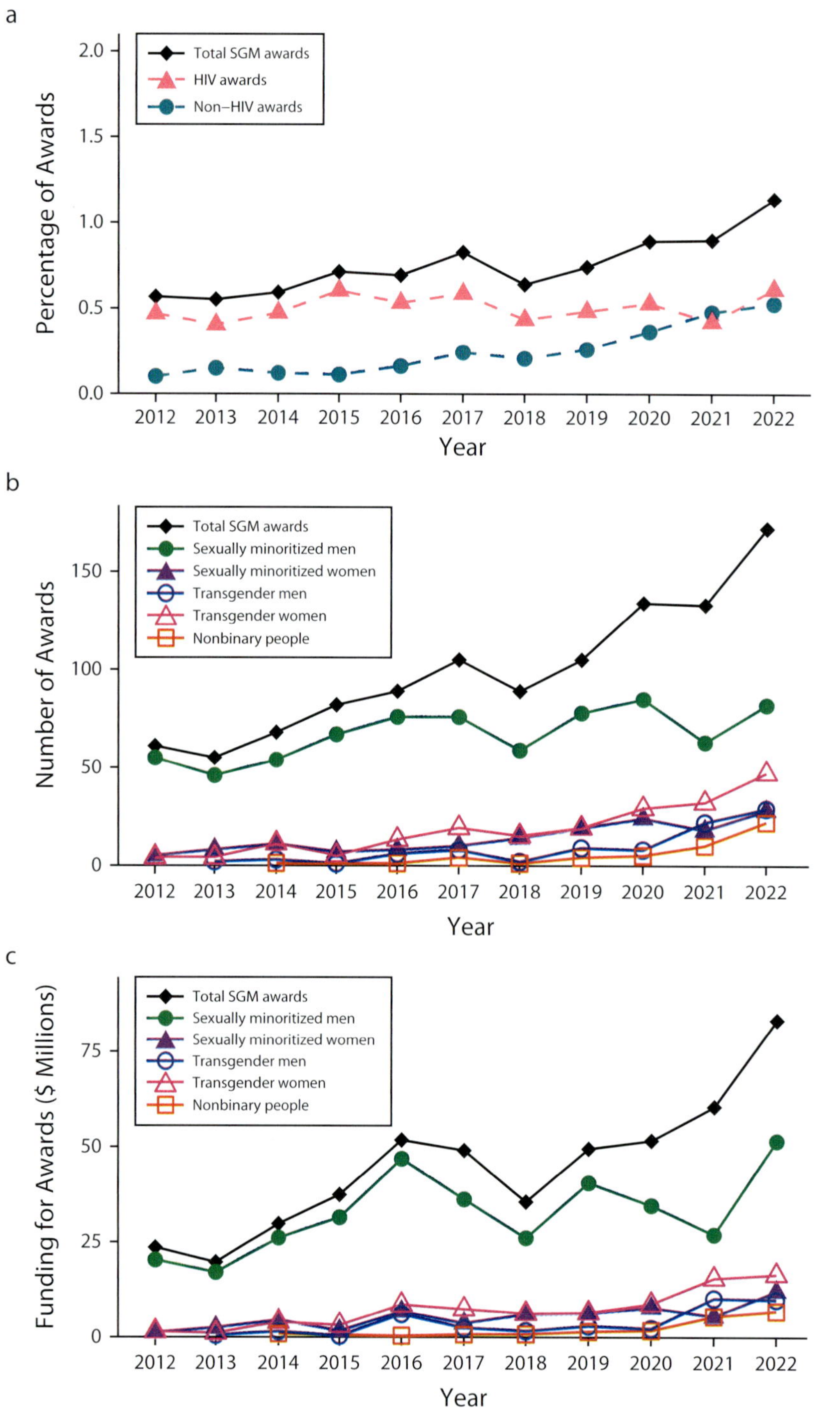

FIGURE 1— **National Institutes of Health–Funded Awards to Research Involving SGM Populations by (a) Percentage, (b) Number, and (c) Funding: United States, 2012–2022**

Note. SGM = sexual and gender minoritized.

TABLE 2— National Institutes of Health–Funded Awards for Research Concerning the Health of SGM Populations Including HIV/AIDS, by Content Area: United States, 2012–2022

	All Awards for Research on SGM Health, Including HIV/AIDS, No. (%), $ in Millions					
Content Area	Total Awards (n = 1093, $ = 491.7 million)	Awards for Research Involving Sexually Minoritized Women (n = 152, $ = 57.6 million)	Awards for Research Involving Sexually Minoritized Men (n = 741, $ = 357.9 million)	Awards for Research Involving Transgender Women (n = 198, $ = 77.6 million)	Awards for Research Involving Transgender Men (n = 90, $ = 37.6 million)	Awards for Research Involving Nonbinary People (n = 48, $ = 17.6 million)
Alcohol use	132 (12.1), 47.1	37 (24.3), 11.8	84 (11.3), 34.1	18 (9.1), 6.5	9 (10.0), 2.5	4 (8.3), 0.8
Cancer	46 (4.2), 19.3	8 (5.3), 1.9	29 (3.9), 15.0	7 (3.5), 2.2	6 (6.7), 1.9	6 (12.5), 2.1
Cardiovascular	32 (2.9), 21.2	3 (2.0), 2.0	13 (1.8), 13.3	12 (6.1), 4.9	6 (6.7), 2.8	3 (6.2), 1.0
Cost-effectiveness and other health financing	39 (3.6), 20.8	0 (0), 0	24 (3.2), 14.7	6 (3.0), 1.2	3 (3.3), 0.8	3 (6.2), 0.8
Couple and family health	61 (5.6), 25.4	23 (15.1), 5.4	48 (6.5), 21.3	4 (2.0), 1.4	2 (2.2), 0.6	1 (2.1), 0.3
COVID-19	15 (1.4), 6.9	5 (3.3), 3.5	8 (1.1), 4.1	1 (0.5), 0.2	1 (1.1), 0.2	1 (2.1), 0.2
Dental/oral health	1 (0.1), 0.7	0 (0), 0	1 (0.1), 0.7	0 (0), 0	0 (0), 0	0 (0), 0
Environmental health	39 (3.6), 24.3	6 (3.9), 8.8	30 (4.0), 22.0	2 (1.0), 5.2	1 (1.1), 4.5	1 (2.1), 0.7
Ethical issues	12 (1.1), 4.2	1 (0.7), 0.6	7 (0.9), 3.2	4 (2.0), 2.0	3 (3.3), 1.1	2 (4.2), 0.5
Exercise	2 (0.2), 0.4	0 (0), 0	1 (0.1), 0.2	1 (0.5), 0.2	0 (0), 0	0 (0), 0
Gender-affirming care	138 (12.6), 53.8	10 (6.6), 8.5	15 (2.0), 10.6	103 (52.0), 41.4	56 (62.2), 25.2	27 (56.2), 10.7
Genetics	49 (4.5), 19.9	3 (2.0), 1.0	32 (4.3), 12.6	14 (7.1), 7.5	8 (8.9), 3.7	3 (6.2), 1.4
Health policy	28 (2.6), 10.6	10 (6.6), 3.7	19 (2.6), 9.0	5 (2.5), 1.7	3 (3.3), 0.7	2 (4.2), 0.7
Health services	205 (18.8), 92.5	32 (21.1), 19.8	127 (17.1), 67.5	53 (26.8), 19.4	24 (26.7), 11.6	13 (27.1), 3.4
Hepatitis	5 (0.5), 2.4	0 (0), 0	5 (0.7), 2.4	1 (0.5), 0.5	0 (0), 0	0 (0), 0
HIV/AIDS	716 (65.5), 339.8	22 (14.5), 13.8	592 (79.9), 295.5	129 (65.2), 52.4	24 (26.7), 12.3	6 (12.5), 1.5
Homelessness	6 (0.5), 6.8	2 (1.3), 5.2	3 (0.4), 5.9	2 (1.0), 4.8	1 (1.1), 4.5	0 (0), 0
Homophobia	181 (16.6), 80.1	61 (40.1), 24.7	136 (18.4), 62.3	24 (12.1), 9.8	10 (11.1), 4.5	5 (10.4), 1.2
Illicit drug use	218 (19.9), 105.6	23 (15.1), 8.9	164 (22.1), 88.9	34 (17.2), 11.5	14 (15.6), 4.8	5 (10.4), 1.5
Immigration	8 (0.7), 3.0	1 (0.7), 0.5	4 (0.5), 1.0	1 (0.5), 0.4	0 (0), 0	0 (0), 0
Infrastructure for researchers of SGM health	187 (17.1), 120.1	30 (19.7), 18.5	118 (15.9), 82.7	41 (20.7), 20.3	21 (23.3), 11.5	10 (20.8), 3.0
Intersectionality	94 (8.6), 37.5	16 (10.5), 7.1	57 (7.7), 23.7	24 (12.6), 7.9	12 (13.3), 3.7	10 (20.8), 3.0
Intervention	436 (39.9), 219.2	30 (19.7), 19.4	332 (44.8), 176.6	81 (40.9), 36.4	16 (17.8), 13.9	9 (18.8), 6.0
Measurement validation or testing of sampling methods	126 (11.5), 46.9	19 (12.5), 6.3	66 (8.9), 25.0	26 (13.1), 7.9	19 (21.1), 5.5	11 (22.9), 3.1
Mental health	322 (29.5), 134.3	85 (55.9), 31.6	183 (24.7), 79.4	63 (31.8), 24.9	37 (41.1), 16.3	19 (39.6), 9.0
Neurologic disorders	23 (2.1), 17.3	6 (3.9), 3.7	14 (1.9), 8.9	2 (1.0), 0.6	2 (2.2), 0.6	2 (4.2), 0.6
Nutrition, food, and dietary habits	6 (0.5), 1.7	4 (2.6), 0.8	4 (0.5), 1.4	0 (0), 0	0 (0), 0	0 (0), 0

Continued

TABLE 2— Continued

Content Area	Total Awards (n = 1093, $ = 491.7 million)	All Awards for Research on SGM Health, Including HIV/AIDS, No. (%), $ in Millions: Awards for Research Involving Sexually Minoritized Women (n = 152, $ = 57.6 million)	Awards for Research Involving Sexually Minoritized Men (n = 741, $ = 357.9 million)	Awards for Research Involving Transgender Women (n = 198, $ = 77.6 million)	Awards for Research Involving Transgender Men (n = 90, $ = 37.6 million)	Awards for Research Involving Nonbinary People (n = 48, $ = 17.6 million)
Sexual health, excluding HIV/AIDS	186 (17.0), 83.9	19 (12.5), 6.5	136 (18.4), 67.8	32 (16.2), 9.4	16 (17.8), 5.0	8 (16.7), 1.8
Racism	77 (7.0), 43.5	18 (11.8), 9.2	58 (7.8), 29.6	15 (7.6), 8.7	8 (8.9), 5.4	5 (10.4), 4.2
Reproductive health, including maternal and child health	21 (1.9), 9.4	7 (4.6), 1.3	2 (0.3), 3.7	6 (3.0), 2.2	7 (7.8), 2.4	3 (6.2), 0.7
Screening	64 (5.9), 24.9	10 (6.6), 2.6	48 (6.5), 21.4	17 (8.6), 4.4	9 (10.0), 1.6	8 (16.7), 1.8
Structural analysis	162 (14.8), 84.2	26 (17.1), 12.9	107 (14.4), 56.9	37 (18.7), 16.2	15 (16.7), 7.2	11 (22.9), 6.6
Tobacco	34 (3.1), 10.5	16 (10.5), 5.6	19 (2.6), 6.4	3 (1.5), 1.3	3 (3.3), 1.3	2 (4.2), 0.8
Transphobia	111 (10.2), 39.7	28 (18.4), 13.8	37 (5.0), 19.2	67 (33.8), 19.7	27 (30.0), 9.0	15 (31.2), 4.5
Tuberculosis	3 (0.3), 1.6	0 (0), 0	2 (0.3), 1.4	1 (0.5), 0.3	1 (1.1), 0.3	0 (0), 0
Vaccines or Immunizations	12 (1.1), 6.2	3 (2.0), 0.7	7 (0.9), 4.3	1 (0.5), <0.1	1 (1.1), <0.1	1 (2.1), <0.1
Violence	95 (8.7), 37.5	25 (16.4), 9.8	47 (6.3), 21.1	24 (12.1), 6.3	10 (11.1), 3.3	5 (10.4), 1.8
Weight related	11 (1.0), 3.4	8 (5.3), 2.0	4 (0.5), 0.5	1 (0.5), 0.5	1 (1.1), 0.5	1 (2.1), 0.5

Note. SGM = sexual and gender minoritized. All dollar amounts are inflation adjusted using the Biomedical Research and Development Price Index to represent purchasing power in 2022.

Native Hawaiian/Pacific Islander (3; 0.3%; $2.6 million). Excluding awards related to HIV/AIDS, those noting race/ethnicity in the abstract decreased to 40.8%, those noting Black people decreased to 9.8%, and those noting Hispanic/Latino/a/x/e people decreased to 6.4%.

A total of 207 (18.9%; $110.5 million) awards explicitly mentioned people younger than 18 years in their NIH RePORTER abstracts, and 36 (3.3%; $17.5 million) mentioned people 50 years or older. Excluding HIV/AIDS–related awards, 94 (24.9%) mentioned people younger than 18 years, and 22 (5.8%) mentioned people 50 years or older.

Awards focusing on populations outside the United States numbered 157 (14.4%; $54.9 million). Excluding HIV/AIDS–related awards, 16 (4.2%; $6.7 million) involved populations outside the United States.

Historical Changes

From 2012 to 2022, the number of NIH awards for SGM-related research went from 61 to 172, increasing from 0.6% to 1.1% of all NIH awards, and SGM-related research funding increased from $23.6 to $83.2 million (Figure 1). The percentage increase in SGM-related research awards was driven by a proportional increase in non-HIV/AIDS–related awards (0.1% in 2012 to 0.5% in 2022); research involving HIV/AIDS and SGM people consistently received about 0.5% of all NIH awards from 2012 to 2022. Sexually minoritized men were included in the bulk of awards for SGM research, with awards increasing from 55 ($20.3 million) in 2012 to 82 ($51.6 million) in 2022. Sexually minoritized women, transgender women and men, and nonbinary people were explicitly mentioned in fewer

TABLE 3— National Institutes of Health–Funded Awards for Research on the Health of SGM Populations Excluding HIV/AIDS, by Content Area: United States, 2012–2022

Content Area	Awards for SGM Health Research Excluding HIV/AIDS, No. (%), $ in Millions					
	Total Awards (n = 377, $ = 151.9 million)	Research Involving Sexually Minoritized Women (n = 130, $ = 43.7 million)	Research Involving Sexually Minoritized Men (n = 149, $ = 62.4 million)	Research Involving Transgender Women (n = 69, $ = 25.2 million)	Research Involving Transgender Men (n = 66, $25.3 million)	Research Involving Nonbinary People (n = 42, $ = 16.1 million)
Alcohol use	62 (16.4), 18.3	30 (23.1), 9.1	23 (15.4), 8.1	8 (11.6), 2.3	8 (12.1), 2.3	4 (9.5), 0.8
Cancer	31 (8.2), 8.8	7 (5.4), 1.9	15 (10.1), 5.3	6 (8.7), 1.9	6 (9.1), 1.9	6 (14.3), 2.1
Cardiovascular	20 (5.2), 9.3	3 (2.3), 2.0	5 (3.4), 2.7	8 (11.6), 3.5	6 (9.1), 2.8	3 (7.1), 1.0
Cost-effectiveness and other health financing	8 (2.1), 3.9	0 (0), 0	0 (0), 0	3 (4.3), 0.8	3 (4.5), 0.8	3 (7.1), 0.8
Couples and family health	30 (8.0), 7.9	22 (16.9), 5.2	27 (18.1), 4.9	1 (91.4), 0.3	1 (1.5), 0.3	1 (2.4), 0.3
COVID-19	12 (3.2), 6.7	5 (3.8), 3.5	6 (4.0), 3.8	1 (1.4), 0.2	1 (1.5), 0.2	1 (2.4), 0.2
Dental/oral health	0 (0), 0	0 (0), 0	0 (0), 0	0 (0), 0	0 (0), 0	0 (0), 0
Environmental health	13 (3.4), 4.9	3 (2.3), 1.5	6 (4.0), 3.2	0 (0), 0	0 (0), 0	0 (0), 0
Ethical issues	5 (1.3), 1.7	0 (0), 0	2 (1.3), 1.0	0 (0), 0	0 (0), 0	0 (0), 0
Exercise	2 (0.5), 0.4	0 (0), 0	1 (0.7), 0.2	1 (1.4), 0.2	0 (0), 0	0 (0), 0
Gender-affirming care	73 (19.4), 27.6	7 (5.4), 3.2	7 (4.7), 3.2	42 (60.9), 16.8	43 (65.2), 16.7	25 (59.5), 10.4
Genetics	17 (4.5), 6.8	3 (2.3), 1.0	4 (2.7), 0.9	6 (8.7), 3.4	6 (9.1), 3.2	3 (7.1), 1.4
Health policy	13 (3.4), 3.7	8 (6.2), 2.5	5 (3.4), 2.1	2 (2.9), 0.7	2 (3.0), 0.7	2 (4.8), 0.7
Health services	69 (18.3), 28.4	22 (16.9), 10.8	27 (18.1), 13.3	23 (33.3), 6.2	17 (25.8), 5.0	12 (28.6), 3.2
Hepatitis	1 (0.3), 0.2	0 (0), 0	1 (0.7), 0.2	0 (0), 0	0 (0), 0	0 (0), 0
Homelessness	2 (0.5), 1.4	0 (0), 0	1 (0.7), 0.7	0 (0), 0	0 (0), 0	0 (0), 0
Homophobia	85 (22.5), 35.9	53 (40.8), 19.7	49 (32.9), 20.9	7 (10.1), 2.7	9 (13.6), 3.9	3 (7.1), 1.0
Illicit drug use	45 (11.9), 16.1	14 (10.8), 4.7	20 (13.4), 8.1	9 (13.0), 2.5	7 (10.6), 2.2	5 (11.9), 1.5
Immigration	4 (1.1), 2.1	1 (0.8), 0.5	1 (0.7), 0.5	0 (0), 0	0 (0), 0	0 (0), 0
Infrastructure for researchers of SGM health	74 (19.6), 44.9	25 (19.2), 11.2	29 (19.5), 18.8	16 (23.2), 4.9	16 (24.2), 5.2	9 (21.4), 2.8
Intersectionality	38 (10.1), 17.0	13 (10.0), 4.3	14 (9.4), 6.3	9 (13.0), 2.3	10 (15.2), 3.1	9 (21.4), 2.7
Intervention	75 (19.9), 36.4	23 (17.7), 11.9	34 (2.8), 16.5	11 (15.9), 6.0	8 (12.1), 5.6	7 (16.7), 5.6
Measurement validation or testing of sampling methods	65 (17.2), 22.2	17 (13.1), 5.3	18 (12.1), 5.1	15 (21.7), 4.7	16 (24.2), 4.9	11 (26.2), 3.1
Mental health	62 (16.4), 69.9	30 (23.1), 25.8	23 (15.4), 25.1	33 (47.8), 15.1	32 (48.5), 14.9	18 (42.9), 8.7
Neurologic disorders	13 (3.4), 11.9	6 (4.6), 3.7	6 (4.0), 3.7	2 (2.9), 0.6	2 (3.0), 0.6	2 (4.8), 0.6
Nutrition, food, and dietary habits	6 (1.6), 1.7	4 (3.1), 0.8	4 (2.7), 1.4	0 (0), 0	0 (0), 0	0 (0), 0
Sexual health, excluding HIV/AIDS	64 (17.0), 25.9	13 (10.0), 3.5	39 (26.2), 17.8	8 (11.6), 2.6	10 (15.2), 2.9	7 (16.7), 1.6
Racism	31 (8.2), 21.6	15 (11.5), 6.4	18 (12.1), 8.8	6 (8.7), 5.1	6 (9.1), 5.1	5 (11.9), 4.2

Continued

TABLE 3— Continued

	Awards for SGM Health Research Excluding HIV/AIDS, No. (%), $ in Millions					
Content Area	**Total Awards (n = 377, $ = 151.9 million)**	**Research Involving Sexually Minoritized Women (n = 130, $ = 43.7 million)**	**Research Involving Sexually Minoritized Men (n = 149, $ = 62.4 million)**	**Research Involving Transgender Women (n = 69, $ = 25.2 million)**	**Research Involving Transgender Men (n = 66, $25.3 million)**	**Research Involving Nonbinary People (n = 42, $ = 16.1 million)**
Reproductive health, including maternal and child health	20 (5.3), 9.1	7 (5.4), 1.3	2 (1.3), 3.7	5 (7.2), 2.0	6 (9.1), 2.2	3 (7.1), 0.7
Screening	26 (6.9), 9.6	8 (6.2), 1.8	14 (9.4), 7.2	11 (15.9), 2.5	7 (10.6), 1.3	8 (19.0), 1.8
Structural analysis	52 (13.8), 29.0	21 (16.2), 8.6	21 (14.1), 10.4	11 (15.9), 6.4	11 (16.7), 6.6	8 (19.0), 5.5
Tobacco	30 (8.0), 8.8	16 (12.3), 5.6	16 (10.7), 5.6	3 (4.3), 1.3	3 (4.5), 1.3	2 (4.8), 0.8
Transphobia	60 (15.9), 20.6	21 (16.2), 9.2	19 (12.8), 9.0	25 (36.2), 7.9	21 (31.8), 7.3	13 (31.0), 4.2
Tuberculosis	1 (0.3), 0.3	0 (0), 0	0 (0), 0	1 (1.4), 0.3	1 (1.5), 0.3	0 (0), 0
Vaccines or Immunizations	10 (2.7), 4.6	3 (2.3), 0.7	7 (4.7), 4.3	1 (1.4), <0.1	1 (1.5), <0.1	1 (2.4), <0.1
Violence	53 (14.1), 19.1	22 (16.9), 7.7	19 (12.8), 6.2	9 (13.0), 2.5	7 (10.6), 2.8	4 (9.5), 1.5
Weight related	11 (2.9), 3.4	8 (6.2), 2.0	5 (3.4), 0.5	1 (1.4), 0.5	1 (1.5), 0.5	1 (2.4), 0.5

Note. SGM = sexual and gender minoritized. All dollar amounts are inflation adjusted using the Biomedical Research and Development Price Index to represent purchasing power in 2022.

than 5 NIH RePORTER abstracts receiving awards in 2012, each award totaling less than $1.5 million. Awards mentioning these subgroups steadily increased over the study period; in 2022, 47 ($16.3 million) involved transgender women, 28 ($12.0 million) involved sexually minoritized women, 29 ($9.9 million) involved transgender men, and 22 ($6.7 million) involved nonbinary people.

Health Content Areas

Of the total 1093 awards for SGM-related research, the most common areas of health research awarded were HIV/AIDS (716 awards; 65.5%; $339.8 million), mental health (322 awards; 29.5%; $134.3 million), illicit drug use (218 awards; 19.9%; $105.6 million), sexual health other than HIV/AIDS (186 awards; 17.0%; $83.9 million), and alcohol use (132 awards; 12.1%; $47.1 million). Specific content areas by SGM subpopulations are reported in Table 2. A substantial number of awards went to research that planned to deliver health services (205 awards; 18.8%; $92.5 million), build SGM research infrastructure (187 awards; 17.1%; $120.1 million), or validate measures or sampling methods (126 awards; 11.5%; $46.9 million). Intersectionality (94 awards; 8.4%; $37.5 million), structural factors (162 awards; 14.8%; $84.2 million), homophobia (181 awards; 16.6%; $80.1 million), transphobia (111 awards; 10.2%; $39.7 million), and racism (77 awards; 7.0%; $43.5 million) were also recurrent content areas. Intersectionality appeared in just 258 (0.2%) of 140 627 non-SGM abstracts. Our validation showed that 6 (1.7%) of 344 linked articles reporting SGM research that received awards in 2014 met the intersectionality criteria, comparable to our 2.8% estimate for intersectionality that year.

Content areas varied by SGM subgroups. Relative to the distribution of all awards for SGM research, awards involving sexually minoritized women more often focused on mental health (85 awards; 55.95; $31.6 million), homophobia (61 awards; 40.1%; $24.7 million), alcohol use (37 awards; 24.3%; $11.8 million), violence (25 awards; 16.4%; $9.8 million), and couples and family health (23 awards; 15.1%; $5.4 million). The awards for research involving sexually minoritized women infrequently focused on HIV/AIDS (22 awards; 14.5%; $13.8 million). Content areas for awards involving sexually minoritized men were similar to the total sample but more likely to focus on HIV/AIDS (592 awards; 79.9%; $295.5 million). HIV/AIDS was also a common focus in awards for SGM research involving transgender women (129 awards; 65.2%; $52.4 million) but much less so for awards involving transgender men (24 awards; 26.7%; $12.3 million) and nonbinary people (6 awards; 12.5%; $1.5 million). More than half of awards involving transgender women, transgender men, and nonbinary people focused on gender-affirming care, and almost a third focused on transphobia.

Content areas by SGM subpopulation for research awards excluding HIV/AIDS are included in Table 3. Overall, 377 awards excluding HIV/AIDS commonly focused on mental health (40 awards; 53.3%; $21.8 million), sexual health (18 awards; 24.0%; $6.8 million), alcohol (14 awards; 18.7%; $5.4 million), cancer (12 awards; 16.0%; $4.0 million), or violence (11 awards; 14.7%; $4.2 million).

Appendix 3 (available as a supplement to the online version of this article at http://www.ajph.org) contains intervention research breakdowns to supplement the analyses of Coulter et al.

DISCUSSION

We found a significant increase in the number and percentage of awards and the amount of funding awarded for SGM health research from 2012 (61 awards; 0.6%; $23.6 million) to 2022 (172 awards; 1.1%; $83.2 million). We found that 1093 NIH awards (0.8%; $491.7 million) for research focused on SGM health from 2012 to 2022. Coulter et al. reported that 628 (0.5%) NIH awards went to research focused on SGM health from 1989 to 2011.[12] Whereas the 1989 to 2011 increase in awards to SGM-focused studies was primarily attributable to HIV/AIDS research receiving more awards,[12] the increase in percentage of awards to SGM-focused studies since 2011 appear to have been driven by non-HIV/AIDS research. These funding increases are consistent with NIH efforts to address SGM health disparities since the 2011 Institute of Medicine report.[1–4]

Although awards to SGM-focused studies have nearly tripled from 2012 to 2022, the increase in SGM health research funding may not be sufficient to achieve SGM health equity. An important insight of our study is that the funding for SGM health research remains highly disproportionate to SGM population size in the United States. National growth in the proportion of people who report SGM identities (3.2% in 2012 to 7.1% in 2022)[13,19] has outpaced the increase in the proportion of NIH awards to SGM health–focused studies since 2011 (0.6% in 2012 to 1.1% in 2022). Furthermore, SGM population growth has been highest among chronically understudied SGM subpopulations (i.e., sexually minoritized women and transgender or nonbinary people).[14] Funding from 2012 to 2022 confirms that SGM health remains on the periphery of the NIH research portfolio. This is an example of a structural driver that sustains SGM health inequities, consistent with the principles of intersectionality.[6] Our key conclusion is that NIH must redouble efforts to invest considerably more in research for all SGM populations. Our second key recommendation is to prioritize the SGM communities who experience multiple forms of oppression (e.g., sexism, transphobia, racism) and for whom research is lacking by prioritizing intersectionality in research.

Although NIH funding for SGM health research has increased, sexually minoritized women and transgender and nonbinary people have remained relatively understudied. Since 2011, most funding (including awards for HIV/AIDS–focused studies) has been directed to sexually minoritized men (67.8%; $357.9 million), which far exceeds the funding for any other subgroup: transgender women (18.1%; $77.6 million), sexually minoritized women (13.9%; $57.6 million), transgender men (8.2%; $37.6 million), and nonbinary people (4.4%; $17.6 million). To combat the HIV/AIDS pandemic in these high-risk SGM subgroups, much needed resources have been directed to sexually minoritized men, with some resources also directed to transgender women, albeit to a lesser extent.[20] This has advanced research on HIV/AIDS prevention and treatment, as well as on intersecting health conditions and experiences (e.g., substance use) for these subgroups. Transgender men and nonbinary people also exhibit higher HIV risk than does the general population. Our findings highlight the gap in funding for HIV/AIDS-inclusive research for these subgroups.[21,22]

After excluding awards for HIV/AIDS–related research, we found that sexually minoritized men were still the most frequently included subgroup (39.5%; $62.7 million) compared with sexually minoritized women (34.5%; $43.7 million), transgender women (18.3%; $25.2 million), transgender men (17.5%; $25.3 million), and nonbinary people (11.1%; $16.1 million). Furthermore, sexually minoritized men were regularly studied alone, whereas other subgroups were often studied in combination, splitting funding among them (Appendix B). Altogether, these results attest that sexually minoritized cisgender men have been studied far more than have transgender and nonbinary people or sexually minoritized women. The research disparity has narrowed somewhat since Coulter et al. demonstrated that for SGM studies receiving NIH awards between 1989 and 2011 involved sexually minoritized men (86.1%) far more than they involved sexually minoritized women (13.5%) and transgender people (6.8%). Yet, as the NIH strategic plan calls for research on understudied SGM subgroups,[4] our study highlights the persistent lack of funding for sexually minoritized women and transgender and nonbinary people—a critical gap given the size and growth of people self-reporting these subgroup identities nationally.

Furthermore, intersectionality research on SGM health appears limited. From 2012 to 2022, only 8.6% of NIH abstracts related to SGM health mentioned intersectionality. Only 14.8% of abstracts mentioned structural factors. Less than half (42.2%) of abstracts explicitly mentioned race or ethnicity, an improvement from the 31.4% found by Coulter et al. Across abstracts, only 7.8% mentioned racism. A minority of awards centered racially minoritized SGM people: Black (20.4%), Hispanic/Latino/a/x/e (9.9%), Asian (1.3%), American Indian/Alaska Native (0.3%), and Native Hawaiian/Pacific Islander (0.3%). Excluding awards for HIV/AIDS research, the percentage of awards that centered Black (9.8%) and Hispanic/Latino/a/x/e (6.4%) people decreased.

There is substantial evidence of racial inequities in research enrollment and NIH grant distribution,[23–27] with NIH acknowledging that racially minoritized people are not included in studies as often as White people despite federal reporting requirements for racial/ethnic identity in NIH research.[28] Our analysis suggests similar inequities in SGM research, which is concerning given the burden of health inequities in SGM communities of color,[1,3,29] who now make up nearly half of the SGM population in the United States and are growing.[29,30] Since 2011, NIH has emphasized intersectionality in SGM research,[1,3,4] but our analysis highlights its limited presence, including key dimensions of race and racism, in NIH funding for SGM health research from 2011 to 2022. Fidelity to intersectionality's roots and praxis demands a recognition of structural oppression and especially systemic racism as fundamental drivers of health inequities.[6,31,32] These also appear to be underresearched.

This analysis can serve as a tool for NIH and researchers in general to identify additional intersectional needs and track progress for SGM health research. For example, there is a lack of research on older SGM populations, with only 3.3% of awards explicitly involving people aged 50 years or older. This is consistent with how the NIH strategic plan has identified aging as a key consideration for future SGM health research.[4] Additionally, bisexual+ people are the largest group in the LGBTQ (lesbian, gay, bisexual, transgender, queer or questioning) community in the United States[14] but remain understudied. NIH has acknowledged this gap in its strategic plan and issued a notice of special interest for research on health disparities in bisexual+ populations.[33]

We have also exposed health content areas that may be underfunded given their burden in SGM communities, for example, cancer (4.2%; $19.3 million) and violence (8.7%; $37.5 million). Our findings increase the transparency of the funding patterns in NIH-funded SGM health research, including research on SGM subpopulations and health areas that have received marginal funding, to equip both researchers and NIH to urge that resources be allocated to support SGM health in our shared mission of health equity.

Limitations

Because our study replicated the methods of Coulter et al., it was subject to similar limitations.[12] We evaluated only new NIH awards and first-year funding, excluding supplementary grants and continuations, and collapsed 4 award mechanisms, which may differ systematically in content and focus. Some NIH abstracts in the RePORTER system may not include SGM search terms, even if they examined SGM health, because of the omission of these terms when the political landscape was particularly hostile to SGM research or because the scope changed after funding.[34]

Additionally, given that NIH abstracts are limited to 30 lines, the detail investigators can provide is restricted.

We, therefore, may have underestimated both the number of NIH awards related to SGM health and the frequency of content areas (e.g., intersectionality) in SGM research receiving awards. Future studies should consider evaluating differences between NIH abstracts and linked publications in the RePORTER system, which may offer insights into how funding was used (e.g., study inclusion of SGM subpopulations or racially minoritized people). Furthermore, studies should consider evaluating the distribution of NIH awards for SGM research among researchers with minoritized backgrounds, who may experience inequities and face barriers to obtaining NIH funding.[25,35]

Public Health Implications

Funding for SGM health research increased at NIH from 2012 to 2022, consistent with NIH efforts to build SGM research infrastructure and increase grant support for SGM research activities. However, the funding increase appears insufficient to achieve SGM health equity given the size and growth of SGM communities and the persistence of SGM health disparities. Our findings suggest persistent inequities in NIH funding for studies of sexually minoritized women, transgender or nonbinary people, and racially minoritized SGM people.

Intersectionality is an indispensable framework for SGM health research. Honoring intersectionality's historical emphasis on power, structural inequality, and social justice necessitates that we examine and address how systems of oppression are embedded in our public health institutions and shape the flow of institutional funding for SGM research detailed herein. Doing so benefits all public health research. AJPH

ABOUT THE AUTHORS

Ben C. D. Weideman, Alexandra M. Ecklund, Rhea Alley, and B. R. Simon Rosser are with the Division of Epidemiology & Community Health, School of Public Health, University of Minnesota, Minneapolis. G. Nic Rider is with the Eli Coleman Institute for Sexual and Gender Health, Department of Family Medicine and Community Health, University of Minnesota Medical School, Minneapolis.

CORRESPONDENCE

Correspondence should be sent to B. R. Simon Rosser, PhD, MPH, LP, 1300 S. 2nd St #300, Minneapolis, MN 55454 (e-mail: rosser@umn.edu). Reprints can be ordered at https://www.ajph.org by clicking the "Reprints" link.

PUBLICATION INFORMATION

Full Citation: Weideman BCD, Ecklund AM, Alley R, Rosser BRS, Rider GN. Research funded by National Institutes of Health concerning sexual and gender minoritized populations: a tracking update for 2012 to 2022. *Am J Public Health*. 2025;115(3):374–386.

Acceptance Date: October 28, 2024.

DOI: https://doi.org/10.2105/AJPH.2024.307913

ORCID iDs:

Ben C. D. Weideman https://orcid.org/0009-0000-6843-5578

Alexandra M. Ecklund https://orcid.org/0000-0002-8822-701X

Rhea Alley https://orcid.org/0009-0008-8344-1878

B. R. Simon Rosser https://orcid.org/0000-0001-8862-531X

G. Nic Rider https://orcid.org/0000-0002-6730-5613

CONTRIBUTORS

B. C. D. Weideman analyzed the data and drafted and revised the article. B. C. D. Weideman, A. M. Ecklund, R. Alley, and G. N. Rider conceptualized the study and collected and coded the data. A. M. Ecklund, R. Alley, B. R. S. Rosser, and G. N. Rider contributed to the analysis and interpretation of findings and critically reviewed and revised the article. All authors approved the final version of the article.

ACKNOWLEDGMENTS

The research in this article was supported by the National Cancer Institute, National Institutes of Health (NIH; awards R01CA265945-01A1 [primary investigator: B. R. S. R.] and T32CA163184 [coprimary investigators: Michelle Allen and Irina Stepanov]).

Note. The content of this article is solely the responsibility of the authors and does not necessarily represent the official views of NIH.

CONFLICTS OF INTEREST

The authors have no conflicts of interest to report.

HUMAN PARTICIPANT PROTECTION

This study was an analysis of publicly available data and was exempt from review by the University of Minnesota's institutional review board.

REFERENCES

1. Institute of Medicine Committee on Lesbian, Gay, Bisexual, and Transgender Health Issues and Research Gaps and Opportunities. *The Health of Lesbian, Gay, Bisexual, and Transgender People: Building a Foundation for Better Understanding*. Washington, DC: National Academies Press; 2011.
2. Sexual and Gender Minority Research Office. Sexual and gender minority populations in NIH-supported research. August 28, 2019. Available at: https://grants.nih.gov/grants/guide/notice-files/NOT-OD-19-139.html. Accessed March 3, 2023.
3. National Academies of Sciences, Engineering, and Medicine 2020. *Understanding the Well-Being of LGBTQI+Populations*. Washington, DC: National Academies Press; 2020. https://doi.org/10.17226/25877
4. National Institutes of Health. Strategic plan to advance research on the health and well-being of sexual & gender minorities. Available at: https://dpcpsi.nih.gov/sites/default/files/SGM StrategicPlan_2021_2025.pdf. Accessed May 4, 2024.
5. Bowleg L. The problem with the phrase women and minorities: intersectionality-an important theoretical framework for public health. *Am J Public Health*. 2012;102(7):1267–1273. https://doi.org/10.2105/AJPH.2012.300750
6. Bowleg L. Evolving intersectionality within public health: from analysis to action. *Am J Public Health*. 2021;111(1):88–90. https://doi.org/10.2105/AJPH.2020.306031
7. Aguayo-Romero RA. (Re)centering Black feminism into intersectionality research. *Am J Public Health*. 2021;111(1):101–103. https://doi.org/10.2105/AJPH.2020.306005
8. Collins PH. *Black Feminist Thought: Knowledge, Consciousness, and the Politics of Empowerment*. New York, NY: Routledge; 1991.
9. Crenshaw KW. Mapping the margins: intersectionality, identity politics, and violence against women of color. *Stanford Law Rev*. 1991;43(6):1241–1299. https://doi.org/10.2307/1229039
10. Collins PH. *Intersectionality as Critical Social Theory*. Durham, NC: Duke University Press; 2019.
11. National Institutes of Health. About NIH. Available at: https://www.nih.gov/about-nih. Accessed December 27, 2023.
12. Coulter RW, Kenst KS, Bowen DJ. Scout. Research funded by the National Institutes of Health on the health of lesbian, gay, bisexual, and transgender populations. *Am J Public Health*. 2014;104(2):e105–e112. https://doi.org/10.2105/AJPH.2013.301501
13. Gates GJ, Newport F. Special report: 3.4% of US adults identify as LGBT. October 18, 2012.

Available at: https://news.gallup.com/poll/158066/special-report-adults-identify-lgbt.aspx. Accessed January 28, 2024.

14. Jones JM. LGBTQ+ identification in US now at 7.6%. March 13, 2024. Available at: https://news.gallup.com/poll/611864/lgbtq-identification.aspx. Accessed June 4, 2024.
15. Twenge JM, Wells BE, Le J, Rider GN. Increases in self-identifying as transgender among US adults, 2014–2022. *Sex Res Soc Policy*. [Published ahead of print: July 13, 2024]. https://doi.org/10.1007/s13178-024-01001-7
16. National Institutes of Health. Research Portfolio Online Reporting Tools Expenditures and Results (RePORTER) system. Available at: https://reporter.nih.gov. Accessed December 27, 2023.
17. Ashley F, Brightly-Brown S, Rider GN. Beyond the trans/cis binary: introducing new terms will enrich gender research. *Nature*. 2024;630(8016):293–295. https://doi.org/10.1038/d41586-024-01719-9
18. Biomedical Research and Development Price Index (BRDPI). January 2024. Available at: https://officeofbudget.od.nih.gov/gbipriceindexes.html. Accessed April 6, 2024.
19. Jones JM. LGBT identification in US ticks up to 7.1%. Available at: https://news.gallup.com/poll/389792/lgbt-identification-ticks-up.aspx. Accessed May 22, 2023.
20. Poteat T, German D, Flynn C. The conflation of gender and sex: gaps and opportunities in HIV data among transgender women and MSM. *Glob Public Health*. 2016;11(7–8):835–848. https://doi.org/10.1080/17441692.2015.1134615
21. Lemons A, Beer L, Finlayson T, et al. Characteristics of HIV-positive transgender men receiving medical care: United States, 2009–2014. *Am J Public Health*. 2018;108(1):128–130. https://doi.org/10.2105/AJPH.2017.304153
22. Coleman E, Radix AE, Bouman WP, et al. Standards of care for the health of transgender and gender diverse people, version 8. *Int J Transgend Health*. 2022;23(suppl 1):S1–S259. https://doi.org/10.1080/26895269.2022.2100644
23. National Academies of Sciences, Engineering, and Medicine; Policy and Global Affairs; Committee on Women in Science, Engineering, and Medicine; Committee on Improving the Representation of Women and Underrepresented Minorities in Clinical Trials and Research, et al. *Improving Representation in Clinical Trials and Research: Building Research Equity for Women and Underrepresented Groups*. Washington, DC: National Academies Press; 2022.
24. Chen E, Wallace D, Leos C, Merino Y. Examining the White supremacist practices of funding organizations for public health research and practice: a composite narrative from female, BIPOC junior researchers in public health. *Health Promot Pract*. 2023;24(1):45–58. https://doi.org/10.1177/15248399221129864
25. Nguyen M, Chaudhry SI, Desai MM, Dzirasa K, Cavazos JE, Boatright D. Gender, racial, and ethnic and inequities in receipt of multiple national institutes of health research project grants. *JAMA Netw Open*. 2023;6(2):e230855. https://doi.org/10.1001/jamanetworkopen.2023.0855
26. Koch AR, Craemer KA, Garland CE, et al. Federally funded randomized controlled trials increase analysis and reporting of study outcomes by sex, race, and ethnicity. *J Womens Health (Larchmt)*. 2024;33(1):14–19. https://doi.org/10.1089/jwh.2023.0307
27. Maxwell A. Plans and enrollment often fell short for underrepresented groups in a sample of NIH-funded clinical trials. May 2024. Available at: https://oig.hhs.gov/documents/evaluation/9900/OEI-01-21-00320.pdf. Accessed December 4, 2024.
28. Pérez-Stable EJ. Communicating the value of race and ethnicity in research. July 27, 2018. Available at: https://www.nih.gov/about-nih/what-we-do/science-health-public-trust/perspectives/science-health-public-trust/communicating-value-race-ethnicity-research. Accessed June 6, 2024.
29. Williams Institute. Race and well-being among LGBT adults. Available at: https://williamsinstitute.law.ucla.edu/visualization/lgbt-races. Accessed October 11, 2024.
30. Jones JM. Growing LGBT ID seen across major US racial, ethnic groups. Available at: https://news.gallup.com/poll/393464/growing-lgbt-seen-across-major-racial-ethnic-groups.aspx. Accessed October 11, 2024.
31. Phelan JC, Link BG. Is racism a fundamental cause of inequalities in health? *Annu Rev Sociol*. 2015;41:311–330. https://doi.org/10.1146/annurev-soc-073014-112305
32. Hardeman RR, Murphy KA, Karbeah J, Kozhimannil KB. Naming institutionalized racism in the public health literature: a systematic literature review. *Public Health Rep*. 2018;133(3):240–249. https://doi.org/10.1177/0033354918760574
33. National Institutes of Health. Research on the health of bisexual and bisexual+ people. August 11, 2022. Available at: https://grants.nih.gov/grants/guide/notice-files/NOT-OD-22-166.html. Accessed December 4, 2024.
34. Kempner J. The chilling effect: how do researchers react to controversy? *PLoS Med*. 2008;5(11):e222. [Erratum in: *PLoS Med*. 2009;6(1). https://doi.org/10.1371/journal.pmed.1000014]. https://doi.org/10.1371/journal.pmed.0050222
35. Veldhuis CB. Doubly marginalized: addressing the minority stressors experienced by LGBTQ+ researchers who do LGBTQ+ research. *Health Educ Behav*. 2022;49(6):960–974. https://doi.org/10.1177/10901981221116795

Changes in Contraceptive Services During Utah's Family Planning Elevated Contraceptive Access Initiative: A Prospective Assessment of Intervention and Control Sites

Rebecca G. Simmons, PhD, MPH, Alexandra Gero, MPH, Gentry Carter, MS, Jessica N. Sanders, PhD, MSPH, Caitlin Quade, MPH, Jami Baayd, MSPH, Madeline Mullholand, MPA, Sarah Elliott, MPH, Kyl Myers, PhD, Erica Torres, MPH, Justin D. Smith, PhD, and David K. Turok, MD, MPH

See also Riley, p. 259.

Objectives. To assess contraceptive service changes during the Family Planning Elevated (FPE) Contraceptive Access Program in Utah clinics from 2018 to 2023.

Methods. We assessed de-identified electronic health record data on female clients aged 18 to 50 years from intervention and matched control sites. We used comparative interrupted time series analyses comparing total number of contraceptive services and their proportion relative to visits between intervention and control sites before, during, and after FPE.

Results. Intervention sites provided on average 1.76 (95% confidence interval [CI] = 1.17, 2.66) times as many contraceptive services per month as controls during the 24-month intervention period, with no significant decreases in services noted in the postintervention period. The proportions of total visits related to family planning decreased by a factor of 0.70 (95% CI = 0.52, 0.94) during the intervention period. However, this effect was mitigated at intervention sites where proportions of contraceptive services were 1.44 (95% CI = 0.97, 2.14) times greater than control sites and did not significantly decrease after the intervention.

Conclusions. Contraceptive access initiatives have capacity to make meaningful change in communities where they are employed, even after they end. (*Am J Public Health*. 2025;115(3):387–396. https://doi.org/10.2105/AJPH.2024.307917)

AJPH March 2025, Vol. 115, No. 3

Despite the existence of more than 18 different contraceptive methods, many people are not currently using the family planning method they want.[1] Misalignment between preferred methods and actual method use has been associated with dissatisfaction, lower adherence, and contraceptive discontinuation while still wishing to avoid pregnancy.[2] Improving access to preferred contraception requires an ongoing, systemic commitment to address the various barriers people commonly face in obtaining their preferred method over their more than 30 years of reproductive capacity.

Over the past 15 years, contraceptive access initiatives have been implemented across the United States, attempting to address many long-standing barriers to method access within the health care system.[3] The aims and goals of these initiatives have rightly evolved over the years, shifting from a focus on reducing unintended pregnancy solely through the provision of long-acting reversible contraceptives (LARCs; intrauterine devices and implants) to objectives more aligned with reproductive autonomy, allowing all individuals to access all methods of family planning to meet their health and reproductive goals.[4]

To date, however, most research and evaluation on contraceptive access initiatives primarily focus on outcomes of LARC expansion and reducing unintended pregnancy.[5–13] While newer and updated initiatives have shifted in focus,[14,15] impact metrics and evidence supporting this more expansive approach still need to be improved. This article details outcomes from the Family Planning Elevated (FPE) Contraceptive Access Program, a statewide family planning initiative in Utah that sought to improve health system capacity to offer all methods of contraception.[16–19] These analyses assessed the number of contraceptive services provided, the proportion of those services compared with all visits during the intervention, and the sustainment of these changes. We hypothesized that the FPE program would favorably change all 3 of these outcomes.

METHODS

We conducted a comparative interrupted time series analysis (CITSA) where we compared contraceptive service provision at intervention and control sites before, during, and after the intervention by extrapolating preperiod outcome trends to construct postperiod counterfactual outcomes to model differential outcome trends.[16] A key assumption of CITSA is that by assessing both level and trend changes before, during, and after an event, level or trend changes in the outcome variable are presumed to be the same for both the control group and the treatment group, had the treatment group not undergone the intervention.

We standardized time to be a 1- to 48-month time frame where each clinic's first 12 months of contraceptive service provision occurred before FPE implementation, months 13 to 36 occurred during the 2-year intervention, and each clinic's final 12 months (months 37 to 48) of contraceptive service provision occurred after the intervention ended.

Setting

The FPE contraceptive access initiative aimed to improve access to high-quality comprehensive contraceptive services across Utah. FPE had 2 primary goals: (1) to bolster the health system's capacity to provide high-quality, comprehensive contraceptive care to individuals who were newly eligible for Medicaid coverage following the 2018 Medicaid Expansion to Healthy Adults below 138% of the federal poverty level (according to the Department of Health and Human Services) and (2) to offer no-cost contraceptive services to individuals earning between 139% and 250% of the federal poverty level who fell within a contraceptive coverage gap (were uninsured, underinsured [e.g., on an insurance plan that does not cover contraception[20]], or did not qualify for coverage because of documentation status) to demonstrate the need for stronger contraceptive coverage options through a Section 1115 Medicaid Family Planning Waiver. The FPE research team both designed and evaluated the program.

Unlike previous contraceptive access initiatives, the goals of FPE did not specifically involve reducing unintended pregnancy. The initiative was focused on strengthening health system activities and capacities that increased access to all US Food and Drug Administration–approved methods of contraception available in primary care settings. We selected contraceptive provision (number of services provided) as a proxy measure of contraceptive access, based on the hypothesis that addressing barriers to access would lead to increased utilization of contraceptive services that would be evident in service delivery data. We also decentered contraceptive continuation as a goal for this initiative. Clients eligible for no-cost contraceptive service provision through FPE were encouraged to select any method they desired and to switch methods as often as needed throughout the intervention period. Discontinuation and removal of LARC methods at any time was also specifically supported, and individuals who received a LARC method through FPE remained eligible to have it removed at no cost for an additional year after the intervention ended at all intervention sites. No-cost removal remains available through a University of Utah–supported LARC removal initiative. Appendix A (available as a supplement to the online version of this article at https://ajph.org) provides an overview of priority implementation strategies that occurred during the FPE program.

Participants

To be eligible for participation in FPE, interested clinics needed to

1. have the ability to bill Medicaid,
2. primarily serve low-income Utahns,
3. have at least 1 licensed clinician who could be trained to insert and remove intrauterine devices and contraceptive implants,
4. have either an onsite pharmacy or an existing partnership with a community pharmacy where clients could obtain prescription-based contraceptives (i.e., oral contraceptives, contraceptive patches,

vaginal rings, ulipristal acetate emergency contraception), and

5. be enrolled or eligible to enroll in the federal 340B Drug Pricing Program, which allows eligible health care organizations to purchase drugs at lower cost.

Interested clinics also agreed to participate in contraceptive trainings and monitoring and to provide service delivery data to the investigative team for the duration of the intervention. We enrolled FPE clinics into the program over the course of 18 months into 3 cohorts: spring of 2019, fall of 2019, and spring of 2020.

For this study, the research team also recruited control sites to provide comparative service delivery data. We matched control sites to participating FPE sites on rural or urban status (as defined by the Federal Office of Rural Health Policy[21]), the current provision of contraceptive services (yes or no), a similar number of clinicians who could provide family planning at the sites (±2), and the ability to accept Medicaid clients (current billing to Medicaid). Because of inherent differences in organizational structures, we matched intervention and control sites by clinic rather than by health organization. This most often resulted in a 1:1 match between a FPE health organization and a participating control health organization; however, some control organizations offered to provide eligible data for more than 1 clinical site and were thus matched to suitable FPE clinics within participating health organizations (e.g., FPE sites 5a and 5b and control sites 5a and 5b in Table 1). For example,

TABLE 1— Overview of Family Planning Elevated (FPE) Contraceptive Access Program Intervention and Control Sites: Utah, 2018–2023

Cohort and Site	Rural/Urban Designation (RUCA Code)[a]	Clinic Type	No. of Clinicians Able to Provide Family Planning at Site
Cohort 1 (spring 2019)			
FPE clinic 1a	Urban (1)	FQHC	12
Control clinic 1a	Urban (1)	Private	14
FPE clinic 1b	Urban (1)	FQHC	5
Control clinic 1b	Urban (1)	FQHC	5
FPE clinic 2	Urban (1)	FQHC	4
Control clinic 2	Urban (1)	State-run clinic	3
FPE clinic 3	Rural (4)	Private	1.5
Control clinic 3	Rural (4)	Private	3
Cohort 2[b] (fall 2019)			
FPE clinic 4a	Urban (1)	FQHC	6
Control clinic 4a	Urban (1)	Private	5
FPE clinic 5b	Urban (1)	FQHC	7
Control clinic 5b	Urban (1)	Private	6
Cohort 3 (spring 2020)			
FPE clinic 6	Urban (1)	Family planning	2
Control clinic 6	Urban (1)	Family planning	3
FPE clinic 7a	Rural (7)	FQHC	4
Control clinic 7a	Rural (10)	FQHC	7[c]
FPE clinic 7b	Rural (7)	FQHC	3
Control clinic 7b	Rural (10)	FQHC	2

Note. FQHC = federally qualified health center; RUCA = Rural Urban Commuting Area.

[a]Rural/urban designation identified using the Federal Office of Rural Health Policy Defined Rural Areas.

[b]Cohort 2 also included 2 county health departments that are not included in the primary outcome analyses because of the lack of appropriate controls (see Methods section).

[c]The value for control clinic 7a was outside the bound because the control clinic hired more people after agreeing to participate. We discussed and decided to include the correct numbers.

1 family planning–specific organization did not enroll all clinical sites in the FPE intervention. As such, we designated 1 of their comparably sized, nonparticipating sites, located in a different county more than 20 miles from the intervention site, as a control site for this analysis. This approach was selected for this organization as there were no appropriate controls for this type of site (e.g., Title X grantee, family planning organization). A summary of all intervention and control clinics included in our analyses is included as Table 1.

The FPE initiative also included 2 county health departments in Utah, which were the only 2 county health departments that provided the full range of contraceptive services before the intervention. Because of fundamental differences in clinic setup, billing, and reimbursement that occur at county health facilities, they had substantially different service delivery data outputs than other clinical sites and therefore were not matched with control sites. For example, before participating in FPE, 1 of these sites did not have electronic service delivery data and the other site did not bill insurers or other external sources for reimbursement. State block grants primarily fund these county health departments. Such inherent differences made selection of suitable control clinics for these sites impossible, and, thus, they were excluded from the current primary analyses. These were also the smallest clinics and provided a limited number of services throughout the intervention (n = 860 services over the intervention period).

Data Collection

Our analyses focused on exploring the impact of FPE on both the change in total number of contraceptive services provided over time and the change in the proportion of clinic services dedicated to family planning care relative to all care provided among female clients aged 18 to 50 years. For our analyses, FPE sites and matched-control sites reported de-identified electronic service delivery data on all services provided to women between the ages of 18 and 50 years for a total of 48 months. This included 12 months before the intervention, 24 months during the intervention, and 12 months after the intervention.

While FPE did provide reimbursement for vasectomy services, a limited number of participating clinics offered vasectomy services, and, thus, we did not assess contraceptive services among male clients as part of these analyses. While this article uses the terms "female/women" and "male," we acknowledge that not all individuals who need contraceptive services identify as female or male; our terminology for this research is specific to that utilized by the electronic health records systems that provided data for this project. FPE also provided no-cost methods and reimbursement for services for adolescents aged younger than 18 years; however, because of an existing state law that requires state-funded institutions (including the University of Utah) to obtain parental consent for adolescent contraceptive care provision, many clinical organizations did not ultimately use FPE funds for this population. Thus, although we collected data on this population, they were not included in our primary outcome analysis.

We identified all diagnostic (*International Classification of Diseases, 10th Revision* [Geneva, Switzerland: World Health Organization; 1992]) and procedural (Current Procedural Terminology, Healthcare Common Procedure Coding System [https://bit.ly/3PvNQxT]) codes associated with contraception (Appendix B, available as a supplement to the online version of this article at https://ajph.org). Any visit that included at least 1 of the associated codes was counted as a family planning–related visit. For example, if an individual received an intrauterine device and also discussed diabetes management with their provider at a particular visit, that visit was counted as a family planning visit in our analyses.

Analyses

Because of nonnormality, we log-transformed the number of family planning–related visits and the percentage of total services related to family planning at each time point for each clinic and then assessed changes of these 2 outcomes using 2 respective CITSA models, which each accounted for level and trend differences between matched intervention and control clinics over the 3 study periods (preintervention [12 months], intervention [24 months], postintervention [12 months]). Though clinics began and ended the intervention in 3 different cohorts (Table 1), matched intervention and control site data included the same calendar time for preintervention, intervention, and postintervention periods. For these analyses, we then standardized time into the 3 study periods. Further information about analytic models is provided in Appendix C (available as a supplement to the online version of this article at https://ajph.org).

A priori we committed to limiting this analysis to 9 clinical sites and their respective controls, resulting in 18 different facilities.[16] During the COVID-19 pandemic, 1 of the control sites (control clinic 2) closed permanently because of

COVID-19 and another stopped providing service delivery data to the project (control clinic 3). Thus, data from these 2 sites were truncated, with 1 site (control clinic 2) providing 12 months of preintervention data and 18 months of intervention data and the second providing 12 months of preintervention data and 23 months of intervention data (control clinic 3). We accounted for autocorrelation both over time and within each facility's measurements using generalized least squares methods in our CITSA models. Each model accounted for the nonzero amount of correlation between residuals within each facility using an autoregressive moving averages correlation structure with a second-order autoregression and a first-order moving average.

We conducted all analyses with R version 4.3.3.[22] We used the nlme package to apply generalized least squares within our regression models.[23]

RESULTS

Overall, FPE enrolled 8 health care organizations, representing 28 clinical sites that received the FPE intervention. FPE also contracted with 6 control organizations that provided data for 9 clinical sites (Table 1). While all FPE sites provided service delivery data to the FPE program, this primary outcome analysis is limited to 9 FPE sites and their 9 matched control sites, as specified in our protocol paper.[16]

Number of Family Planning Visits

Table 2 presents outcomes from the CITSA model assessing differences in total number of contraceptive services between FPE intervention and control sites. During the preintervention period, FPE sites provided monthly contraceptive visits similarly to control sites (b = 1.42; 95% confidence interval [CI] = 0.31, 6.52). During the intervention period, control sites experienced a nonsignificant average decrease in the number of contraceptive visits (b = 0.76; 95% CI = 0.56, 1.03) compared with the preintervention time frame. However, FPE clinics provided 1.76 times (95% CI = 1.17, 2.66) more contraceptive visits than control sites during the intervention. In the postintervention period, control (b = 1.00; 95% CI = 0.70, 1.41) and FPE sites (b = 1.00; 95% CI = 0.64, 1.56) both showed nonsignificant decreases in the number of contraceptive visits each month. However, contraceptive visits remained higher in FPE sites over the

TABLE 2— Regression Output Assessing Intervention and Time Effects on the Log of Total Contraceptive Visits During Family Planning Elevated Using Interrupted Time Series Analysis: Utah, 2018–2023

Variable	b (95% CI)	Exponentiated b (Exponentiated 95% CI)
(Intercept)	3.53 (2.40, 4.65)	34.06 (11.07, 104.75)
Intervention sites vs control sites	0.35 (−1.18, 1.88)	1.42 (0.31, 6.52)
Preintervention trend effect	0.01 (−0.03, 0.06)	1.01 (0.97, 1.06)
Preintervention trend effect for intervention sites vs control sites	−0.02 (−0.08, 0.04)	0.98 (0.92, 1.04)
Level change for control sites		
During intervention	−0.28 (−0.59, 0.03)	0.76 (0.56, 1.03)
After intervention	0.00 (−0.35, 0.35)	1.00 (0.70, 1.41)
Level change effect for intervention sites vs control sites		
During intervention	0.57 (0.15, 0.98)	1.76 (1.17, 2.66)
After intervention	0.00 (−0.45, 0.45)	1.00 (0.64, 1.56)
Trend effect for control sites		
During intervention	−0.02 (−0.07, 0.04)	0.98 (0.93, 1.04)
After intervention	−0.02 (−0.07, 0.04)	0.98 (0.93, 1.04)
Trend effect for intervention sites vs control sites		
During intervention	0.01 (−0.06, 0.08)	1.01 (0.94, 1.08)
After intervention	−0.01 (−0.08, 0.06)	0.99 (0.92, 1.06)

Note. CI = confidence interval.

course of the study, including after the intervention. Figure 1 provides a graphic overview of monthly contraceptive service provision across study periods.

Proportion of Family Planning Services

Table 3 presents outcomes from the CITSA model assessing the proportion of visits related to contraception among FPE sites compared with their controls. In the preintervention period, FPE sites provided percentages of visits related to contraception similarly to controls

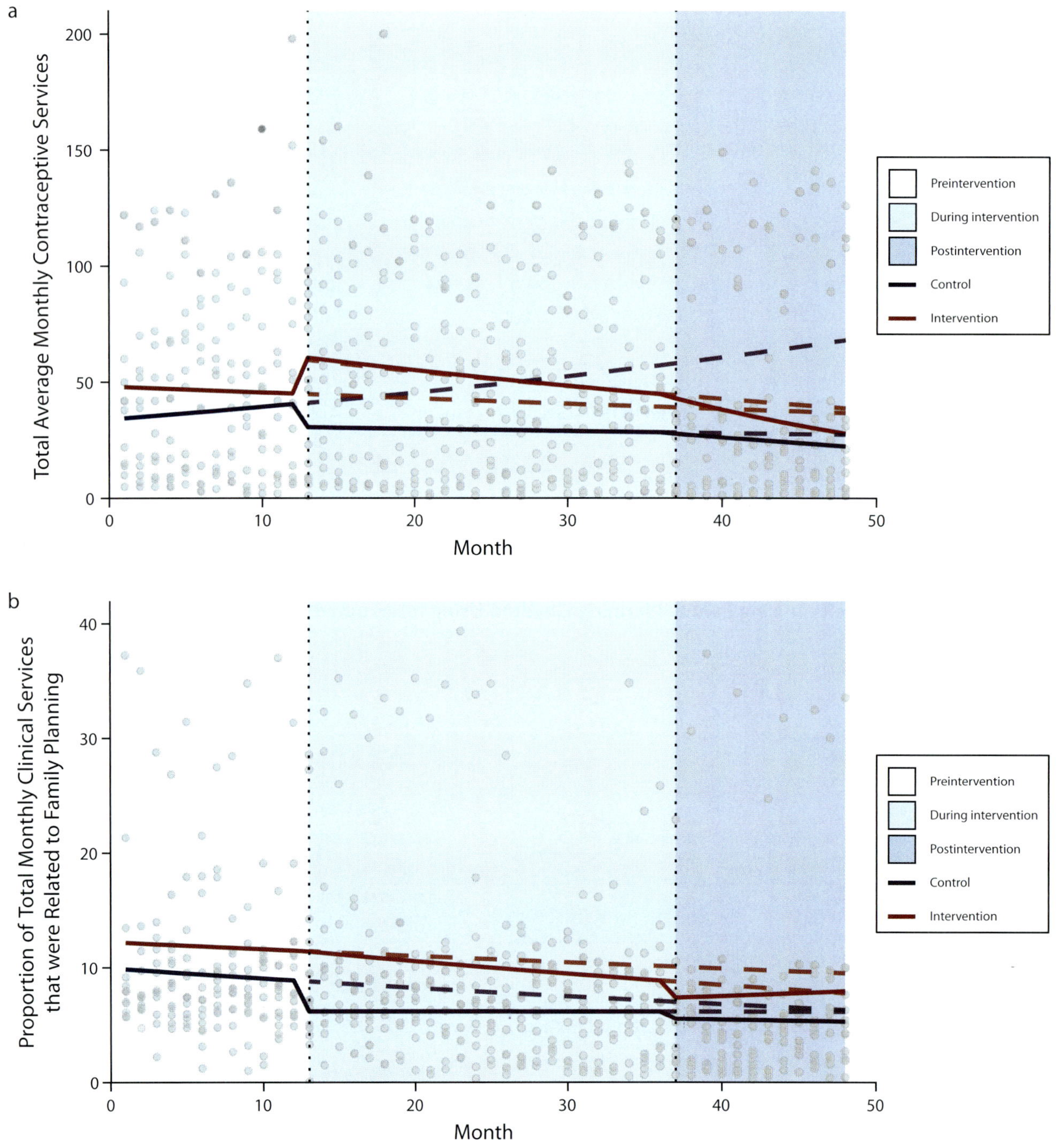

FIGURE 1— **Predicted Outcomes and Counterfactuals Before, During, and After the Family Planning Elevated Contraceptive Access Initiative for (a) the Total Number of Contraceptive Services and (b) the Proportion of Total Clinical Services That Were Related to Contraception: Utah, 2018–2023**

TABLE 3— **Intervention and Time Effects on the Log of Contraceptive Visits' Proportion of Total Visits During Family Planning Elevated Contraceptive Access Program Using Interrupted Time Series Analysis: Utah, 2018–2023**

Variable	b (95% CI)	Exponentiated b (Exponentiated 95% CI)
(Intercept)	2.30 (1.50, 3.10)	9.96 (4.46, 22.24)
Intervention sites vs control sites	0.21 (−0.88, 1.29)	1.23 (0.42, 3.62)
Preintervention trend effect	−0.01 (−0.05, 0.04)	0.99 (0.95, 1.04)
Preintervention trend effect for intervention sites vs control sites	0.00 (−0.06, 0.06)	1.00 (0.95, 1.07)
Level change for control sites		
During intervention	−0.36 (−0.66, −0.06)	0.70 (0.52, 0.94)
After intervention	−0.11 (−0.44, 0.23)	0.90 (0.64, 1.26)
Level change effect for intervention sites vs control sites		
During intervention	0.36 (−0.03, 0.76)	1.44 (0.97, 2.14)
After intervention	−0.08 (−0.51, 0.35)	0.92 (0.60, 1.41)
Trend effect for control sites		
During intervention	0.01 (−0.04, 0.06)	1.01 (0.96, 1.07)
After intervention	0.00 (−0.06, 0.05)	1.00 (0.94, 1.05)
Trend effect for intervention sites vs control sites		
During intervention	−0.01 (−0.09, 0.06)	0.99 (0.92, 1.06)
After intervention	0.02 (−0.05, 0.09)	1.02 (0.95, 1.10)

Note. CI = confidence interval.

(b = 1.23; 95% CI = 0.42, 3.62). During the intervention period, the percentage of visits related to contraception among control sites decreased by a factor of 0.70 (95% CI = 0.52, 0.94). However, among FPE sites during the intervention, the percentage of visits that were contraception-related was larger than that among control sites by a factor of 1.44 (95% CI = 0.97, 2.14). Broadly, the proportion of services related to contraceptive care decreased for both FPE and control sites during and after the intervention period, but the drop was significantly more precipitous for control sites (Figure 1).

DISCUSSION

The FPE intervention led to a significant level increase in the total contraceptive services provided, which was sustained across the intervention period. These shifts were not mirrored by control sites, which saw a moderate, nonsignificant decrease in total contraceptive services during the same period. Importantly, this increase in services occurred during a time of exogenous challenges to contraceptive service provision, including the COVID-19 pandemic, which occurred within 6 months of the FPE start date for 6 of the 9 organizations participating in the intervention. Multiple studies have demonstrated that the pandemic increased barriers to contraceptive services, particularly during the initial months of the pandemic and particularly among people with economic disadvantages.[24–26]

In addition, the FPE intervention began during the same year that Utah's sole Title X grantee (Planned Parenthood of Utah) withdrew from the Title X program, because of the 2019 federal rule change. Studies assessing the impact of the loss of Title X on contraceptive access and preferences have demonstrated clear harms from the rule change, including decreased contraceptive service provision as these sites were forced to increase contraceptive service and method fees to offset the funding losses.[27–29] Our findings show that despite these substantial external challenges, intervention sites increased service provision by 76%, suggesting that participating in FPE largely blunted the impact of these stressors. Though more findings are needed to bolster our work, these findings suggest that contraceptive access initiatives may be an important tool for donors, implementors, and policymakers to consider when facing states or communities with critical stressors to reproductive care.

In addition, while the impact of this initial level increase lasted through the intervention period, FPE sites did not report significant drops in contraceptive service provision after the intervention, though there was a nonsignificant decreasing trend. This suggests a sustained intervention effect, though perhaps one that does not persist indefinitely, as the slopes do trend down nonsignificantly. Unlike other contraceptive access initiatives, such as those conducted in Colorado, Massachusetts, or New Mexico, where state agencies and government act as either progenitors or collaborators in contraceptive access initiatives, FPE was conducted without government partnership, though with an express purpose to demonstrate the need for policy change (increased eligibility for contraceptive services through Medicaid or the Medicaid family planning waiver).[5,9,30] As such, while FPE data did ultimately contribute to policies that increase eligibility for contraception among Utahns,[31] other elements of the initiative (e.g., ongoing access to no-cost methods, media campaigns, cash grants) ended with the intervention. Understanding the longer-term impacts of independent initiatives is an important next step in identifying how contraceptive access initiatives can be leveraged to support sustainable family planning in a variety of contexts, including states with more restrictive reproductive settings.

The total proportion of services related to family planning decreased across both intervention and control sites over time; however, FPE sites were significantly more likely than controls to have visits related to family planning both during and after the intervention period. The overall decrease in proportion of family planning services during the intervention was likely related to the addition of new services, both in response to the COVID-19 pandemic (e.g., COVID-19 testing and treatment) and other challenges to financial viability. For example, the organization participating in FPE that was a Title X recipient lost their Title X grantee status during the FPE intervention period and ultimately expanded their care by offering new acute care services as a way to maintain viability. The addition of new codes and new service types likely increased the number of clinical services provided at sites, contributing to the overall decrease in proportions of contraceptive care relative to total clinical services. Notably, FPE sites maintained a higher proportion of contraceptive service provision during and after the intervention. Though this finding does not reach statistical significance ($P = .07$), it is likely that it has clinical relevance.

Strengths and Limitations

Critical study strengths compared with other contraceptive initiatives include the focus on family planning–related services and all methods of contraception in the context of primary care and family planning–focused settings. Using matched control sites also allowed for real-world comparisons that have not been done previously. FPE was committed to scientific rigor and transparency by publishing protocols and analyzing predetermined primary outcomes.[16]

This implementation study also had several important limitations. The decision to participate in the FPE intervention was organization-driven, and randomizing clinics into the intervention was not feasible. While the incentives and offerings were consistent across sites, organizations had to commit to integrating training into provider schedules and a novel reimbursement system into clinic workflow; therefore, self-selection bias among sites already committed to improving family planning–related care may have contributed to FPE's impact. We also lost 2 control sites during this study because of the pandemic, though our statistical approach attempted to account for this loss. Ultimately, future studies can attempt to replicate FPE findings in times less affected by significant external events. In addition, our inability to measure adolescent access and access to vasectomy in these primary outcome analyses remains a real limitation to the scope of our findings. Finally, although we selected measures of contraceptive provision that approximate access at the clinic level, we acknowledge that these are insufficient to describe all facets of access. Future studies that incorporate other proxy measures, such as the number of days to a scheduled contraceptive appointment, are needed to demonstrate more of this complexity.

FPE occurred during a complex period, with most implementation sites beginning the intervention immediately before or during the COVID-19 pandemic. During this time, Utah also became 1 of 6 states in the nation to lose 100% of its Title X program, divesting more funding and protections for contraceptive care. All told, the impacts of our intervention were inextricably tangled with concurrent environmental complexities. Nonetheless, our outcomes demonstrate that the FPE intervention supported contraceptive service provision despite challenging circumstances.

Public Health Implications

Our findings support the premise that contraceptive access initiatives can play a critical role in contraceptive provision, even under challenging circumstances, and that the impacts of these initiatives extend beyond the intervention itself. AJPH

ABOUT THE AUTHORS

Rebecca G. Simmons, Alexandra Gero, Gentry Carter, Jessica N. Sanders, Caitlin Quade, Jami Baayd, Madeline Mullholand, Sarah Elliott, Kyl Myers, Erica Torres, and David K. Turok are with the Division of Family Planning in the School of Medicine at the University of Utah, Salt Lake City. Justin D. Smith is with the Department of Population Health Sciences at the University of Utah, Salt Lake City.

CORRESPONDENCE

Correspondence should be sent to Rebecca Simmons, 30 Mario Capecchi Dr, Salt Lake City, UT 84112 (e-mail: rebecca.simmons@hsc.utah.edu). Reprints can be ordered at https://www.ajph.org by clicking the "Reprints" link.

PUBLICATION INFORMATION

Full Citation: Simmons RG, Gero A, Carter G, et al. Changes in contraceptive services during Utah's Family Planning Elevated contraceptive access initiative: a prospective assessment of intervention and control sites. *Am J Public Health*. 2025;115(3):387–396.

Acceptance Date: November 4, 2024.

DOI: https://doi.org/10.2105/AJPH.2024.307917

ORCID iDs:

Rebecca G. Simmons https://orcid.org/0000-0003-3516-4585

Alexandra Gero https://orcid.org/0000-0002-0130-0748

Caitlin Quade https://orcid.org/0000-0002-3082-8154

Jami Baayd https://orcid.org/0000-0003-4159-4207

Madeline Mullholand https://orcid.org/0000-0001-5724-803X

Justin D. Smith https://orcid.org/0000-0003-3264-8082

CONTRIBUTORS

All authors contributed to article preparation and writing. R. G. Simmons contributed to study design, analysis plan, data collection, and data analyses. A. Gero contributed to analysis plan, data collection, and data analyses. G. Carter contributed to data analyses. J. N. Sanders contributed to study design, analysis plan, and data analyses. C. Quade, J. Baayd, M. Mullholand, and E. Torres contributed to data collection. S. Elliott contributed to data collection and data analyses. K. Myers contributed to study design, analysis plan, and data collection. D. K. Turok contributed to study design, data collection, and data analyses.

ACKNOWLEDGMENTS

This study was funded by Arnold Ventures, an anonymous foundation, and The Dr Ezekiel R. and Edna Wattis Dumke Foundation. This study received donated devices from Bayer Pharmaceuticals, Cooper Surgical, and Merck/Organon Pharmaceuticals.

The authors would like to extend sincere thanks to all of our clinical partners in this project, Susanna Cohen and Gaby Garcia at the LIFT Lab, and Alan Pruhs at the Association of Utah Community Health.

CONFLICTS OF INTEREST

The authors have no conflicts of interest to disclose.

HUMAN PARTICIPANT PROTECTION

This study was deemed "exempt" by the University of Utah institutional review board (IRB 00117213).

REFERENCES

1. Gomez AM, Bennett AH, Arcara J, et al. Estimates of use of preferred contraceptive method in the United States: a population-based study. *Lancet Reg Health Am*. 2024;30:100662. https://doi.org/10.1016/j.lana.2023.100662
2. Guttmacher Institute. Improving contraceptive use in the United States. Available at: https://www.guttmacher.org/sites/default/files/pdfs/pubs/2008/05/09/ImprovingContraceptiveUse.pdf. Accessed April 25, 2024.
3. Malcolm NM, Patterson KV, Pliska ES, Akbarali S, Moskosky SB, Hart J. A prologue to the *AJPH* supplement: using evidence to expand contraceptive access. *Am J Public Health*. 2022;112(suppl 5):S470–S472. https://doi.org/10.2105/AJPH.2022.306927
4. Malcolm NM, Patterson KV, Pliska ES, Akbarali S, Moskosky SB, Hart J. Scaling up evidence-based practices in contraceptive access initiatives. *Am J Public Health*. 2022;112(suppl 5):S473–S477. https://doi.org/10.2105/AJPH.2022.306824
5. Burapa W, Martinez JR, Daniel KW. Impacts of a statewide effort to expand contraceptive access in New Mexico, 2014–2020. *Am J Public Health*. 2022;112(suppl 5):S541–S544. https://doi.org/10.2105/AJPH.2022.306817
6. Hale N, Lee J, De Jong J, Smith MG, Khoury AJ. Contraceptive method use among a population-based cohort during the South Carolina Choose Well Initiative. *JAMA Netw Open*. 2024;7(4):e248262. https://doi.org/10.1001/jamanetworkopen.2024.8262
7. Smith MG, Hale N, Kelley S, Satterfield K, Beatty KE, Khoury AJ. South Carolina's Choose Well Initiative to Reduce Unintended Pregnancy: rationale, implementation design, and evaluation methodology. *Am J Public Health*. 2022;112(suppl 5):S484–S489. https://doi.org/10.2105/AJPH.2022.306889
8. Boudreaux M, Gifford K, McDuffie MJ, McColl R, Kim T, Knight EK. Delaware Contraceptive Access Now and contraceptive initiation among Medicaid enrollees, 2015–2020. *Am J Public Health*. 2022;112(suppl 5):S537–S540. https://doi.org/10.2105/AJPH.2022.306938
9. Romer SE, Kennedy KI. The Colorado Initiative to Reduce Unintended Pregnancy: contraceptive access and impact on reproductive health. *Am J Public Health*. 2022;112(suppl 5):S532–S536. https://doi.org/10.2105/AJPH.2022.306891
10. Lindo JM, Packham A. How much can expanding access to long-acting reversible contraceptives reduce teen birth rates? *Am Econ J Econ Policy*. 2017;9(3):348–376. https://doi.org/10.1257/pol.20160039
11. Sanders JN, Myers K, Gawron LM, Simmons RG, Turok DK. Contraceptive method use during the community-wide HER Salt Lake contraceptive initiative. *Am J Public Health*. 2018;108(4):550–556. https://doi.org/10.2105/AJPH.2017.304299
12. Lassar M, Tao K, Thiede K. Advancing reproductive health equity through a new contraceptive access initiative. *Am J Public Health*. 2022;112(suppl 5):S500–S503. https://doi.org/10.2105/AJPH.2022.306899
13. McColl R, Gifford K, McDuffie MJ, Boudreaux M. Same-day long-acting reversible contraceptive utilization after a statewide contraceptive access initiative. *Am J Obstet Gynecol*. 2023;228(4):451.e1–451.e8. https://doi.org/10.1016/j.ajog.2022.12.304
14. Cadena DS, Chaudhri A, Scott C. Contraceptive care using reproductive justice principles: beyond access. *Am J Public Health*. 2022;112(suppl 5):S494–S499. https://doi.org/10.2105/AJPH.2022.306915
15. Axelson SM, Sealy GA, McDonald-Mosley RE. Reproductive well-being: a framework for expanding contraceptive access. *Am J Public Health*. 2022;112(suppl 5):S504–S507. https://doi.org/10.2105/AJPH.2022.306898
16. Simmons RG, Myers K, Gero A, et al. Evaluating a longitudinal cohort of clinics engaging in the family planning elevated contraceptive access program: study protocol for a comparative interrupted time series analysis. *JMIR Res Protoc*. 2020;9(10):e18308. https://doi.org/10.2196/18308
17. Simmons RG, Baayd J, Gero A, et al. Implementation and monitoring of the Family Planning Elevated Contraceptive Access Program, Utah, 2018–2019. *Am J Public Health*. 2022;112(suppl 5):S528–S531. https://doi.org/10.2105/AJPH.2022.306935
18. Baayd J, Simmons RG. Protocol for a process evaluation of Family Planning Elevated: a statewide initiative to improve contraceptive access in Utah (USA). *BMJ Open*. 2020;10(10):e038049. https://doi.org/10.1136/bmjopen-2020-038049
19. Cohen SR, Baayd J, García G, et al. Facility-based simulation as a programmatic tool for implementing a statewide contraceptive initiative. *BMC Health Serv Res*. 2022;22(1):965. https://doi.org/10.1186/s12913-022-08332-4
20. Sonfield A. A fragmented system: ensuring comprehensive contraceptive coverage in all US health insurance plans. *Guttmacher Policy Review*. 2021;24. Available at: https://www.guttmacher.org/sites/default/files/article_files/gpr2400121.pdf. Accessed October 24, 2024.
21. Rural Health Information Hub. Am I rural? – Tool. Available at: https://www.ruralhealthinfo.org/am-i-rural. Accessed April 29, 2024.
22. R: A language and environment for statistical computing. 2024. Available at: https://www.R-project.org. Accessed August 25, 2024.

23. Pinheiro J, Bates D. R Core Team. nlme: linear and nonlinear mixed effects models. 2023. Available at: https://CRAN.R-project.org/package=nlme. Accessed August 25, 2024.
24. Curtis KM, Kulkarni AD, Nguyen AT, et al. Changes in commercial insurance claims for contraceptive services during the beginning of the COVID-19 pandemic—United States, January 2019–September 2020. *Womens Health Issues*. 2024;34(2):186–196. https://doi.org/10.1016/j.whi.2023.10.004
25. Steenland MW, Geiger CK, Chen L, et al. Declines in contraceptive visits in the United States during the COVID-19 pandemic. *Contraception*. 2021;104(6):593–599. https://doi.org/10.1016/j.contraception.2021.08.003
26. Diamond-Smith N, Logan R, Marshall C, et al. COVID-19's impact on contraception experiences: exacerbation of structural inequities in women's health. *Contraception*. 2021;104(6):600–605. https://doi.org/10.1016/j.contraception.2021.08.011
27. Easter R, Friedrich-Karnik A, Kavanaugh ML. Any restrictions on reproductive health care harm reproductive autonomy: evidence from four states. New York, NY: Guttmacher Institute; 2024. https://doi.org/10.1363/2024.300471
28. Kavanaugh ML, Leong E, Haas M. Measuring the relationship between the 2019 Title X Final Rule and patients' sexual and reproductive health care access and behavior in Iowa using a difference-in-difference approach. *Sex Res Soc Policy*. 2024;21(2):598–615. https://doi.org/10.1007/s13178-023-00876-2
29. Smith CW, Kreitzer RJ, Kane KA, Saunders TM. Contraception deserts: the effects of Title X rule changes on access to reproductive health care resources. *Polit Gend*. 2022;18(3):672–707. https://doi.org/10.1017/S1743923X2100009X
30. White KO, Lerner NM, LeRoy L, Decker E, Clark J. Massachusetts initiative to improve contraceptive services: a tale of two programs. *Am J Public Health*. 2022;112(suppl 5):S478–S483. https://doi.org/10.2105/AJPH.2022.306905
31. Utah Department of Health and Human Services. State of Utah's Medicaid Reform 1115 Demonstration. 2023. Available at: https://medicaid.utah.gov/Documents/pdfs/Family%20Planning%20Services.pdf. Accessed August 3, 2024.

Changes to Parental Consent Requirements for Abortion in Massachusetts and Impact on Timeliness of Care for Adolescents Aged 16 to 17 Years

Isabel Fulcher, PhD, Kara Kimball, MD, Zarah Rosen, MD, Jennifer Fortin, MPH, Namita Arunkumar, MD, Danielle Gelfand, BA, Elizabeth Janiak, ScD, and Luu Ireland, MD, MPH

See also Rosen, p. 262.

Objectives. To measure the effect of the ROE Act, which eliminated parental consent requirements for abortion for individuals ages 16 to 17 years, on abortion timing for adolescents in this age group in Massachusetts.

Methods. The primary outcome was gestational duration at abortion for individuals aged 16 to 19 years at Planned Parenthood League of Massachusetts from 2017 to 2022. Our control group included abortions among those aged 18 to 19 years. In our primary analysis, we used a comparative interrupted time series with a linear model to capture temporal trends, seasonality, whether an abortion was undergone during the acute phase of the COVID-19 pandemic, previous abortion, and race/ethnicity categories.

Results. Minors aged 16 to 17 years underwent 749 abortions during the study. Individuals aged 18 to 19 years underwent 2773 abortions. The ROE Act resulted in a 5.46-day decrease in gestational duration at abortion among minors (95% confidence interval = −11.82, 0.91).

Conclusions. Removal of the parental involvement requirement for adolescents aged 16 to 17 years in Massachusetts led to minors undergoing abortions at earlier gestational durations, highlighting the importance of potential impacts of similar legislation to decrease barriers to abortion access for minors.
(*Am J Public Health*. 2025;115(3):397–402. https://doi.org/10.2105/AJPH.2024.307918)

AJPH March 2025, Vol. 115, No. 3

In June 2022, the US Supreme Court removed federal protections for abortion access in *Dobbs v. Jackson Women's Health Organization*,[1] exacerbating the existing crisis in abortion access.[2] Inequities in abortion access are long-standing and include younger people's access to care.[3] Each year, adolescents aged 15 to 17 years receive approximately 3%, and adolescents younger than 15 years approximately 0.2%, of all abortions in the United States.[4] Adolescents face more barriers to abortion care than do their adult counterparts, both because of logistical challenges and as a direct result of additional consent requirements.[5] As of September 2024, there are 14 states with total abortion bans. An additional 4 states ban abortion at 6 weeks gestation, effectively making it unavailable to most individuals. Abortion remains more broadly legal in 33 states. Of these, 23 have parental involvement laws in effect.[6,7]

In 1979, the Supreme Court ruling in *Bellotti v. Baird* (443 US 622) upheld the constitutionality of state laws requiring parental involvement, through consent or notification, for minors seeking abortion. The *Bellotti* case was a challenge to the oldest and one of the strictest parental involvement laws in the United States in Massachusetts. The *Bellotti* decision upheld the right of states to require parental consent for abortion as long as there was an alternative process for those who could not obtain parental consent. In response, most states implemented a form of judicial bypass, allowing those younger than 18 years to seek approval for abortion through a judge.[8] Although judicial bypass was intended as a safeguard, it introduces significant delays, drives up abortion costs, and disproportionately affects youths who are of low income and are a Black, Indigenous, or other person of color.[9–12]

These negative effects of parental involvement laws have been documented over a course of decades and in many states, including Massachusetts.[13–16] Our previous research demonstrated that in Massachusetts, minors who were able to obtain parental consent underwent an abortion on average 8.6 days after initial contact with their abortion provider, whereas those who needed to obtain judicial bypass waited 14.8 days.[9] Delays force minors into later gestational durations, increasing the cost of abortion care and limiting options, often meaning the difference between accessing medication abortion or requiring a procedural abortion. Delayed access to abortion also causes more time missed from school or work as well as increased travel and other costs.[10,17] Even more critical is the uncertainty of the outcome of judicial bypass, which has exhibited increased abortion denial rates.[18,19]

In December 2020, the Massachusetts state legislature removed the requirement for parental consent for abortion care for pregnant adolescents aged 16 to 17 years as part of a legislative package known as the ROE Act.[20] This legislation did not alter the required parental consent for minors aged 15 years or younger. We sought to determine how this policy change affected timeliness of abortion care. We hypothesized that the removal of the parental consent requirement for this age group would decrease the average gestational duration at time of abortion for minors aged 16 to 17 years.

METHODS

We extracted information on all abortions among individuals aged 16 to 19 years at Planned Parenthood League of Massachusetts from May 1, 2017, through June 30, 2022. Planned Parenthood League of Massachusetts operates 3 abortion care facilities across the state, located in Boston, Worcester, and Springfield, Massachusetts.

Our primary analysis was a comparative interrupted time series that modeled average gestational duration in days among affected minors and a control group before versus after the removal of the parental consent requirement, which went into effect January 1, 2021. In comparative interrupted time series analyses, information from a baseline period (i.e., parental consent requirement) and a control group that was not exposed to the intervention (i.e., abortions not impacted by the parental consent requirement) were leveraged to estimate the impact of an intervention at an aggregate level. Our control group consisted of abortions among those aged 18 and 19 years at Planned Parenthood League of Massachusetts. We chose this group because they were closest in age to minors but unaffected by parental consent requirements. The baseline period included abortions between May 1, 2017, and December 31, 2020; the post–parental consent period included abortions between January 1, 2021 and June 30, 2022. We excluded post-*Dobbs* data, considering the increased number of patients traveling into Massachusetts from out of state to seek abortion care and the potential to confound results.[21]

Our primary outcome of interest was gestational duration at abortion in days. The patient-level covariates we extracted were age, number of previous abortions, race and Hispanic ethnicity category, payment type used for abortion (i.e., private insurance, public insurance, support from abortion funds, or self-payment), and abortion type (medication or procedural). We extracted data using SQL (Structured Query Language) queries of the Athena medical and Epic medical record systems. Two independent reviewers manually abstracted gestational duration in weeks and days from the patient's medical chart for each record.

We report summary statistics of the primary outcome and all covariates stratified by age group (minors vs older individuals) and time period (before and after the ROE Act). For the primary comparative interrupted time series analysis, we used a linear model with terms to capture temporal trends, seasonality, confounders of race and Hispanic ethnicity, and having had a previous abortion. Notably, we did not adjust for payment type used on date of service or abortion type, as these variables are potential mediators (not confounders) of the effect of the removal of parental consent requirements on gestational duration at abortion. We used GEE (generalized estimating equations) with an independent working correlation structure to account for multiple abortions per patient during the study period. The mean model formula for the comparative interrupted time series model was as follows:

$$\begin{aligned} Y_t = {} & \beta_0 + \beta_1 t + \beta_2 ROE + \beta_3 minor \\ & + \beta_4 (t * minor) + \beta_5 (ROE * minor) \\ & + \sum_j \beta_{6,j} month_j + \sum_k \beta_{7,k} race_k \\ & + \beta_8 covid + \beta_9 prior, \end{aligned} \quad (1)$$

where t indicates number of months since May 1, 2017, Y_t is the gestational duration in days at abortion in month *t*, and *ROE* and *minor* are binary indicators of the abortion occurring in the post-ROE period and among a minor, respectively. The main effect of interest is β_5, which is the mean change in gestational duration at abortion attributable to the removal of parental involvement requirements for persons aged 16 and 17 years. *Prior* and *covid* are indicator variables for whether the patient ever had a previous abortion and whether the abortion occurred during the acute phase of the COVID-19 pandemic (March 15, 2020–December 31, 2020), respectively.[22] *Month* and *race* are categorical variables, with January and non-Hispanic White as respective reference levels.

RESULTS

We extracted information on 749 abortions among persons aged 16 and 17 years with 524 abortions during the parental consent period and 225 abortions after this period for those aged 16 or 17 years. Comparing the pre- and post-ROE Act periods, the average gestational duration dropped from 62.0 to 58.3 days ($P = .020$; Table 1). The use of medication abortion increased from 39.3% to 51.1% ($P = .003$). The use of abortion funding significantly increased from 6.5% to 11.6% ($P = .002$). The proportion of Hispanic White individuals aged 16 or 17 years seeking abortion increased from 5.2% to 15.6% ($P < .001$).

For our primary analysis, we extracted information on 2773 abortions among older individuals for use as a control group (descriptive statistics are in Table 1). Comparing the pre- and

TABLE 1— Distribution of Key Variables Among Persons Receiving Abortion at Planned Parenthood League of Massachusetts, Stratified by Period and Age Group: 2017–2022

	Minors, Mean ±SD or No. (%)		Young Adults, Mean ±SD or No. (%)		
Variable	During Parental Consent Era[a] (n = 524)	After Parental Consent Removed[b] (n = 225)	During Parental Consent Era[a] (n = 2026)	After Parental Consent Removed[b] (n = 747)	P^c
Gestational duration at abortion, days	62.0 ±22.5	58.3 ±18.6	58.1 ±20.9	56.7 ±19.6	.02
Race and Hispanic ethnicity					<.001
Non-Hispanic White	155 (29.6)	64 (28.4)	761 (37.6)	262 (35.1)	
Non-Hispanic Black	119 (22.7)	50 (22.2)	390 (19.2)	139 (18.6)	
Hispanic	104 (19.8)	37 (16.4)	381 (18.8)	126 (16.9)	
Hispanic White	27 (5.2)	35 (15.6)	123 (6.1)	77 (10.3)	
Hispanic Black	20 (3.8)	10 (4.4)	64 (3.2)	55 (7.4)	
Non-Hispanic Asian	17 (3.2)	1 (0.4)	98 (4.8)	21 (2.8)	
Grouped[d]	27 (5.2)	13 (5.8)	116 (5.7)	29 (3.9)	
Unknown	55 (10.5)	15 (6.7)	93 (4.6)	38 (5.1)	
Previous abortion					.96
0	417 (79.6)	176 (78.2)	1461 (72.1)	528 (70.7)	
≥1	105 (20.0)	43 (19.1)	563 (27.8)	197 (26.4)	
Missing	2 (0.4)	6 (2.7)	2 (0.1)	22 (2.9)	
Service type					.003
Medication	206 (39.3)	115 (51.1)	1007 (49.7)	440 (58.9)	
Surgical	315 (60.1)	108 (48.0)	1016 (50.1)	304 (40.7)	
Missing	3 (0.6)	2 (0.9)	3 (0.1)	3 (0.4)	
Insurance type on date of service					.002
Abortion fund	34 (6.5)	26 (11.6)	89 (4.4)	38 (5.1)	
Private	287 (54.8)	101 (44.9)	1119 (55.2)	366 (49.0)	
Public	166 (31.7)	68 (30.2)	463 (22.9)	212 (28.4)	
Self-pay	37 (7.1)	30 (13.3)	355 (17.5)	131 (17.5)	

[a]May 1, 2017–December 31, 2022.
[b]January 1, 2021–June 30, 2022.
[c]Wilcoxon rank sum test used for continuous variables; χ^2 test used for categorical variables.
[d]Grouped includes patients identifying as American Indian and Alaska Native, Other Pacific Islander, and Other.

TABLE 2— Results From Comparative Interrupted Time Series Model, Including Age Group and Time Period Terms: Massachusetts, 2017–2022

	b (95% CI)
Intercept	59.79 (56.50, 63.08)
Time, among young adults	−0.04 (−0.13, 0.05)
After ROE Act vs before ROE Act, among young adults	−0.08 (−3.88, 3.71)
Minors vs young adults in May 2017	1.43 (−2.61, 5.47)
Interaction: time, minor	0.09 (−0.06, 0.25)
Interaction: ROE Act, minor	−5.46 (−11.82, 0.90)

Note. CI = confidence interval; ROE Act = An Act to Remove Obstacles and Expand Abortion Access.[20] Parameter estimates for COVID-19 period, month, race/ethnicity, and prior abortion categories are excluded for ease of exposition.

post-ROE Act periods as was done in the intervention group, the average gestational duration dropped from 58.1 to 56.7 days ($P = .020$; Table 1). The final comparative interrupted time series model included 3522 abortions among 3226 unique patients.

We found that the elimination of parental consent for persons aged 16 or 17 years led to these youths receiving their abortions an average of 5.46 days sooner than when parental consent was required (95% confidence interval [CI] = −11.82, 0.91; Table 2). Although not statistically significant, these results highlight an important trend in which minors obtain abortions at earlier gestational durations when they are not required to obtain parental consent or judicial bypass. Figure 1 is a visual representation of these findings in which the gap in gestational duration at abortion decreased after the removal of the parental involvement requirement on January 1, 2021.

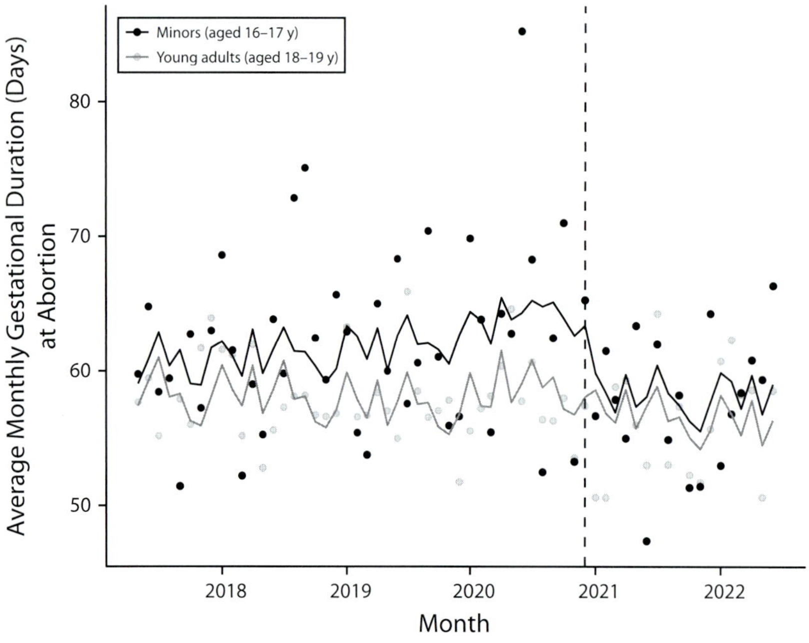

FIGURE 1— Average Gestational Duration (in Days) at Abortion by Month Before Versus After Removal of Parental Consent Requirement for Those Aged 16 or 17 years: Massachusetts, 2017–2022

DISCUSSION

Removal of the parental consent requirement resulted in a trend toward earlier gestational duration at abortion for individuals aged 16 or 17 years in Massachusetts. Although our study does not establish causality, it indicates that legislative measures may influence minors' access to abortion. Notably, the average decrease in gestational duration of 5.46 days corresponds almost exactly to the average time to obtain judicial bypass in our 2019 study (5.2 days adjusted difference).[9] However, it is possible that the removal of the parental involvement requirement expedites access to abortion both for young people who would have otherwise been required to access judicial bypass and for young people with parental support. By eliminating the parental consent requirement, the state enabled young persons to choose who can accompany them for their care, rather than being forced to wait until a custodial parent's work schedule or other obligations permits them to take the minor to an abortion appointment so that they may consent to care on their child's behalf.

In addition to our primary outcome, a number of additional noteworthy findings occurred. We found an increase in the proportion of medication abortion. It is possible that decreased gestational duration at abortion for minors following the removal of the parental consent requirement increased eligibility and preference for medication over

AJPH March 2025, Vol. 115, No. 3

procedural abortion. However, changes in health care utilization related to the COVID-19 pandemic, such as protocols that decreased in-person visits, may also be responsible, as there was a 27% increase in the rate of requests for medication abortion nationwide during the first month of the pandemic, March 2020.[23] We also observed an increase in support from abortion funds and self-paid care and a concomitant decrease in the use of private insurance. Future research is merited to explore the reason for this change in funding for abortion care.

We observed an increase in the proportion of abortion patients who identify as Hispanic ethnicity and White race, alongside a decrease in the proportion whose race and ethnicity were unknown. We hypothesize that these shifts represent a change in the completeness of self-report of race/ethnicity rather than a true demographic shift in the population of patients served to include more Hispanic individuals. We know of no specific policy change or other event that would differentially affect Hispanic-identified individuals in this period.

Limitations

The greatest limitation of this study is our relatively small sample size. Although results appear to show a decrease in gestational duration at abortion after the parental involvement requirement was removed, this difference is not statistically significant at traditionally accepted levels ($P < .05$). Because of the limited number of abortions among minors younger than 16 years, we were unable to compare this group with minors aged 16 to 17 years, limiting our ability to interpret access to abortion care for minors in this younger age group.

Unfortunately, we were not able to extend our study period because of the potential for significant confounding by the *Dobbs* decision on June 24, 2022. Specifically, parallel research has shown an increase in overall abortion volume and in interstate travel for abortion into Massachusetts after the *Dobbs* decision, which could plausibly result in abortion delay for in-state residents and later average gestational duration at coming in for care among out-of-state travelers.[21]

Furthermore, given the broad state by state variability in abortion access, our findings may not be generalizable beyond Massachusetts. Studies of the effect of removing parental involvement laws in other states that have recently done so, such as Illinois and Minnesota, will provide further data on the range of possible consequences of this policy change.

An additional limitation of our study was our inability to include data from additional clinics in the area, which may have served different patient populations. Future studies should explore the possibility of incorporating these clinics to capture a broader and more representative sample.

Public Health Implications

The removal of the parental involvement requirement for adolescents aged 16 to 17 years in Massachusetts was associated with an average 5.46-day decrease in gestational duration at abortion among this age group. The results support our hypothesis that mandated parental consent results in a delay in care for minors obtaining abortions. Although medical and procedural abortions are safe, with low complication rates at all stages of gestation, the risk of complications increases by approximately 38% for each additional week beyond 8 weeks.[24]

These results are relevant in evaluating the potential impact of similar legislation and in supporting the critical need to advocate fewer barriers in minors' access to abortion. Our data support other states working to remove medically unnecessary restrictions and suggest that removing parental consent for minors aged 15 years and younger in Massachusetts could also help ensure expeditious access to abortion care. AJPH

ABOUT THE AUTHORS

Isabel Fulcher is with the Department of Global Health and Social Medicine, Harvard Medical School, Boston, MA. Isabel Fulcher, Jennifer Fortin, Namita Arunkumar, Danielle Gelfand, Elizabeth Janiak, and Luu Ireland are with Planned Parenthood League of Massachusetts, Boston. Kara Kimball, Zarah Rosen, and Luu Ireland are with the Obstetrics and Gynecology Department, UMass Memorial Health, Worcester. Elizabeth Janiak is with Social and Behavioral Sciences, Harvard T. H. Chan School of Public Health, Boston, MA.

CORRESPONDENCE

Correspondence should be sent to Zarah Rosen, Planned Parenthood League of Massachusetts, 1055 Commonwealth Avenue, Boston, MA 02215 (e-mail: zarah.rosen@umassmemorial.org). Reprints can be ordered at https://www.ajph.org by clicking the "Reprints" link.

PUBLICATION INFORMATION

Full Citation: Fulcher I, Kimball K, Rosen Z, et al. Changes to parental consent requirements for abortion in Massachusetts and impact on timeliness of care for adolescents aged 16 to 17 years. *Am J Public Health*. 2025;115(3):397–402.

Acceptance Date: November 4, 2024.

DOI: https://doi.org/10.2105/AJPH.2024.307918

ORCID iD:
Luu Ireland https://orcid.org/0000-0001-6856-9226

CONTRIBUTORS

I. Fulcher, K. Kimball, J. Fortin, N. Arunkumar, D. Gelfand, E. Janiak, and L. Ireland collected the data. I. Fulcher, E. Janiak, and L. Ireland conceptualized and planned the research and edited the article. K. Kimball, J. Fortin, N. Arunkumar, and D. Gelfand collated the data. Z. Rosen coordinated article submission and wrote the article.

ACKNOWLEDGMENTS

The authors thank Youri Hwang, PhD, for assistance with querying the medical record.

Note. The findings and conclusions in this article are those of the authors and do not necessarily reflect the views of the Planned Parenthood Federation of America, Inc.

CONFLICTS OF INTEREST

We have no conflicts of interest to disclose.

HUMAN PARTICIPANT PROTECTION

The University of Massachusetts Medical School institutional review board approved this study (ID H00023917).

REFERENCES

1. *Dobbs v. Jackson Women's Health Organization*, 597 US 215 (2022).
2. Kaufman R, Brown R, Martínez Coral C, Jacob J, Onyango M, Thomasen K. Global impacts of *Dobbs v. Jackson Women's Health Organization* and abortion regression in the United States. *Sex Reprod Health Matters*. 2022;30(1):2135574. https://doi.org/10.1080/26410397.2022.2135574
3. Finer LB, Frohwirth LF, Dauphinee LA, Singh S, Moore AM. Timing of steps and reasons for delays in obtaining abortions in the United States. *Contraception*. 2006;74(4):334–344. https://doi.org/10.1016/j.contraception.2006.04.010
4. Jerman J, Jones RK, Onda T. Characteristics of US abortion patients in 2014 and changes since 2008. May 2016. Available at: https://www.guttmacher.org/report/characteristics-us-abortion-patients-2014. Accessed December 27, 2024.
5. Reddy DM. Effect of mandatory parental notification on adolescent girls' use of sexual health care services. *JAMA*. 2002;288(6):710–714. https://doi.org/10.1001/jama.288.6.710
6. Kaiser Family Foundation. Abortion policy: gestational limits and exceptions. Available at: https://www.kff.org/womens-health-policy/state-indicator/gestational-limit-abortions. Accessed December 27, 2024.
7. Kaiser Family Foundation. Parental consent/notification for minors seeking abortion. September 2024. Available at: https://www.kff.org/womens-health-policy/state-indicator/parental-consent notification. Accessed December 27, 2024.
8. *Bellotti v. Baird*, 443 US 622 (1979).
9. Janiak E, Fulcher IR, Cottrill AA, et al. Massachusetts' parental consent law and procedural timing among adolescents undergoing abortion. *Obstet Gynecol*. 2019;133(5):978–986. https://doi.org/10.1097/AOG.0000000000003190
10. Gilbert AL, Fulcher IR, Cottrill AA, Janiak E. The financial burden of antiquated laws: the case of Massachusetts' parental involvement law for abortion. *Womens Health Rep (New Rochelle)*. 2021;2(1):550–556. https://doi.org/10.1089/whr.2021.0002
11. Ralph LJ, King E, Belusa E, Foster DG, Brindis CD, Biggs MA. The impact of a parental notification requirement on Illinois minors' access to and decision-making around abortion. *J Adolesc Health*. 2018;62(3):281–287. https://doi.org/10.1016/j.jadohealth.2017.09.031
12. Dennis A, Henshaw SK, Joyce TJ, Finer LB, Blanchard K. The impact of laws requiring parental involvement for abortion: a literature review. March 2009. Available at: https://www.guttmacher.org/sites/default/files/pdfs/pubs/ParentalInvolvementLaws.pdf. Accessed December 27, 2024.
13. Cartoof VG, Klerman LV. Parental consent for abortion: impact of the Massachusetts law. *Am J Public Health*. 1986;76(4):397–400. https://doi.org/10.2105/AJPH.76.4.397
14. MacAfee L, Castle J, Theiler RN. Association between the New Hampshire parental notification law and minors undergoing abortions in northern New England. *Obstet Gynecol*. 2015;125(1):170–174. https://doi.org/10.1097/AOG.0000000000000585
15. Henshaw SK. The impact of requirements for parental consent on minors' abortions in Mississippi. *Fam Plann Perspect*. 1995;27(3):120–122. https://doi.org/10.2307/2136110
16. Rogers JL, Boruch RF, Stoms GB, DeMoya D. Impact of the Minnesota parental notification law on abortion and birth. *Am J Public Health*. 1991;81(3):294–298. https://doi.org/10.2105/AJPH.81.3.294
17. Coleman-Minahan K, Stevenson AJ, Obront E, Hays S. Young women's experiences obtaining judicial bypass for abortion in Texas. *J Adolesc Health*. 2019;64(1):20–25. https://doi.org/10.1016/j.jadohealth.2018.07.017
18. Stevenson AJ, Coleman-Minahan K. Use of judicial bypass of mandatory parental consent to access abortion and judicial bypass denials, Florida and Texas, 2018–2021. *Am J Public Health*. 2023;113(3):316–319. https://doi.org/10.2105/AJPH.2022.307173
19. White K, Narasimhan S, Hartwig SA, et al. Parental involvement policies for minors seeking abortion in the Southeast and quality of care. *Sex Res Social Policy*. 2022;19(1):264–272. https://doi.org/10.1007/s13178-021-00539-0
20. An Act to Remove Obstacles and Expand Abortion Access, S.1209, 191st Gen. Ct. (Mass. 2020). Available at: https://malegislature.gov. Accessed December 27, 2024.
21. Keefe-Oates B, Fulcher I, Fortin J, et al. Use of abortion services in Massachusetts after the Dobbs decision among in-state vs out-of-state residents. *JAMA Netw Open*. 2023;6(9):e2332400. https://doi.org/10.1001/jamanetworkopen.2023.32400
22. Fulcher IR, Onwuzurike C, Goldberg AB, Cottrill AA, Fortin J, Janiak E. The impact of the COVID-19 pandemic on abortion care utilization and disparities by age. *Am J Obstet Gynecol*. 2022;226(6):819.e1–819.e15. https://doi.org/10.1016/j.ajog.2022.01.025
23. Tschann M, Ly ES, Hilliard S, Lange HLH. Changes to medication abortion clinical practices in response to the COVID-19 pandemic. *Contraception*. 2021;104(1):77–81. https://doi.org/10.1016/j.contraception.2021.04.010
24. Paul M, Lichtenberg ES, Borgatta L, Grimes DA, Stubblefield PG, Creinin MD, eds. *Management of Unintended and Abnormal Pregnancy: Comprehensive Abortion Care*. Chichester, UK: Blackwell Publishing; 2009. https://doi.org/10.1002/9781444313031

Impact of Gender Identity Field in the Veterans Health Administration Electronic Health Record, 2016–2023

Sarah M. Leder, MSW, A. Alex McConnell, PhD, Shane Lamba, MPH, Chava Sonnier, MSOD, Alexis R. Matza, PhD, Wyatt E. Meriwether, PhD, George R. Brown, MD, Jillian C. Shipherd, PhD, Michael R. Kauth, PhD, and Kenneth T. Jones, PhD

See also Patterson, p. 268.

Objectives. To distinguish differences in physical and mental health between transgender and gender-diverse (TGD) veterans identified via diagnostic codes, self-identification, and their combination.

Methods. We used sociodemographic characteristics and physical and mental health diagnoses for TGD veterans receiving care in Veterans Health Administration (VHA).

Results. Among the cohort of 12 745 TGD veterans, 69.3% were identified solely using self-reported gender identity data, 23.4% were identified using only TGD-related diagnostic codes, and 7.2% had both TGD-related diagnostic codes and gender identity data in their medical record. TGD veterans identified using self-reported gender identity data were younger and more racially and ethnically diverse compared with those identified with only diagnostic codes. Across nearly all independently examined health conditions, TGD veterans identified via self-reported gender identity were at lower risk compared with those identified via diagnostic codes.

Conclusions. Inferences drawn from studies of TGD veteran health may be significantly impacted by choice of methodology for defining the TGD veteran cohort. New analyses using self-reported gender identity data, as opposed to diagnostic codes, are critical to understand the health of this population within VHA. (*Am J Public Health*. 2025;115(3):403–413. https://doi.org/10.2105/AJPH.2024.307920)

AJPH March 2025, Vol. 115, No. 3

Transgender and gender-diverse (TGD) persons are overrepresented in military and veteran populations, which makes the Veterans Health Administration (VHA) one of the largest integrated health care providers for TGD adults in the United States.[1–3] However, TGD veterans have historically been invisible in most VHA quality improvement efforts and research.[4] Self-reported gender identity information has only recently been included in the VHA electronic health record (EHR) and has been slow to populate, despite self-reporting being the gold standard for identifying TGD people.[5] Quality improvement and research activities have relied on outdated, stigmatizing TGD-related *International Classification of Diseases, Ninth* or *Tenth Revisions, Clinical Modification* (Hyattsville, MD: National Center for Health Statistics; 1980 and 2015) codes (hereafter referred to as diagnostic codes or *ICD* codes) to identify TGD veterans because of the historical lack of gender identity data in VHA administrative systems.[6] We examined how estimates of TGD veteran demographics and health differ when using self-reported gender identity data, TGD-related diagnostic codes, or their combination to identify TGD veterans in VHA.

USING DIAGNOSTIC CODES TO INFER GENDER

Few studies have used survey data with gender identity[7,8] to study the health and health care use of TGD veterans. In contrast, much of the literature has relied on diagnostic codes to identify presumably transgender veterans accessing VHA health care.[9] In most studies, veterans who lack these diagnoses, either because they do not meet the criteria or have never been evaluated for these diagnoses, are used as controls and assumed to be cisgender, a sometimes erroneous assumption given that not all TGD people experience gender dysphoria or disclose such experiences to their health care providers.[6] These studies have consistently shown higher rates of psychiatric conditions among TGD veterans, including posttraumatic stress disorder (PTSD), depression, and serious mental illness, compared with veterans without such diagnostic codes in their medical records.[10,11] TGD veterans identified using diagnostic codes also have high rates of suicide,[10,12] elevated alcohol and nonalcohol substance use disorders,[10,11,13,14] and high rates of social risk factors such as history of military sexual trauma, homelessness, economic insecurity, and incarceration.[15–17]

Physical health disparities are also apparent, though relatively underresearched compared with psychiatric disparities. VHA researchers[10] found that TGD veterans are at 1.5 to 2 times higher risk for health conditions, including heart attack, benign prostatic hyperplasia, stroke, chronic obstructive pulmonary disease, congestive heart failure, diabetes, high cholesterol, high blood pressure, obesity, and kidney disease. The rate of HIV diagnosis was 5 times higher compared with controls.[10]

IMPLICATIONS OF THE DIAGNOSTIC APPROACH

While the diagnostic approach has historically been the primary means to leverage EHR data to understand the population-level health of TGD veterans using VHA services, it has multiple methodological limitations.[6] First, it is inherently pathologizing and could inflate estimates of illness, particularly in the domain of mental health. Specifically, TGD veterans identified solely by a gender dysphoria diagnosis must have, by definition, received a diagnosis that requires clinically significant distress or impairment to be present,[18] which may also be associated with more comorbidities or severe dysphoria.[19] As such, veterans identified via self-reported gender identity data may appear comparatively healthier. Second, not all TGD people experience distress related to their gender identity or seek medical interventions to facilitate their transition. Therefore, veterans with related diagnostic codes represent only a subset of TGD veterans, precluding accurate estimates of the size, characteristics, and health of TGD veterans receiving services in VHA. Finally, there have been repeated calls by TGD people, advocates, researchers, and policymakers to better understand intragroup differences.[19] For example, using the diagnostic approach does not distinguish nonbinary individuals or reliably differentiate transgender women from transgender men in analyses without additional data such as hormone therapy prescriptions[20] or surgical history,[21] which also rely on assumptions and may promote misclassification.

GENDER IDENTITY IN VHA RECORDS

VHA created an optional self-reported gender identity data field in its EHR in 2017, which was not initially visible to providers nor well populated. As a consequence, researchers continued to rely on TGD-related diagnostic codes to identify the TGD veteran population in the EHR. Further complicating the picture, veterans can update their birth sex to align with their gender identity in the EHR. However, there is no established method to determine whether the change was intentionally made to reflect gender identity or to fix a data entry error. The gender identity field became visible to VHA providers in 2021 to increase the provision of affirming care. Since then, VHA developed multiple paths for veterans to enter and update their gender identity information in the medical record system. The gender identity field is a self-reported field and can be completed by veterans by editing their profile information on VA.gov, completing form 10-10EZ or 10-10EZR, or by requesting that an eligibility and enrollment staff member update the information. However, it should be noted that veterans have to initiate this change and may be unaware that they can do so, contributing to a high level of missingness in this data field. Despite these barriers to entry, 2.3 million of approximately 6 million active VHA health care users have gender identity data recorded.

In the current study, we sought to understand how estimates of TGD veterans' demographic characteristics and health conditions vary based on different methods of defining the sample cohort to inform future analyses of TGD veteran health and well-being.

METHODS

Data were from VHA's corporate data warehouse, which contains health record information from the EHR.

Participants

Veterans included in this analysis were confined to those with at least 1 VHA outpatient visit between fiscal years 2017 and 2023 (October 1, 2016, to September 30, 2023), ensuring an opportunity for data collection. We adapted our inclusion criteria regarding medical diagnostic codes from Brown and Jones's 2016 study on transgender veterans[10] and previous validation work.[22]

We defined a TGD veteran as a patient with at least 1 of the 3 following criteria present in their EHR: TGD-related *ICD* codes, an entry in the gender identity field indicating a TGD identity, or a gender identity entry discrepant from the birth sex field.[23] We used the following *ICD* codes to create the TGD veteran cohort: 302.3 (transvestic fetishism), 302.5X (trans-sexualism), 302.6 (gender identity disorder in children), and 302.85 (gender identity disorder in adolescents or adults) from *ICD-9-CM*, and F64.X (gender identity disorders), F65.1 (transvestic fetishism), and Z87.890 (personal history of sex reassignment) from *ICD-10-CM*.[22] Gender identity options were "Man," "Woman," "Transgender Man," "Transgender Woman," "Non-binary," "Prefer not to answer," or "A gender not listed here." For this study, veterans were considered TGD if they responded, "Transgender Man," "Transgender Woman," "Nonbinary," or "A gender not listed here," or if they selected "Man" or "Woman" and had a discordant value in the birth sex field (e.g., gender identity selected was "Woman" while birth sex indicated male).

Measures

Sociodemographic characteristics. Once the cohort of TGD veterans was established, we used unique identifiers to pull sociodemographic characteristics, service, and enrollment information from the corporate data warehouse. When veterans had more than 1 entry for any characteristic in their EHR, the most recent entry was used.

Age was calculated using the birthdate documented in their EHR. We used race and ethnicity codes from the EHR. Race groups included American Indian/Alaska Native, Asian, Black or African American, Native Hawaiian or other Pacific Islander, and White.[24] If a veteran had more than 1 race recorded, they were classified as "More than one race." Ethnicity was categorized as a dichotomous variable—Hispanic/Latino and not Hispanic/Latino.[24] Veterans who identified as Hispanic/Latino were categorized as Hispanic/Latino regardless of race. When race and ethnicity information was missing, veterans were classified as "Unknown."

Service-connected disability was collapsed into 3 categories: "No Rating," "0%–50% Rating," and "51%–100% Rating." We assessed military sexual trauma and coded it as "Yes" or "No." If a veteran identified a religion or spiritual affiliation in the corporate data warehouse, they were considered religious. If religious affiliation was missing or "atheist," veterans were categorized as not religious.[10] Rurality of residence was based on VHA's location file for veterans and, for the purposes of this article, we used 3 groups: "Urban," "Rural," or "Highly Rural."[25] Sexual orientation response options were "Lesbian or Gay," "Straight or Heterosexual," "Bisexual," "Queer," "Don't Know," "Another option not listed here," "Prefer not to answer," and "Defer for this visit." Veterans' periods of service options were World War II, the Korean Conflict, the Vietnam Era, the Gulf War (August 2, 1990–present), and unknown. The most recently recorded enrollment priority group was used as a proxy for socioeconomic status or disability and collapsed into the following categories: a rating of 50% or higher service-connected disability, catastrophically disabled, low income, and other.[10]

Physical and mental health conditions. Dichotomous indicator variables determined if veterans had a health condition. If a relevant *ICD* code was ever present in their EHR, they were considered to have the corresponding condition (Appendix A, available as a supplement to the online version of this article at https://ajph.org).

Statistical Analysis

We performed all analyses in R version 4.3.2 (R Studio for Statistical Computing, Vienna, Austria). First, we constructed 3 comparison groups: (1) those with only diagnoses indicative of TGD-related *ICD* codes (*ICD* group), (2) TGD veterans who self-reported using the gender identity field and lacked a TGD-related diagnosis (GI group), and (3) veterans with both a TGD-related *ICD* diagnosis and reported as transgender in the gender identity field (both group).

We assessed descriptive statistics for sociodemographic characteristics and physical and mental health diagnoses by the 3 TGD veteran groups (*ICD* group, GI group, and both group). We calculated means and standard deviations for age and analyzed them using the Kruskal–Wallis rank sum test. We tested counts and percentages of categorical variables by using the Pearson χ^2 and Fisher exact test. The a priori statistical significance for this study was set and is reported at $P < .05$. Although physical and mental health conditions were examined individually and independently, we conducted posthoc Bonferroni corrections for the physical health conditions ($P < .004$) and mental health conditions ($P < .005$) to reduce the chance of type I error, though this may increase type II error.[26]

We ran multiple logistic regression models to assess the association between health conditions and group membership, using the *ICD* group as the referent based on previous research. Regression coefficients are represented as odds ratios (ORs) with 95% confidence intervals (CIs). Age (continuous), race/ethnicity, marital status, rurality, and priority group, based on similar research,[10,27,28] were covariates. Multicollinearity was evaluated using variance inflation factors to assess the strength of predictors on the main outcomes. We present only the main effects of the logistic regression models.

RESULTS

We identified 12 745 TGD veterans in our study. The majority self-reported using the gender identity field and did not have a TGD-related *ICD* code: GI group, 69.3% (n = 8833); *ICD* group, 23.4% (n = 2988); and both group was the minority at 7.2% (n = 924).

Sociodemographic Characteristics

Compared with the *ICD* group, TGD veterans in the GI group were younger and more likely to be from a racial/ethnic minority group, married, live in urban areas, and have a service-connected disability (Table 1). Compared with the *ICD* group, the GI group was less likely to be considered low-income. The both group was more likely to have a service-connected disability compared with the *ICD* group. Significant differences existed across all sociodemographic characteristics ($P < .001$), except for military sexual trauma ($P = .05$).

Physical and Mental Health Conditions

Table 2 reports the frequencies and percentages of physical and mental health diagnoses among TGD veterans across the 3 groups and the overall sample. Unadjusted ORs and adjusted ORs (AORs) representing the association of study group with physical health conditions are reported in Table 3. In adjusted models, compared with the *ICD* group, the GI group was less likely to have acute myocardial infarction (AOR = 0.45; 95% CI = 0.34, 0.60), cerebrovascular accident (AOR = 0.54; 95% CI = 0.50, 0.66), cirrhosis (AOR = 0.49; 95% CI = 0.34, 0.69), congestive heart failure (AOR = 0.53; 95% CI = 0.44, 0.63), diabetes (AOR = 0.53; 95% CI = 0.47, 0.59), HIV (AOR = 0.18; 95% CI = 0.12, 0.27), hypercholesterolemia (AOR = 0.46; 95% CI = 0.42, 0.51), hypertension (AOR = 0.54; 95% CI = 0.48, 0.60), ischemic heart disease (AOR = 0.51; 95% CI = 0.44, 0.60), obesity (AOR = 0.51; 95% CI = 0.46, 0.56), chronic renal disease (AOR = 0.46; 95% CI = 0.40, 0.54), end-stage renal disease (AOR = 0.46; 95% CI = 0.40, 0.54), and traumatic brain injury (AOR = 0.61; 95% CI = 0.52, 0.70; all $Ps < .001$). The likelihood of cardiac arrest was also significantly lower in the GI group compared to the *ICD* group (AOR = 0.38; 95% CI = 0.19, 0.76; $P = 0.006$). Notably, in the adjusted models, there were no significant differences between the *ICD* group and the both group.

Table 4 reports the unadjusted ORs and AORs of the relationship between study groups and mental health conditions. In adjusted models, compared with the *ICD* group, the TGD GI group was less likely to have affective disorders (AOR = 0.54; 95% CI = 0.48, 0.60), major depressive disorders (AOR = 0.34; 95% CI = 0.31, 0.38), other depression disorders (AOR = 0.25; 95% CI = 0.23, 0.28), eating disorders (AOR = 0.53; 95% CI = 0.41, 0.68), generalized anxiety disorder (AOR = 0.69; 95% CI = 0.62, 0.77), panic disorder (AOR = 0.57; 95% CI = 0.49, 0.66), PTSD (AOR = 0.52; 95% CI = 0.47, 0.58), serious mental illness (AOR = 0.46; 95% CI = 0.41, 0.51), suicide (AOR = 0.24; 95% CI = 0.18, 0.30), and suicidal ideation (AOR = 0.50; 95% CI = 0.45, 0.56; all $Ps < .001$). Notably, relative to the *ICD* group, the both group was significantly more likely to have affective disorders (AOR = 1.19; 95% CI = 1.01, 1.39; $P = .035$), generalized anxiety disorder (AOR = 1.20; 95% CI = 1.02, 1.41; $P = .026$), panic disorder (AOR = 1.31; 95% CI = 1.13, 1.57; $P = .011$), PTSD (AOR = 1.33; 95% CI = 1.13, 1.57; $P = .001$), and suicidal ideation (AOR = 1.20; 95% CI = 1.02, 1.42; $P = .028$).

DISCUSSION

Because of limitations in available data, previous investigations of TGD veterans' population-level health in VHA relied almost exclusively on TGD-related diagnostic codes.[9] With increased availability of GI data in VHA administrative systems, we sought to understand the impact of this methodological approach on conclusions regarding TGD veterans' demographic characteristics, physical health, and mental health. These analyses revealed that veterans identified by self-reported gender identity represent a different subset of the TGD veteran population than those solely identified using TGD-related diagnostic codes. These veterans appear to be younger

TABLE 1— The Sociodemographic Variables for Transgender and Gender-Diverse (TGD) Veterans Using Veterans Health Administration Data: United States, 2016–2023

	Overall (n = 12 745), No. (%) or Mean ±SD	*ICD* Group[a] (n = 2 988), No. (%) or Mean ±SD	Both Group[b] (n = 924), No. (%) or Mean ±SD	GI Group[c] (n = 8 833), No. (%) or Mean ±SD
Age, y	50 ±17.3	60 ±14.3	56 ±14.3	46 ±17.1
Deceased	794 (6.2)	421 (14.1)	46 (5.0)	327 (3.7)
Birth sex				
Female	5 885 (46.2)	1 445 (48.4)	323 (35.0)	4 117 (46.6)
Male	6 860 (53.8)	1 543 (51.6)	601 (65.0)	4 716 (53.4)
Combined race and ethnicity				
American Indian or Alaska Native	140 (1.1)	43 (1.4)	11 (1.2)	86 (1.0)
Asian	219 (1.7)	37 (1.2)	4 (0.4)	178 (2.0)
Black or African American	1 723 (13.5)	167 (5.6)	72 (7.8)	1 484 (16.8)
Hispanic or Latino	981 (7.7)	148 (5.0)	50 (5.4)	783 (8.9)
More than 1 race	229 (1.8)	34 (1.1)	18 (1.9)	177 (2.0)
Native Hawaiian or other Pacific Islander	120 (0.9)	24 (0.8)	6 (0.6)	90 (1.0)
White	8 247 (64.7)	2 362 (79.0)	712 (77.1)	5 173 (58.6)
Unknown	1 086 (8.5)	173 (5.8)	51 (5.5)	862 (9.8)
Grouped self-identified gender[d]				
Woman	3 200 (25.1)	430 (14.4)	373 (40.4)	2 397 (27.1)
Gender minority	4 162 (32.7)	0 (0.0)	277 (30.0)	3 885 (44.0)
Man	2 956 (23.2)	286 (9.6)	119 (12.9)	2 551 (28.9)
Unknown	2 427 (19.0)	2 272 (76.0)	155 (16.8)	0 (0.0)
Sexual orientation[e]				
Sexual minority	2 643 (20.7)	559 (18.7)	204 (22.1)	1 880 (21.3)
Straight or heterosexual	2 975 (23.3)	541 (18.1)	110 (11.9)	2 324 (26.3)
Unknown	7 127 (55.9)	1 888 (63.2)	610 (66.0)	4 629 (52.4)
Married or partnered status				
Married	3 972 (31.2)	681 (22.8)	223 (24.1)	3 068 (34.7)
Separated or divorced	3 961 (31.1)	1 250 (41.8)	376 (40.7)	2 335 (26.4)
Single	3 971 (31.2)	907 (30.4)	279 (30.2)	2 785 (31.5)
Widowed	341 (2.7)	101 (3.4)	27 (2.9)	213 (2.4)
Unknown	500 (3.9)	49 (1.6)	19 (2.1)	432 (4.9)
Religion				
No	594 (4.7)	10 (0.3)	1 (0.1)	583 (6.6)
Yes	12 151 (95.3)	2 978 (99.7)	923 (99.9)	8 250 (93.4)
Rurality				
Urban	9 439 (74.1)	2 125 (71.1)	655 (70.9)	6 659 (75.4)
Rural	3 082 (24.2)	815 (27.3)	257 (27.8)	2 010 (22.8)
Highly rural	103 (0.8)	30 (1.0)	8 (0.9)	65 (0.7)
Unknown	121 (0.9)	18 (0.6)	4 (0.4)	99 (1.1)
Enrollment priority group				
Catastrophically disabled	107 (0.8)	39 (1.3)	9 (1.0)	59 (0.7)
SCD rating ≥ 50%	7 234 (56.8)	1 432 (47.9)	496 (53.7)	5 306 (60.1)
Low income	2 777 (21.8)	949 (31.8)	248 (26.8)	1 580 (17.9)
Other	2 627 (20.6)	568 (19.0)	171 (18.5)	1 888 (21.4)

Continued

TABLE 1— Continued

	Overall (n = 12 745), No. (%) or Mean ±SD	*ICD* Group[a] (n = 2 988), No. (%) or Mean ±SD	Both Group[b] (n = 924), No. (%) or Mean ±SD	GI Group[c] (n = 8 833), No. (%) or Mean ±SD
War time period served				
World War II	33 (0.3)	0 (0.0)	0 (0.0)	33 (0.4)
Vietnam	3 604 (28.3)	1 561 (52.2)	391 (42.3)	1 652 (18.7)
Korean	187 (1.5)	39 (1.3)	4 (0.4)	144 (1.6)
Persian Gulf	8 761 (68.7)	1 387 (46.4)	527 (57.0)	6 847 (77.5)
Unknown	160 (1.3)	1 (0.0)	2 (0.2)	157 (1.8)
Combat veteran				
Yes	241 (1.9)	6 (0.2)	1 (0.1)	234 (2.6)
No	12 504 (98.1)	2 982 (99.8)	923 (99.9)	8 599 (97.4)
SCD rating				
No SCD rating	3 473 (27.2)	1 049 (35.1)	260 (28.1)	2 164 (24.5)
0%–50%	2 443 (19.2)	614 (20.5)	201 (21.8)	1 628 (18.4)
51%–100%	6 829 (53.6)	1 325 (44.3)	463 (50.1)	5 041 (57.1)
Military sexual trauma				
Yes	3 063 (24.0)	721 (24.1)	252 (27.3)	2 090 (23.7)
No	9 682 (76.0)	2 267 (75.9)	672 (72.7)	6 743 (76.3)

Note. SCD = service-connected disability. All variables were statistically significant, $P < .001$ based on Kruskal–Wallis (continuous), Pearson χ^2, and Fisher exact test (categorical).
[a]*ICD* group = veterans with transgender-related *International Classification of Diseases* (*ICD*) codes without TGD self-reported gender identity information.
[b]Both group = veterans with transgender-related *ICD* codes and TGD self-reported gender identity.
[c]GI group = veterans with TGD self-reported gender identity without transgender-related *ICD* codes.
[d]Gender minority category includes "Transgender Man," "Transgender Woman," "Non-binary," and "A gender not listed here."
[e]Sexual minority category includes "Lesbian and Gay," "Bisexual," "Queer," and "Another option not listed here."

and more racially and ethnically diverse, on average, compared with veterans represented in past studies, as well as physically and mentally healthier. Conversely, veterans identified with both diagnostic codes and gender identity information in their EHR are at greater risk for several mental health conditions relative to those identified only using TGD-related diagnostic codes.

TGD veterans with gender identity data and no associated diagnostic codes had a lower risk of 13 out of 14 physical health conditions, compared with the *ICD* group, even after we adjusted for sociodemographic factors such as age, race and ethnicity, socioeconomic status, and rurality. Similarly, the GI group had a lower adjusted risk of all mental health conditions even when we controlled for age, socioeconomic status, and rurality. Instead, several potential explanations for these findings are plausible. First, while all TGD veterans are vulnerable to the pernicious effects of gender minority stress on health,[19,29,30] those experiencing more significant distress related to their gender identity (i.e., those with diagnoses associated with transgender experience) may be more physically and mentally impacted by this stress, potentially leading to elevated rates of physical and mental health conditions. Indeed, some recent evidence suggests that gender dysphoria may itself act as a proximal minority stressor.[31] This is further supported by finding relatively higher rates of some mental health conditions among the both group whereas the GI group did not demonstrate such differences.

Differences between the *ICD* and GI groups may also be at least partly attributable to differences in care experiences or care needs by veterans in different groups. For example, veterans willing to document their gender identity in their medical record may have had more positive health care experiences (and, subsequently, greater willingness to include their gender identity in their medical record) than veterans who disclosed their identity to a provider to receive gender-affirming medical interventions but chose not to document their gender identity. Veterans willing to document their gender identity may have more trust in the health care system and, therefore, may access appropriate care and have better health outcomes. Alternatively, veterans in the both group, at relatively higher

TABLE 2— **Descriptive Statistics of Physical and Mental Health Conditions for Transgender and Gender-Diverse (TGD) Veterans: United States, 2016–2023**

	Overall (n = 12 745), No. (%)	ICD Group[a] (n = 2 988), No. (%)	Both Group[b] (n = 924), No. (%)	GI[c] Group (n = 8 833), No. (%)
Physical health conditions				
Acute myocardial infarction	263 (8.1)	133 (4.5)	33 (3.6)	97 (1.1)
Cardiac arrest	46 (0.4)	23 (0.8)	7 (0.8)	16 (0.2)
Cerebrovascular accident	648 (5.1)	286 (9.6)	87 (9.4)	275 (3.1)
Cirrhosis	179 (1.4)	85 (2.8)	25 (2.7)	69 (0.8)
Diabetes	2 482 (19.5)	996 (33.3)	281 (30.4)	1 205 (13.6)
Heart failure	698 (5.5)	325 (10.9)	87 (9.4)	286 (3.2)
HIV	146 (1.1)	77 (2.6)	24 (2.6)	45 (0.5)
Hypercholesterolemia	6 322 (49.6)	2 158 (72.2)	633 (68.5)	3 531 (40.0)
Hypertension	5 006 (39.3)	1 813 (60.7)	529 (57.3)	2 664 (30.2)
Ischemic heart disease	1 598 (12.5)	732 (24.5)	182 (19.7)	684 (7.7)
Obesity	4 846 (38.0)	1 581 (52.9)	501 (54.2)	2 764 (31.3)
Renal disease, chronic	1 127 (8.8)	515 (17.2)	144 (15.6)	468 (5.3)
Renal disease, end stage	997 (7.8)	456 (15.3)	128 (13.9)	413 (4.7)
Traumatic brain injury	1 350 (10.6)	386 (12.9)	141 (15.3)	823 (9.3)
Mental health conditions				
Affective disorders	2 930 (23.0)	880 (29.5)	316 (34.2)	1 734 (19.6)
Depression, major	7 812 (61.3)	2 194 (73.4)	710 (76.8)	4 908 (55.6)
Depression, other	3 823 (30.0)	1588 (53.1)	485 (52.5)	1 750 (19.8)
Eating disorders	404 (3.2)	128 (4.3)	43 (4.7)	233 (2.6)
Generalized anxiety disorder	3 308 (26.0)	830 (27.8)	308 (33.3)	2 170 (24.6)
Panic disorder	1 294 (10.2)	377 (12.6)	155 (16.8)	762 (8.6)
Posttraumatic stress disorder	6 229 (48.9)	1 585 (53.0)	573 (62.0)	4 071 (46.1)
Serious mental illness	2 679 (21.0)	885 (29.6)	309 (33.4)	1 485 (16.8)
Suicidal ideation	2 664 (20.9)	792 (26.5)	293 (31.7)	1 579 (17.9)
Suicide	423 (3.3)	211 (7.1)	70 (7.6)	142 (1.6)

[a]*ICD* group = veterans with transgender-related *International Classification of Diseases (ICD)* codes without TGD self-reported gender identity information.
[b]Both group = veterans with transgender-related *ICD* codes and TGD self-reported gender identity.
[c]GI group = veterans with TGD self-reported gender identity without transgender-related *ICD* codes.

risk for certain mental health conditions (e.g., PTSD), may have greater health needs and document gender identity to ensure they get the most affirming care.

Limitations

Although use of gender identity data in a nationwide EHR study represents a significant improvement in understanding population-level health of TGD veterans in VHA, several limitations exist. We included in the analyses any documentation of the *ICD* codes for conditions of interest across time. Observed mental and physical health conditions documented in the past may have been addressed or resolved but were still included in our analyses.

Beginning in 2011, VHA policies allow patients to modify their birth sex in their records. As such, the value entered as a patient's birth sex is not always accurate—for instance, if a TGD veteran changed their sex to align with their gender identity and entered "man" or "woman" as their gender identity without other identifying characteristics in their record, they may have been inadvertently excluded from this cohort. TGD veterans without a TGD-related *ICD* code who also have not shared their gender identity may also have been omitted or miscategorized in this study.

These findings should be interpreted considering missing data issues in the

TABLE 3— The Unadjusted and Adjusted Odds Ratios of Physical Health Conditions for Transgender and Gender-Diverse (TGD) Veterans as Compared With TGD Veterans Identified by *ICD* Codes Using Veterans Health Administration Data: United States, 2016–2023

	Both Group[a] (n = 924)		GI[b] Group (n = 8833)	
Physical Health Conditions	**OR (95% CI)**	**AOR[c] (95% CI)**	**OR (95% CI)**	**AOR[c] (95% CI)**
Acute myocardial infarction	0.80 (0.53, 1.16)	...	0.24 (0.18, 0.31)	0.45 (0.34, 0.60)
Cardiac arrest	0.98 (0.39, 2.19)	...	0.23 (0.12, 0.44)	0.38* (0.19, 0.76)
Cerebrovascular accident	0.98 (0.76, 1.26)	...	0.30 (0.26, 0.36)	0.54 (0.45, 0.66)
Cirrhosis	0.95 (0.59, 1.47)	...	0.27 (0.19, 0.37)	0.49 (0.34, 0.69)
Congestive heart failure	0.85 (0.66, 1.09)	...	0.27 (0.23, 0.32)	0.53 (0.44, 0.63)
Diabetes	0.87 (0.74, 1.02)	...	0.32 (0.29, 0.35)	0.53 (0.47, 0.59)
HIV	1.01 (0.62, 1.58)	...	0.19 (0.13, 0.28)	0.18 (0.12, 0.27)
Hypercholesterolemia	0.84* (0.71, 0.98)	0.97 (0.82, 1.16)	0.26 (0.23, 0.28)	0.46 (0.42, 0.51)
Hypertension	0.87 (0.75, 1.01)	...	0.28 (0.26, 0.31)	0.54 (0.48, 0.60)
Ischemic heart disease	0.76 (0.63, 0.91)	0.93 (0.76, 1.13)	0.26 (0.23, 0.29)	0.51 (0.44, 0.58)
Obesity	1.05 (0.91, 1.22)	...	0.41 (0.37, 0.44)	0.51 (0.46, 0.56)
Renal disease, chronic	0.89 (0.72, 1.08)	...	0.27 (0.24, 0.31)	0.46 (0.40, 0.54)
Renal disease, end stage	0.89 (0.72, 1.10)	...	0.27 (0.24, 0.31)	0.46 (0.40, 0.54)
Traumatic brain injury	1.21 (0.98, 1.49)	...	0.69 (0.61, 0.79)	0.61 (0.52, 0.70)

Note. AOR = adjusted odds ratio; CI = confidence interval; *ICD* = *International Classification of Diseases;* OR = unadjusted odds ratio. Referent group = transgender veterans with transgender-related *ICD* codes and without self-reported gender identity information (OR = 1). Models were multiple logistic regressions, with each physical health condition analyzed individually in a separate model, and only main effects are presented.
[a]Both group = veterans with transgender-related *ICD* codes and TGD self-reported gender identity.
[b]GI group = veterans with TGD self-reported gender identity without transgender-related *ICD* codes.
[c]Models adjusted for age, race/ethnicity, marital status, rurality, and priority groups. Adjusted models were only run on health conditions with statistically significant ORs in the unadjusted models.
*Logistic regression model was not significant when we conducted a posthoc Bonferroni correction (new $P = .004$).

data fields used for this study. Because of the optional nature of the self-report gender identity field, approximately two thirds of active VHA users remain without recorded gender identity. This degree of missingness may have impacted the patterns observed. In addition, missing diagnostic information limits the data as there is no way to differentiate those who do not meet criteria for TGD-related diagnoses from those who have never been evaluated.

Lastly, after applying a posthoc Bonferroni correction to the logistic regression models, findings regarding the GI group remained unaffected. However, for the both group, several associations related to mental health conditions became nonsignificant (e.g., affective disorders, major depression disorders, and serious mental illness). The finding for PTSD remained significant after correction. Following the posthoc Bonferroni correction on physical health conditions, the unadjusted OR for hypercholesterolemia ($P = .029$) and the AOR for cardiac arrest ($P = .006$) were nonsignificant for the both and GI groups, respectively. The relatively small size of the both group may have been particularly sensitive to the Bonferroni correction because of its conservative nature.[32] As the gender identity field in the VHA EHR becomes more well-populated, future VHA research should re-examine the relation between the both group and mental health conditions.

Implications and Future Directions

Given the stark differences in health profiles between TGD veterans identified with self-report data versus diagnostic data, future analyses of TGD veteran health should carefully consider the impact of cohort definitions. While self-report data are the gold standard, until the gender identity field is better populated within VHA, it may be necessary to utilize multiple methods (e.g., diagnostic codes and self-reported data) to yield a more complete picture of the population. Future work investigating the care utilization patterns and health care experiences of TGD veterans identified

TABLE 4— The Unadjusted and Adjusted Odds Ratios of Mental Health Conditions for Transgender and Gender-Diverse (TGD) Veterans as Compared With TGD Veterans Identified by *ICD* Codes Using Veterans Health Administration Data: United States, 2016–2023

	Both Group[a] (n = 924)		GI[b] Group (n = 8833)	
Mental Health Conditions	OR (95% CI)	AOR[c] (95% CI)	OR (95% CI)	AOR[c] (95% CI)
Affective disorders	1.25* (1.06, 1.46)	1.19* (1.01, 1.39)	0.59 (0.53, 0.64)	0.54 (0.48, 0.60)
Depression, major	1.20* (1.01, 1.43)	1.10 (0.92, 1.31)	0.45 (0.41, 0.50)	0.34 (0.31, 0.38)
Depression, other	0.97 (0.84, 1.13)	. . .	0.22 (0.20, 0.24)	0.25 (0.23, 0.28)
Eating disorders	1.09 (0.76, 1.54)	. . .	0.61 (0.49, 0.76)	0.53 (0.41, 0.68)
Generalized anxiety disorder	1.30 (1.11, 1.52)	1.20* (1.02, 1.41)	0.85 (0.77, 0.93)	0.69 (0.62, 0.77)
Panic disorder	1.40 (1.14, 1.71)	1.31* (1.06, 1.61)	0.65 (0.57, 0.75)	0.57 (0.49, 0.66)
Posttraumatic stress disorder	1.45 (1.24, 1.68)	1.33 (1.13, 1.57)	0.76 (0.70, 0.82)	0.52 (0.47, 0.58)
Serious mental illness	1.19* (1.02, 1.40)	1.15 (0.98, 1.35)	0.48 (0.44, 0.53)	0.46 (0.41, 0.51)
Suicidal ideation	1.29 (1.10, 1.51)	1.20* (1.02, 1.42)	0.60 (0.55, 0.67)	0.50 (0.45, 0.56)
Suicide	1.08 (0.81, 1.42)	. . .	0.22 (0.17, 0.27)	0.24 (0.18, 0.30)

Note. AOR = adjusted odds ratio; CI = confidence interval; *ICD* = *International Classification of Diseases;* OR = unadjusted odds ratio. Referent group = transgender veterans with transgender-related *ICD* codes and without self-reported gender identity information (OR = 1). Models were multiple logistic regressions, with each mental health condition analyzed individually in a separate model, and only main effects are presented.
[a]Both group = veterans with transgender-related *ICD* codes and TGD self-reported gender identity.
[b]GI group = veterans with TGD self-reported gender identity without transgender-related *ICD* codes.
[c]Models adjusted for age, race/ethnicity, marital status, rurality, and priority groups. Adjusted models were only run on health conditions with statistically significant ORs in the unadjusted models.
*Logistic regression model was not significant when we conducted a posthoc Bonferroni correction (new *P* = .005).

via diagnostic codes compared with self-reported gender identity could also shed light on the implications of each method—for example, examining if veterans identified via diagnostic codes utilize more health care (and, thus, are more likely to have diagnoses of any kind in the health record) or whether those with solely gender identity data have more positive experiences of health care.

Future work should re-evaluate gender-related disparities in many of the physical and mental health conditions examined by comparing self-reported cisgender veterans to self-reported TGD veterans. Indeed, while a direct comparison cannot be drawn from the current data, rates of many conditions among the self-reported TGD cohort appear lower in the current study than rates among the (presumed) cisgender veterans in past studies, despite using nearly identical methodologies.[10]

Finally, a significant limitation of past research and of the current study was the aggregation of transgender men, transgender women, and nonbinary individuals into a single group. As more veterans choose to share their gender identity with VHA, understanding the nuanced needs and experiences of subpopulations of TGD veterans may be possible. This would aid future policy and programming decisions.

Conclusion

Conclusions drawn from previous research on the health and well-being of TGD veterans receiving care in VHA may have been impacted by a reliance on TGD-related diagnostic codes. This subset of the population appears to differ in important ways from those who self-report a TGD identity. Future research should use the newly available gender identity field to reinvestigate disparities between self-reported cisgender and TGD veterans in VHA. Public health programmers and policymakers should consider ways to increase completeness of the gender identity data field to better understand the TGD veteran population utilizing VHA health care services. AJPH

ABOUT THE AUTHORS

Sarah M. Leder, Shane Lamba, Chava Sonnier, and Kenneth T. Jones are with the Veterans Health Administration (VHA) Office of Health Equity, Washington, DC. A. Alex McConnell, Alexis R. Matza, Wyatt E. Meriwether, Jillian C. Shipherd, and Michael R. Kauth are with the VHA Lesbian, Gay, Bisexual, Transgender, and Queer+ (LGBTQ+) Health Program, Washington, DC. George R. Brown is with the East Tennessee State University, Department of Psychiatry, Johnson City, TN.

Note. The views, opinions, and content of this publication are those of the authors and do not necessarily reflect the views, opinions, or policies of the academic affiliations, the Department of Veterans Affairs (VA), or the US government.

CORRESPONDENCE

Correspondence should be sent to Sarah M. Leder, MSW, 810 Vermont Ave NW, Room 778, Washington, DC 20420 (e-mail: sarah.leder@va.gov). Reprints can be ordered at https://www.ajph.org by clicking the "Reprints" link.

PUBLICATION INFORMATION

Full Citation: Leder SM, McConnell AA, Lamba S, et al. Impact of gender identity field in the Veterans Health Administration electronic health record, 2016–2023. *Am J Public Health*. 2025;115(3):403–413.

Acceptance Date: November 5, 2024.

DOI: https://doi.org/10.2105/AJPH.2024.307920

ORCID iDs:

Sarah M. Leder https://orcid.org/0000-0003-4256-3963

A. Alex McConnell https://orcid.org/0000-0002-1786-7538

Shane Lamba https://orcid.org/0000-0002-7598-2278

Chava Sonnier https://orcid.org/0009-0008-3922-3590

Alexis R. Matza https://orcid.org/0000-0002-1692-7797

Wyatt E. Meriwether https://orcid.org/0000-0002-5666-1321

Jillian C. Shipherd https://orcid.org/0000-0001-6742-7912

Michael R. Kauth https://orcid.org/0000-0002-0766-8404

Kenneth T. Jones https://orcid.org/0000-0001-5206-897X

CONTRIBUTORS

S. M. Leder, S. Lamba, C. Sonnier, and K. T. Jones conceptualized and designed the study. S. M. Leder and A. A. McConnell drafted the article. C. Sonnier, A. R. Matza, W. E. Meriwether, G. Brown, J. C. Shipherd, M. R. Kauth, and K. T. Jones reviewed and edited the article. S. M. Leder, S. Lamba, and C. Sonnier obtained and analyzed data. All authors provided significant input, review, and editing and read and approved the final version of the article.

ACKNOWLEDGMENTS

Data from this article were presented at Academy Health's Annual Research Meeting in June 2024 in Baltimore, MD.

The authors would like to thank all members of the Office of Health Equity and the LGBTQ+ Health Program for their support and input throughout this project.

CONFLICTS OF INTEREST

The authors do not have any potential or actual conflicts of interest to disclose.

HUMAN PARTICIPANT PROTECTION

This project is part of ongoing quality improvement and evaluation efforts within the VHA Office of Health Equity and LGBTQ+ Health Program Office. As such, current analyses were designated as nonresearch and did not undergo review by the VA institutional review board.

REFERENCES

1. Blosnich JR, Brown GR, Shipherd JC, Kauth M, Piegari RI, Bossarte RM. Prevalence of gender identity disorder and suicide risk among transgender veterans utilizing Veterans Health Administration care. *Am J Public Health*. 2013;103(10):e27–e32. https://doi.org/10.2105/AJPH.2013.301507
2. Gates GJ, Herman JL. Transgender military service in the United States. The Williams Institute at UCLA School of Law. Available at: https://www.jstor.org/stable/resrep35579. Accessed February 29, 2024.
3. Shipherd JC, Mizock L, Maguen S, Green KE. Male-to-female transgender veterans and VA health care utilization. *Int J Sex Health*. 2012;24(1):78–87. https://doi.org/10.1080/19317611.2011.639440
4. Kondo K, Low A, Everson T, et al. Health disparities in veterans: a map of the evidence. *Med Care*. 2017;55(suppl 2):S9–S15. https://doi.org/10.1097/MLR.0000000000000756
5. Burgess C, Kauth MR, Klemt C, Shanawani H, Shipherd JC. Evolving sex and gender in electronic health records. *Fed Pract*. 2019;36(6):271–277.
6. Blosnich JR. Costs of (in)visibility: issues of disclosure and data for health equity research with sexual and gender minority veterans. *Health Equity*. 2023;7(1):338–341. https://doi.org/10.1089/heq.2023.0005
7. Beckman K, Shipherd J, Simpson T, Lehavot K. Military sexual assault in transgender veterans: results from a nationwide survey. *J Trauma Stress*. 2018;31(2):181–190. https://doi.org/10.1002/jts.22280
8. Hahn H, Burkitt KH, Kauth MR, Shipherd JC, Blosnich JR. Primary sources of health care among LGBTQ+ veterans: findings from the Behavioral Risk Factor Surveillance System. *Health Serv Res*. 2022;58(2):392–401. https://doi.org/10.1111/1475-6773.14096.
9. Kauth MR, Blosnich JR, Marra J, Keig Z, Shipherd JC. Transgender health care in the US military and Veterans Health Administration facilities. *Curr Sex Health Rep*. 2017;9(3):121–127. https://doi.org/10.1007/s11930-017-0120-7
10. Brown GR, Jones KT. Mental health and medical health disparities in 5135 transgender veterans receiving healthcare in the Veterans Health Administration: a case–control study. *LGBT Health*. 2016;3(2):122–131. https://doi.org/10.1089/lgbt.2015.0058
11. Livingston NA, Lynch KE, Hinds Z, Gatsby E, DuVall SL, Shipherd JC. Identifying posttraumatic stress disorder and disparity among transgender veterans using nationwide Veterans Health Administration electronic health record data. *LGBT Health*. 2022;9(2):94–102. https://doi.org/10.1089/lgbt.2021.0246
12. Boyer TL, Youk AO, Haas AP, et al. Suicide, homicide, and all-cause mortality among transgender and cisgender patients in the Veterans Health Administration. *LGBT Health*. 2021;8(3):173–180. https://doi.org/10.1089/lgbt.2020.0235
13. Frost MC, Blosnich JR, Lehavot K, et al. Disparities in documented drug use disorders between transgender and cisgender US Veterans Health Administration patients. *J Addict Med*. 2021;15(4):334–340. https://doi.org/10.1097/ADM.0000000000000769
14. Williams EC, Frost MC, Rubinsky AD, et al. Patterns of alcohol use among transgender patients receiving care at the Veterans Health Administration: overall and relative to nontransgender patients. *J Stud Alcohol Drugs*. 2021;82(1):132–141. https://doi.org/10.15288/jsad.2021.82.132
15. Jasuja GK, Reisman JE, Rao SR, et al. Social stressors and health among older transgender and gender diverse veterans. *LGBT Health*. 2023;10(2):148–157. https://doi.org/10.1089/lgbt.2022.0012
16. Fletcher OV, Chen JA, van Draanen J, et al. Prevalence of social and economic stressors among transgender veterans with alcohol and other drug use disorders. *SSM Popul Health*. 2022;19:101153. https://doi.org/10.1016/j.ssmph.2022.101153
17. Carter SP, Montgomery AE, Henderson ER, et al. Housing instability characteristics among transgender veterans cared for in the Veterans Health Administration, 2013–2016. *Am J Public Health*. 2019;109(10):1413–1418. https://doi.org/10.2105/AJPH.2019.305219
18. *Diagnostic and Statistical Manual of Mental Disorders*. 5th ed., text rev. Washington, DC: American Psychiatric Association; 2022. https://doi.org/10.1176/appi.books.9780890425787.
19. Valentine SE, Shipherd JC. A systematic review of social stress and mental health among transgender and gender non-conforming people in the United States. *Clin Psychol Rev*. 2018;66:24–38. https://doi.org/10.1016/j.cpr.2018.03.003
20. Streed CG Jr, King D, Grasso C, et al. Validation of an administrative algorithm for transgender and gender diverse persons against self-report data in electronic health records. *J Am Med Inform Assoc*. 2023;30(6):1047–1055. https://doi.org/10.1093/jamia/ocad039
21. Nik-Ahd F, Waller J, De Hoedt AM, et al. Seeing the unseen: how can we best identify transgender women within the Veterans Affairs healthcare system's electronic medical record? *J Sex Med*. 2023;20(4):559–567. https://doi.org/10.1093/jsxmed/qdac033
22. Wolfe HL, Reisman JI, Yoon SS, et al. Validating data-driven methods for identifying transgender individuals in the Veterans Health Administration of the US Department of Veterans Affairs. *Am J Epidemiol*. 2021;190(9):1928–1934. https://doi.org/10.1093/aje/kwab102
23. National Academies of Sciences Engineering and Medicine. *Measuring Sex, Gender Identity, and Sexual Orientation*. Washington, DC: The National Academies Press; 2022.
24. Office of Management and Budget. Revisions to the standards for the classification of federal data on race and ethnicity. *Federal Register*. 1997;62(210):58782.
25. Bukowski LA, Blosnich J, Shipherd JC, et al. Exploring rural disparities in medical diagnoses among veterans with transgender-related

diagnoses utilizing Veterans Health Administration care. *Med Care.* 2017;55(suppl 9 suppl 2): S97–S103. https://doi.org/10.1097/MLR.0000000000000745.
26. García-Pérez MA. Use and misuse of corrections for multiple testing. *Methods in Psychology.* 2023; 8:100120. https://doi.org/10.1016/j.metip.2023.100120
27. Brown GR, Jones KT. Health correlates of criminal justice involvement in 4,793 transgender veterans. *LGBT Health.* 2015;2(4):297–305. https://doi.org/10.1089/lgbt.2015.0052
28. Downing JM, Przedworski JM. Health of transgender adults in the US, 2014–2016. *Am J Prev Med.* 2018;55(3):336–344. https://doi.org/10.1016/j.amepre.2018.04.045
29. Hendricks ML, Testa RJ. A conceptual framework for clinical work with transgender and gender nonconforming clients: an adaptation of the minority stress model. *Prof Psychol Res Pr.* 2012;43(5):460–467. https://doi.org/10.1037/a0029597
30. Tucker RP, Testa RJ, Reger MA, Simpson TL, Shipherd JC, Lehavot K. Current and military-specific gender minority stress factors and their relationship with suicide ideation in transgender veterans. *Suicide Life Threat Behav.* 2019;49(1): 155–166. https://doi.org/10.1111/sltb.12432
31. Lindley L, Galup MP. Gender dysphoria and minority stress: support for inclusion of gender dysphoria as a proximal stressor. *Psychol Sex Orientat Gend Divers.* 2020;7(3):265–275. https://doi.org/10.1037/sgd0000439
32. VanderWeele TJ, Mathur MB. Some desirable properties of the Bonferroni correction: is the Bonferroni correction really so bad? *Am J Epidemiol.* 2019;188(3):617–618. https://doi.org/10.1093/aje/kwy250

Predictors of Persistent COVID-19 Vaccine Refusal Among Previously Infected Patients in Nebraska

He (Julia) Bai, MPH, David Brett-Major, MD, MPH, Yi Du, PhD, MS, Sai Paritala, MPH, PharmD, Edward S. Peters, DMD, DM, SCD, Kendra L. Ratnapradipa, PhD, MSW, and Patrick Maloney, PhD, MPH

Objectives. To identify factors associated with persistent COVID-19 vaccine refusal among Nebraska residents 6 months after an initial COVID-19 diagnosis.

Methods. Using case investigation surveillance data and vaccination records from the Nebraska Department of Health and Human Services, a cohort of 16 344 unvaccinated, COVID-19–confirmed individuals (May 2021–February 2023) were asked for their reason for nonvaccination (RNV), then followed for 6 months to assess subsequent vaccination status. We used a modified Poisson regression to estimate risk of unvaccinated status at follow-up against predictors, including RNV, demographic characteristics, adherence to mitigation measures, hospitalization, and rurality.

Results. Compared with those whose RNV was missed opportunity/lack of convenience, individuals who cited religious exemption (adjusted incidence risk ratio [AIRR = 1.36; 95% confidence interval [CI] = 1.31, 1.41), philosophical objection (AIRR = 1.28; 95% CI = 1.24, 1.34), or institutional confidence/complacency concerns (AIRR = 1.26; 95% CI = 1.19, 1.33) showed greatest risk of nonvaccination. Older age, nonadherence to mitigation measures, and higher rurality are positively associated with nonvaccination. Minority status and hospitalization were correlated with vaccination.

Conclusions. Ideology-centered objections held significant weight among previously infected individuals who displayed sustained reluctance toward COVID-19 vaccination. Distinguishing sources of misinformation among ideologically similar communities could instigate reconsideration for vaccination. (*Am J Public Health*. 2025;115(3):414–424. https://doi.org/10.2105/AJPH.2024.307921)

AJPH March 2025, Vol. 115, No. 3

The World Health Organization declared the COVID-19 pandemic on March 11, 2020, with the first confirmed case of COVID-19 in the United States on January 20, 2020.[1] Initial mitigation measures focused on slowing disease spread using nonpharmaceutical interventions such as stay-at-home orders, social distancing, mask mandates, and travel restrictions.[2,3] However, because of differing public health guidelines among states and territories and geographically diverse demographics, the uneven spread of severe acute respiratory syndrome coronavirus 2 (SARS-CoV-2) within the United States further reinforced the need for interventions that reduce disease severity among all populations.

Announced in May 2020, Operation Warp Speed was funded by the US government to support COVID-19 vaccine candidates in catalyzing the clinical development, manufacturing, and allocation of COVID-19 vaccines in the United States.[4] With the staggered availability of vaccines and, as the pandemic progressed, updated recommendations on vaccine booster doses used to combat new strains of SARS-CoV-2, the concept of being "up to date" with COVID-19 vaccinations was continuously redefined. Compared with national estimates from March 2024, Nebraska has a similar proportion of those aged 18 years and older who are up to date with their COVID-19 vaccination (21.8% Nebraska vs 20.9% United States) but a higher proportion of unvaccinated individuals (22.4% Nebraska vs 19.4% United States).[5]

Concerns related to the perceived risk of COVID-19, distrust in government, and endorsement of vaccine-related misinformation, among other factors, have impacted public willingness to abide by public health vaccination guidance. Vaccine hesitancy, defined as "delay in acceptance or refusal of vaccination despite availability of vaccination services," is influenced by a multitude of factors that collectively affect an individual's willingness to vaccinate.[6(p3)] Sex, minority status, age, rurality, and socioeconomic status are commonly reported predictors in vaccine uptake.[7] The reasons for vaccine hesitancy are commonly grouped into factor clusters using the "3 Cs" model.[6] The model emphasizes 3 main clusters that influence hesitancy: confidence (related to trust in safety or effectiveness of the vaccine, health systems that deliver them, and policymakers that enforce them), complacency (perceived risk of disease and necessity of vaccination as a preventive measure), and convenience (extent to which accessibility, availability, affordability, health literacy, and appeal of services affects uptake).[6]

Vaccine hesitancy can result from complex societal and cultural factors that differ among vaccine-hesitant communities. Within minority and migrant populations, themes related to institutional mistrust, lack of confidence in vaccine and vaccine development, and lack of reliable information or messengers are key components that create barriers to vaccination.[8] Alternatively, rural communities maintain confidence in local authorities and health care institutions, but hesitancy stems from reduced vaccine access and complacency-centered reasons.[9,10] Among certain religious groups, the roots of hesitancy are anchored in biblicism with heavy emphasis in individual liberty and distrust in science and mainstream media.[11,12]

While previous research has primarily focused on the drivers of vaccine hesitancy before COVID-19 diagnosis, few studies have investigated the relationship between previous COVID-19 diagnosis (PCD) and persistent vaccine hesitancy. Studies exploring this topic have generally identified a positive association between PCD and persistent COVID-19 vaccine refusal, defined as continued refusal and delay in acceptance of the COVID-19 vaccine after PCD.[13] Other studies have noted a lack of association between PCD and persistent vaccine refusal.[14] A meta-review synthesizing factors influencing COVID-19 vaccination intention identified history of COVID-19 as a main determinant, though the directionality of the association between PCD and vaccination uptake is conflicting.[15]

Because of the inconsistency in the association between PCD and persistent vaccine refusal, additional research is needed to understand why some individuals remain unvaccinated. Research among recovered COVID-19 patients in China have reported reasons for persistent vaccine refusal, including perceived immunity from future infection, lack of reliable information about vaccines, and negative media reports about the vaccine.[16] Similar reasons were mentioned among recovered patients in Italy with the inclusion of safety concerns and effectiveness of the vaccine.[17] Given the limited research pertaining to reasons behind persistent vaccine refusal among hesitant communities, we aimed to address this gap in knowledge by examining persistent vaccine hesitancy among previously diagnosed COVID-19 patients in the United States. The study objective was to identify factors associated with persistent vaccine refusal among Nebraska residents who remain unvaccinated 6 months after an initial COVID-19 diagnosis.

METHODS

A cohort of unvaccinated Nebraska residents was formed using case investigation data from May 2021 to February 2023. Cases were followed for 6 months from date of case investigation to create a prospective cohort study.

Data Sources

All probable, suspected, and confirmed COVID-19 cases meeting the Centers for Disease Control and Prevention case classification definitions were reported to the local health departments and the Nebraska Department of Health and Human Services.[18] After receiving laboratory confirmation, local health department case investigation was initiated via emailed survey or phone contact, typically within 3 days. Questions addressed infection (e.g., symptoms, hospitalization) and potential exposures (e.g., routes of exposure, adherence to mitigation measures, event attendance, contact with other individuals). Cases without a COVID-19 vaccination record were asked why they were not vaccinated.

Each case investigation report was given a case number. Case investigation data were merged with laboratory data (confirming the detection of the specimen as positive, negative, or inconclusive for SARS-CoV-2) and vaccination records (including how many vaccinations and their administration dates) from the Nebraska State Immunization Information System using the system internal ID, which is associated with case number. If an individual identifier had more than 1 case number, only the earliest case number was used.

Study Population

Inclusion criteria included that, at the time of case investigation, persons must (1) have had a confirmed SARS-CoV-2 infection, (2) have had no COVID-19 vaccination record, and (3) were aged 18 years or older. A cohort of 16 344 unvaccinated, COVID-19–confirmed cases were followed for 6 months from case investigation date to ascertain whether they received a COVID-19 vaccination after infection. Individuals who died within 6 months of case investigation were excluded.

Data Elements

The main predictive variable was the reason for not vaccinating at time of case investigation (RNV), categorized as "apathetic/undecided," "institutional confidence/complacency," "missed opportunity/lack of convenience," "philosophical objection," "refused to respond," "religious exemption," and "research/safety confidence" (Box 1). A flowchart explaining the process of creating the predictor variable is listed in Figure 1. Case investigation (survey or phone) had a prepopulated list of potential reasons for not vaccinating, including an option for "other" with a write-in text field. All free-text responses were evaluated individually and sorted into categories, listed in Table A (available as a supplement to the online version of this article at https://ajph.org). If a response had multiple reasons for nonvaccination, reasons were sequentially sorted into primary, secondary, and tertiary response categories. Both the free-text response categories and the prepopulated list of reasons were then condensed.

The outcome under study was COVID-19 vaccination status 6 months after investigation of initial infection (VSIIF). If an individual had received a single dose of COVID-19 vaccine within 6 months of VSIIF, they were considered to have been vaccinated. All others were categorized as unvaccinated.

We chose additional predictors based on previous known association with vaccine hesitancy and assessed these alongside reasons for nonvaccination. Demographic characteristics included age (18–24, 25–34, 35–49, 50–64, or 65 years or older), race/ethnicity (White, American Indian and Alaska Native/Native Hawaiian and Pacific Islander/Asian, Black, Hispanic), and sex (male, female). Facemask use (always/almost always, sometimes/rarely, never, unknown) and attendance of public events (no, yes, unknown) were also included as an indicator of adherence to mitigation measures. The residential zip code was matched with the Rural–Urban Commuting Area code from the US Department of Agriculture Economic Research Service to classify the rurality of the individual's residence (metropolitan, micropolitan, small town, rural).[19]

BOX 1— Definitions of Reasons for Nonvaccination

Final Category	Final Category Definition
Apathetic/undecided	• Reasons that indicate lack of priority for vaccination • General fear for vaccination • Fear of physical aspects related to immunization such as needles • Generally unsure about vaccination without specification of what aspect of vaccination they are unsure about
Institutional confidence/complacency	• Reduced confidence in vaccines overall • Reduced confidence in research, government, or other health care institutions • Comments related to propaganda and other conspiratorial concerns • Complacency because of a perceived lack of risk of disease • Reduction in confidence for vaccines to prevent disease • Distrust in vaccination because of information gathered from news sources or personal life
Missed opportunity/lack of convenience	• Desire for vaccination is evident in the response, but vaccine not received because of illness, lack of time, or convenience-related barriers, such as accessibility
Philosophical objection	• Comments regarding individual freedom or personal choice involving vaccination
Refused to respond	• Refused to answer or disclose reason
Religious exemption	• Religion-based reasons
Research/safety confidence	• Lack of confidence because of safety concerns, novelty of vaccines, lack of information on side effects and long-term effects • Lack of confidence in safety of vaccines because of pregnancy or medical history

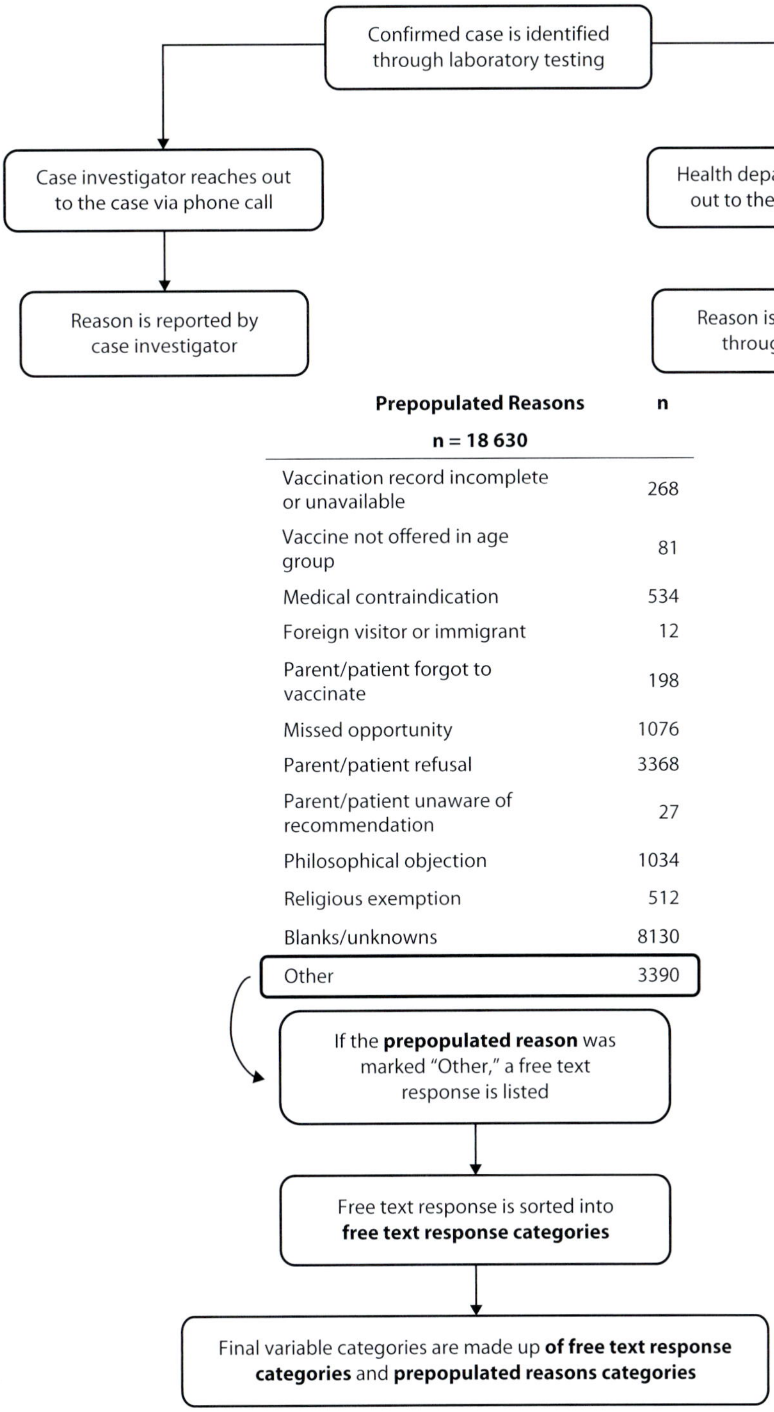

Prepopulated Reasons n = 18 630	**n**
Vaccination record incomplete or unavailable	268
Vaccine not offered in age group	81
Medical contraindication	534
Foreign visitor or immigrant	12
Parent/patient forgot to vaccinate	198
Missed opportunity	1076
Parent/patient refusal	3368
Parent/patient unaware of recommendation	27
Philosophical objection	1034
Religious exemption	512
Blanks/unknowns	8130
Other	3390

FIGURE 1— Predictor Variable "Reasons for Not Vaccinating" Creation Guide

Postinvestigation hospitalization events (yes, no) were also included as an indicator of COVID-19 severity. "Days until interview" indicates number of days between laboratory confirmation and initiation of case investigation. If the date of laboratory confirmation was missing, specimen submission date and first positive COVID-19 laboratory result date were used instead. Cases exceeding 150 days were omitted to reduce outliers.

Statistical Analysis

Frequency and percentage distribution of demographic and behavioral characteristics describe the cohort. We used a modified Poisson regression to test the association between vaccination status and predictors, calculating incidence risk ratios (IRRs) and 95% confidence intervals (CIs). We fitted bivariate and multivariable models to account for potential confounding between predictive variables and the outcome. We conducted a sensitivity analysis to assess for the influence of confounding on the main model by days until interview. We used manual selection to select predictors for inclusion in the final model, though all predictors were included because of their significance. We performed all statistical analyses with SAS version 9.4 (SAS Institute, Cary, NC).

RESULTS

Table 1 describes the cohort stratified by VSIIF. Of the 16 344 cases, 86% remained unvaccinated 6 months after the investigation. Most of the cohort refused to respond to the RNV question (63.3% vaccinated VSIIF vs 73.6% unvaccinated VSIIF). Among those who were vaccinated VSIIF, the most common RNV was missed opportunity/lack of convenience (18.7%), followed by apathetic/undecided toward vaccination (7.3%), and philosophical objection (4.9%) Similar results were seen among the unvaccinated VSIIF, with philosophical objection (8.3%), missed opportunity/lack of convenience (6.8%), and religious exemption (3.4%). Of those who responded to frequency of facemask use, most vaccinated VSIIF individuals answered that they always or almost always wear them (30.5%) while most unvaccinated VSIIF indicated they sometimes or rarely wore facemasks (26.5%). The cohort was predominantly aged younger than 65 years (89.1%), female (54.8%), and White (76.5%); were not hospitalized (93.2%); did not attend public events (61.9%); and lived within a metropolitan zip code (51.7%).

Table B (available as a supplement to the online version of this article at https://ajph.org) shows the distribution of demographic characteristics stratified by age. There was a greater proportion of individuals aged 65 years or older compared with those aged younger than 65 years who never wore a facemask (13.8% vs 12.8%), were hospitalized (20.1% vs 4.4%), were non-Hispanic White (92.9% vs 74.4%), and lived in rural (23.5% vs 12.4%) or small town (18.9% vs 15.4%) designated zip codes. Table C (available as a supplement to the online version of this article at https://ajph.org) characterizes the cohort distribution by responsiveness to RNV. The proportion of nonresponders to responders is higher for unvaccinated VSIIF (87.9% vs 81.7%), non-Hispanic Whites (79.6% vs 68.2%) and among those who lived in rural (15.9% vs 7.6%) or small town (19.7% vs 5.7%) designated zip codes. Figure D (available as a supplement to the online version of this article at https://ajph.org) depicts the 3 eras of predominant SARS-CoV-2 variants during the study period and the distribution of RNV during each era. The Delta variant (June 2021–November 2021) had the largest number of case investigations (10 744), followed by the *o* variant (December 2021–ongoing) with 4717 observations and α variant (March 2021–May 2021) with 853 observations. Aside from refusal to answer, the most common RNV was missed opportunity/lack of convenience during α (15.7%) and Delta (8.7%), and philosophical objection during *o* (10.1%).

Table 2 depicts the crude IRRs and adjusted IRRs (AIRRs) of the risk factors for having an unvaccinated VSIIF. In the final model, compared with those whose RNV was missed opportunity/lack of convenience, the risk of unvaccinated VSIIF was greatest among those who cited their RNV as being religious exemption (AIRR = 1.36; 95% CI = 1.31, 1.41), philosophical objection (AIRR = 1.28; 95% CI = 1.24, 1.34), or institutional confidence/complacency–driven concerns (AIRR = 1.26; 95% CI = 1.19, 1.33). Apathy/undecided toward vaccination (AIRR = 1.05, 95% CI = 0.99, 1.12) had the lowest risk of nonvaccination VSIIF.

The risk of having an unvaccinated VSIIF was greater among those aged 65 years or older (AIRR = 1.02; 95% CI = 1.00, 1.05) and those who attended public events (AIRR = 1.02; 95% CI = 1.00, 1.03). Compared with non-Hispanic White individuals, those of minority races/ethnicities were more likely to be vaccinated, with Hispanic individuals being most likely to be vaccinated (AIRR = 0.89; 95% CI = 0.87, 0.91). There was a positive association between rurality and nonvaccinated VSIIF, with increased risk in nonvaccination correlating with increased rurality of residential zip code. Compared with those who resided in a metropolitan zip code, those who resided in rural zip codes had a 7% greater risk of being nonvaccinated at follow-up (AIRR = 1.07; 95% CI = 1.05, 1.09). Reduced and limited facemask use was associated with nonvaccination, with the risk of unvaccinated VSIIF being greater for those who sometimes or rarely mask (AIRR = 1.03; 95% CI = 1.02, 1.05) and for those who never mask (AIRR = 1.05; 95% CI = 1.03, 1.08) compared with those who always or almost always mask. Hospitalization was associated with reduced risk of nonvaccination (AIRR = 0.93; 95% CI = 0.91, 0.96). There was no difference between males and females in the risk of nonvaccination VSIIF.

TABLE 1— Demographic Characteristics of Unvaccinated COVID-19 Cases by Vaccination Status at 6-Month Follow-Up: Nebraska, May 2021–February 2023

Characteristics	Total (n = 16 344), No. (%)	Vaccinated (n = 2261), No. (%)	Unvaccinated (n = 14 083), No. (%)
Reason for not vaccinating at baseline			
Missed opportunity/lack of convenience	1 376 (8.4)	422 (18.7)	954 (6.8)
Apathetic/undecided	591 (3.6)	164 (7.3)	427 (3.0)
Institutional confidence/complacency	289 (1.8)	31 (1.4)	258 (1.8)
Philosophical objection	1 283 (7.9)	110 (4.9)	1 173 (8.3)
Religious exemption	490 (3.0)	17 (0.8)	473 (3.4)
Research/safety confidence	516 (3.2)	87 (3.9)	429 (3.1)
Refused to respond	11 799 (72.2)	1 430 (63.3)	10 369 (73.6)
Age category, y			
18–24	1 899 (11.6)	283 (12.5)	1 616 (11.5)
25–34	4 220 (25.8)	638 (28.2)	3 582 (25.4)
35–49	5 159 (31.6)	775 (34.3)	4 384 (31.1)
50–64	3 286 (20.1)	416 (18.4)	2 870 (20.4)
≥ 65	1 780 (10.9)	149 (6.6)	1 631 (11.6)
Sex			
Male	7 382 (45.2)	1 000 (44.2)	6 382 (45.3)
Female	8 962 (54.8)	1 261 (55.8)	7 701 (54.7)
Race/ethnicity			
White	12 495 (76.5)	1 358 (60.1)	11 137 (79.1)
AIAN/NHPI/Asian	377 (2.3)	87 (3.9)	290 (2.1)
Black	1 307 (8.0)	305 (13.5)	1 002 (7.1)
Hispanic	2 165 (13.3)	511 (22.6)	1 654 (11.7)
Facemask use			
Always/almost always	3 868 (23.7)	689 (30.5)	3 179 (22.6)
Sometimes/rarely	4 198 (25.7)	470 (20.8)	3 728 (26.5)
Never	2 109 (12.9)	185 (8.2)	1 924 (13.7)
Unknown	6 169 (37.7)	917 (40.6)	5 252 (37.3)
Attend public events			
No	10 108 (61.9)	1 497 (66.2)	8 611 (61.1)
Yes	3 658 (22.4)	445 (19.7)	3 213 (22.8)
Unknown	2 578 (15.8)	319 (14.1)	2 259 (16.0)
Hospitalized			
No	15 349 (93.2)	2 088 (92.4)	13 261 (94.2)
Yes	995 (6.1)	173 (7.7)	822 (5.8)
RUCA census tract designation			
Metropolitan	8 449 (51.7)	1 494 (66.1)	6 955 (49.4)
Micropolitan	3 090 (18.9)	356 (15.8)	2 734 (19.4)
Small town	2 576 (15.8)	240 (10.6)	2 336 (16.6)
Rural	2 229 (13.6)	171 (7.6)	2 058 (14.6)

Note. AIAN = American Indian and Alaska Native; NHPI = Native Hawaiian and Pacific Islander; RUCA = Rural–Urban Commuting Area Codes.

TABLE 2— Risk Factors for Nonvaccination 6 Months After Having COVID-19 Among Nonvaccinated Individuals: Nebraska, May 2021–February 2023

Risk Factors	IRR (95% CI)	
	Crude	Adjusted
Reason for not vaccinating at baseline		
Missed opportunity/lack of convenience (Ref)	1	1
Apathetic/undecided	1.04 (0.98, 1.11)	1.05 (0.99, 1.12)
Institutional confidence/complacency	1.29 (1.22, 1.36)	1.26 (1.19, 1.33)
Philosophical objection	1.32 (1.27, 1.37)	1.28 (1.24, 1.34)
Religious exemption	1.39 (1.34, 1.45)	1.36 (1.31, 1.41)
Research/safety confidence	1.20 (1.14, 1.26)	1.17 (1.11, 1.24)
Refused to respond	1.27 (1.22, 1.31)	1.22 (1.18, 1.27)
Age category, y		
18–24 (Ref)	1	1
25–34	1.00 (0.98, 1.02)	0.99 (0.97, 1.01)
35–49	1.00 (0.98, 1.02)	0.98 (0.96, 1.00)
50–64	1.03 (1.00, 1.05)	0.99 (0.97, 1.01)
≥ 65	1.08 (1.05, 1.10)	1.02 (1.00, 1.05)
Sex		
Male (Ref)	1	1
Female	0.99 (0.98, 1.01)	1.00 (0.98, 1.01)
Race/ethnicity		
White (Ref)	1	1
AIAN/NHPI/Asian	0.86 (0.82, 0.91)	0.90 (0.85, 0.95)
Black	0.86 (0.83, 0.89)	0.91 (0.88, 0.94)
Hispanic	0.86 (0.84, 0.88)	0.89 (0.87, 0.91)
Facemask use		
Always/almost always (Ref)	1	1
Sometimes/rarely	1.08 (1.06, 1.10)	1.03 (1.02, 1.05)
Never	1.11 (1.09, 1.13)	1.05 (1.03, 1.08)
Unknown	1.04 (1.02, 1.05)	1.06 (1.04, 1.08)
Attend public events		
No (Ref)	1	1
Yes	1.03 (1.02, 1.05)	1.02 (1.00, 1.03)
Unknown	1.03 (1.01, 1.05)	0.99 (0.97, 1.01)
Hospitalized		
No (Ref)	1	1
Yes	0.96 (0.93, 0.98)	0.93 (0.91, 0.96)
RUCA census tract designation		
Metropolitan (Ref)	1	1
Micropolitan	1.07 (1.06, 1.09)	1.05 (1.03, 1.07)
Small town	1.10 (1.08, 1.12)	1.06 (1.04, 1.08)
Rural	1.12 (1.10, 1.14)	1.07 (1.05, 1.09)

Note. AIAN = American Indian and Alaska Native; CI = confidence interval; IRR = incidence risk ratio; NHPI = Native Hawaiian and Pacific Islander; RUCA = Rural–Urban Commuting Area. The sample size was n = 16 344.

Table E (available as a supplement to the online version of this article at https://ajph.org) shows the risk factors for having an unvaccinated VSIIF stratified by predominant SARS-CoV-2 variant. We observed similar patterns of association with the final model across all variant periods. To assess whether time between laboratory confirmation and case investigation was a confounding factor on VSIIF, we ran a sensitivity analysis on 16 199 cases detailed in Table F (available as a supplement to the online version of this article at https://ajph.org) by including days until interview into the final model. The average number of days until interview was 2.7 (SE = 4.16), and it did not confound the results of our model.

DISCUSSION

More than 80% of the study population remained unvaccinated 6 months after the investigation. Previous studies using a national sample of US respondents observed greater odds of vaccine hesitancy among those with PCD.[20] In addition, research exploring vaccination intent observed a decline in the percentage of individuals who were vaccine-hesitant over time, yet the percentage of individuals identified as strongly hesitant remained unchanged.[21] Our observation that the risk of nonvaccination was highest among those with institutional confidence/complacency–driven concerns and ideology-centered objections may explain this phenomenon. Experiencing asymptomatic or mild symptoms can further drive complacency, reinforcing perception of lower threat of disease, which could impact their likelihood of vaccinating in the future.[16] Individuals who prefer acquiring natural immunity through infection over vaccination may also continue to be vaccine-hesitant after PCD because of increased complacency. However, hospitalization could be an indicator of severe or prolonged COVID-19 outcomes, thus elevating an individual's perceived threat of disease and reducing the risk of nonvaccination as seen in our results.

Furthermore, studies related to religion and COVID-19 have found a negative association between religiosity and intention to vaccinate, which we also identified.[12,22] Research has indicated that attitudes and beliefs related to COVID-19 skepticism and vaccine hesitancy could be associated with some political or religious affiliations and were not mitigated through personal experiences from COVID-19.[14] Philosophical exemption, on the other hand, serves as a catch-all for other ideology-based reasons for objection. Alternatively, the number of US adults who prefer to "wait and see" declined over several months, with hesitancy stemming from concerns over safety/lack of research.[23] In our study, the risk of being nonvaccinated was lowest among those who were apathetic/undecided and those who expressed research/safety confidence–related concerns. Our results indicate that among those who elected not to receive a vaccination 6 months after the investigation, individuals who were apathetic/undecided or concerned regarding safety/research could be receptive to changing uptake behavior whereas those who had ideology-centered concerns were more strongly hesitant.

Race and ethnicity have played a pivotal role in influencing attitudes toward vaccination within the United States. Minorities have been disproportionally impacted by the COVID-19 pandemic through severity of clinical presentation, rates of hospitalization, and increased morbidity and mortality.[7,24] Gaps in access to health care and worsening socioeconomic disparities also exacerbated the social and economic impact of the pandemic on minorities. Belief-based predictors of hesitancy among non-Hispanic African Americans and Hispanics include medical and institutional mistrust, history of discrimination, exposure to misinformation, lack of reliable information or messengers, and safety- or efficiency-related concerns.[8] Race has been a well-established determining factor of vaccine uptake and hesitancy.[7] Nevertheless, previous research indicates rates of vaccine hesitancy decreased and vaccine intention increased among minorities compared with non-Hispanic White populations over time.[25] Our study also emphasizes the reduced risk of persistent nonvaccination among minorities compared with non-Hispanic Whites with PCD despite their greater rate of hesitancy compared with the general population. Greater severity of illness among minorities could also reduce complacency and increase perceived risk of disease, further encouraging vaccination.

Similarly, we observed that with an increase in rurality, there is a small but significant increase in the risk of persistent nonvaccination. Concerns regarding vaccine efficacy, social stigma, access to vaccines, and fear over vaccine safety were indicated as reasons for hesitancy among rural residents in previous studies.[26] Rural communities are also more likely to believe the vaccine was unsafe and exhibit lower health literacy rates.[27] Though the most trusted sources of information among rural Nebraskans include interpersonal acquaintances, Public Broadcasting Service, and local news or newspapers, trust in local and state news sources overall has declined significantly since 2017.[28] Alienation from trusted sources of information because of poor health literacy could drive individuals to consume digestible but inaccurate information instead.[27]

We noted a surprisingly elevated risk of nonvaccinated VSIIF among older adults that can be further explained once stratifying the demographics by age group. The older population displayed a greater proportion of ideology-centered reasons for nonvaccination, rural or small-town residency, and non-Hispanic White race/ethnicity. Because of the association between the listed determinants with persistent vaccine refusal, we can conclude that the older population within our cohort was highly vaccine-resistant.

Our results indicate noncompliance to mitigation measures such as facemasks and public event attendance were associated with greater risk of nonvaccination. Similar results have been seen on the national scale, where respondents with low vaccination intention were also less likely to report engaging in COVID-19 prevention behaviors.[29] Such observations are not surprising; distrust in vaccines and in the government is a high risk predictor of nonvaccination; thus, aversion to government mandates can influence compliance behavior toward all mitigation measures, including vaccination, mask wearing, and social distancing.[30] Furthermore, reasons for opposition against government mandates, such as concerns over restrictions on personal liberty and right to choose, could be used to abstain from both vaccination and other mitigation measures.[31]

Limitations

Our study was subject to several limitations. Lack of information regarding method of investigation administration occludes if there is differentiation and subsequent bias in the responses. Case investigations conducted by investigators may be subject to reporter bias. Survey-based case investigations were subject to social desirability bias by potentially conforming to acceptable norms regarding vaccination. Out-of-state immunizations must be individually reported and could lead to inaccurate reporting of vaccination status. The fluctuation of COVID-19 cases within Nebraska led to delayed case investigation initiation in some local health departments, which would have excluded from our study anyone who vaccinated between time of infection and case investigation. This could skew participation toward those with negative VSIIF status.

Prepopulated responses incorporated into the final RNV categories did not have associated free text and therefore lack the detail of "other" responses. Because of the incomplete nature of symptom reporting, severity of symptoms could not be inferred. Lack of information on comorbidities, medical history, occupation, and income has reduced our understanding related to socioeconomic status, potential frequency of exposure, and immunocompromised status.

Our study also excluded individuals who utilized at-home test kits to confirm their infection positivity without subsequent laboratory testing, subjecting our research to bias if the reason for nonvaccination differed between at-home and laboratory test users. Individuals who died before 6-month follow-up were excluded (< 5% of the cohort), producing a slim potential for selection bias. The most recently available Rural–Urban Commuting Area data set was from 2010, potentially leading to bias in the assignment of urbanicity. Finally, there was a large proportion of individuals who refused to respond to why they were not vaccinated, subjecting our analysis to potential underestimation of the strength of association, reducing our statistical power, and limiting the generalizability of our results.

Public Health Implications

The implications of our findings can be used to identify highly resistant communities that may show elevated contention and limited adherence to public health–related mitigation strategies suggested by individuals outside of their community. Thus, advocating for intervention may require endorsements from those they trust within the community. Previous strategies involving partnerships with members of the community, such as religious leaders among faith communities and copartisan politicians among partisan communities, have been successful in promoting vaccination.[32,33] Findings also identified populations that are receptive toward vaccination despite initial hesitancy. Public health leaders can strengthen confidence in vaccines by addressing the main causes of hesitancy from audiences that could be persuaded to vaccinate, including minority populations. Persistent vaccine refusal among rural communities must be further assessed in Nebraska, given the large population living in nonmetropolitan areas.

Conclusions

Our study observed ideology and reduced institutional confidence/complacency–centered objections, older age, low adherence to mitigation measures, and rurality as risk factors for persistent COVID-19 vaccine refusal. Future research related to these topics should further prioritize partisanship, occupation, and religiosity as determinants of interest given their relationship with vaccination intent and hesitancy, as well as identify differences in RNV based on COVID-19 diagnosis status to better understand its role in cultivating vaccination decision-making. Sources of misinformation among different unvaccinated groups should also be reevaluated to better understand what strategies could be implemented among the highly vaccine-resistant. AJPH

ABOUT THE AUTHORS

He (Julia) Bai, David Brett-Major, Yi Du, Sai Paritala, Edward S. Peters, Kendra L. Ratnapradipa, and Patrick Maloney are with the College of Public Health, University of Nebraska Medical Center, Omaha.

CORRESPONDENCE

Correspondence should be sent to He (Julia) Bai, 984395 Nebraska Medical Center, Omaha, NE 68198-4395 (e-mail: julia.bai@unmc.edu). Reprints can be ordered at https://www.ajph.org by clicking the "Reprints" link.

PUBLICATION INFORMATION

Full Citation: Bai He (Julia), Brett-Major D, Du Y, et al. Predictors of persistent COVID-19 vaccine refusal among previously infected patients in Nebraska. *Am J Public Health*. 2025;115(3):414–424.

Acceptance Date: November 5, 2024.

DOI: https://doi.org/10.2105/AJPH.2024.307921

ORCID iDs:

He (Julia) Bai https://orcid.org/0000-0001-5022-4289

David Brett-Major https://orcid.org/0000-0002-7583-8495

Yi Du https://orcid.org/0000-0003-4044-1989

Edward S. Peters https://orcid.org/0000-0003-4928-6532

Kendra L. Ratnapradipa https://orcid.org/0000-0003-0265-2400

Patrick Maloney https://orcid.org/0000-0003-2376-9819

CONTRIBUTORS

H. Bai conceptualized the study, cleaned and modified the data set, conducted the data analysis, and wrote the article. P. Maloney supervised the data analysis and contributed support to concept, design, and interpretation of results. All authors aided in the interpretation of the analysis and provided critical feedback and review of the contents.

ACKNOWLEDGMENTS

The authors would like to thank their partners at the Nebraska Department of Health and Human Services for their continued support.

CONFLICTS OF INTEREST

The authors have no disclosures related to potential and actual conflicts of interest.

HUMAN PARTICIPANT PROTECTION

The study is exempt from institutional review board review because of the use of de-identified information.

REFERENCES

1. David J. Sencer CDC Museum. CDC Museum COVID-19 timeline. Centers for Disease Control and Prevention. August 4, 2021. Available at: https://stacks.cdc.gov/view/cdc/110786. Accessed February 28, 2023.
2. Mat Daud AA. Five common misconceptions regarding flattening-the-curve of COVID-19. *Hist Philos Life Sci*. 2022;44(3):41. https://doi.org/10.1007/s40656-022-00522-x
3. Guzman-Cottrill JA, Malani AN, Weber DJ, et al. Local, state and federal face mask mandates during the COVID-19 pandemic. *Infect Control Hosp Epidemiol*. 2021;42(4):455–456. https://doi.org/10.1017/ice.2020.1403
4. Lancet Commission on COVID-19 Vaccines and Therapeutics Task Force Members. Operation Warp Speed: implications for global vaccine security. *Lancet Glob Health*. 2021;9(7):e1017–e1021. https://doi.org/10.1016/S2214-109X(21)00140-6
5. National Center for Immunization and Respiratory Diseases. COVID-19 vaccination coverage and vaccine confidence among adults. Centers for Disease Control and Prevention. March 31, 2024. Available at: https://www.cdc.gov/vaccines/imz-managers/coverage/covidvaxview/interactive/adults.html. Accessed May 11, 2024.
6. MacDonald NE. Vaccine hesitancy: definition, scope and determinants. *Vaccine*. 2015;33(34):4161–4164. https://doi.org/10.1016/j.vaccine.2015.04.036
7. Yasmin F, Najeeb H, Moeed A, et al. COVID-19 vaccine hesitancy in the United States: a systematic review. *Front Public Health*. 2021;9:770985. https://doi.org/10.3389/fpubh.2021.770985
8. Shearn C, Krockow EM. Reasons for COVID-19 vaccine hesitancy in ethnic minority groups: a systematic review and thematic synthesis of initial attitudes in qualitative research. *SSM Qual Res Health*. 2023;3:100210. https://doi.org/10.1016/j.ssmqr.2022.100210
9. Kirzinger A, Sparks G, Brodie M. KFF COVID-19 Vaccine Monitor—rural America. KFF. April 9, 2021. Available at: https://www.kff.org/coronavirus-covid-19/poll-finding/kff-covid-19-vaccine-monitor-rural-america. Accessed May 11, 2024.
10. Koskan AM, LoCoco IE, Daniel CL, Teeter BS. Rural Americans' COVID-19 vaccine perceptions and willingness to vaccinate against COVID-19 with their community pharmacists: an exploratory study. *Vaccines (Basel)*. 2023;11(1):171. https://doi.org/10.3390/vaccines11010171
11. Whitehead AL, Perry SL. How culture wars delay herd immunity: Christian nationalism and anti-vaccine attitudes. *Socius*. 2020;6:2378023120977727. https://doi.org/10.1177/2378023120977727
12. Corcoran KE, Scheitle CP, DiGregorio BD. Christian nationalism and COVID-19 vaccine hesitancy and uptake. *Vaccine*. 2021;39(45):6614–6621. https://doi.org/10.1016/j.vaccine.2021.09.074
13. Limbu YB, Gautam RK, Pham L. The health belief model applied to COVID-19 vaccine hesitancy: a systematic review. *Vaccines (Basel)*. 2022;10(6):973. https://doi.org/10.3390/vaccines10060973
14. Levin J, Bradshaw M. Determinants of COVID-19 skepticism and SARS-CoV-2 vaccine hesitancy: findings from a national population survey of US adults. *BMC Public Health*. 2022;22(1):1047. https://doi.org/10.1186/s12889-022-13477-2
15. Limbu YB, Gautam RK. The determinants of COVID-19 vaccination intention: a meta-review. *Front Public Health*. 2023;11:1162861. https://doi.org/10.3389/fpubh.2023.1162861
16. Huang Y, Zhang L, Fu J, et al. COVID-19 vaccine hesitancy among patients recovered from COVID-19 infection in Wuhan, China: cross-sectional questionnaire study. *JMIR Public Health Surveill*. 2023;9:e42958. https://doi.org/10.2196/42958
17. Gerussi V, Peghin M, Palese A, et al. Vaccine hesitancy among Italian patients recovered from COVID-19 infection towards influenza and SARS-CoV-2 vaccination. *Vaccines (Basel)*. 2021;9(2):172. https://doi.org/10.3390/vaccines9020172
18. Centers for Disease Control and Prevention. Coronavirus disease 2019 (COVID-19) 2023 case definition. February 28, 2023. Available at: https://ndc.services.cdc.gov/case-definitions/coronavirus-disease-2019-2023. Accessed May 31, 2024.
19. Economic Research Service. Rural-Urban Commuting Area Codes. US Department of Agriculture. July 3, 2019. Available at: https://www.ers.usda.gov/data-products/rural-urban-commuting-area-codes.aspx. Accessed March 20, 2023.
20. Do DP, Frank R. Prior COVID-19 infection: an underappreciated factor in vaccine hesitancy in the USA. *J Public Health (Oxf)*. 2022;44(2):471–474. https://doi.org/10.1093/pubmed/fdab404
21. Beleche T, Ruhter J, Kolbe A, Marus J, Bush L, Sommers B. COVID-19 vaccine hesitancy: demographic factors, geographic patterns, and changes over time. 2021. Available at: https://aspe.hhs.gov/sites/default/files/migrated_legacy_files/200816/aspe-ib-vaccine-hesitancy.pdf. Accessed April 11, 2024.
22. Olagoke AA, Olagoke OO, Hughes AM. Intention to vaccinate against the novel 2019 coronavirus disease: the role of health locus of control and religiosity. *J Relig Health*. 2021;60(1):65–80. https://doi.org/10.1007/s10943-020-01090-9
23. Hamel L, Lopes L, Sparks G, Stokes M, Brodie M. KFF COVID-19 vaccine monitor: April 2021. KFF.

April 2021. Available at: https://www.kff.org/coronavirus-covid-19/poll-finding/kff-covid-19-vaccine-monitor-april-2021. Accessed April 11, 2024.

24. Tai DBG, Sia IG, Doubeni CA, Wieland ML. Disproportionate impact of COVID-19 on racial and ethnic minority groups in the United States: a 2021 update. *J Racial Ethn Health Disparities*. 2022;9(6):2334–2339. https://doi.org/10.1007/s40615-021-01170-w

25. Padamsee TJ, Bond RM, Dixon GN, et al. Changes in COVID-19 vaccine hesitancy among Black and White individuals in the US. *JAMA Netw Open*. 2022;5(1):e2144470. https://doi.org/10.1001/jamanetworkopen.2021.44470

26. Robinson R, Nguyen E, Wright M, et al. Factors contributing to vaccine hesitancy and reduced vaccine confidence in rural underserved populations. *Humanit Soc Sci Commun*. 2022;9(1):416. https://doi.org/10.1057/s41599-022-01439-3

27. Kricorian K, Civen R, Equils O. COVID-19 vaccine hesitancy: misinformation and perceptions of vaccine safety. *Hum Vaccin Immunother*. 2022;18(1):1950504. https://doi.org/10.1080/21645515.2021.1950504

28. Vogt B. Changes in trust in media in rural Nebraska. Institute of Agriculture and Natural Resources. July 27, 2022. Available at: https://digitalcommons.unl.edu/ruralpoll/13. Accessed May 31, 2024.

29. Latkin CA, Dayton L, Yi G, Colon B, Kong X. Mask usage, social distancing, racial, and gender correlates of COVID-19 vaccine intentions among adults in the US. *PLoS One*. 2021;16(2):e0246970. https://doi.org/10.1371/journal.pone.0246970

30. Ramirez MD, Wood RM. Authoritarian opposition? Authoritarian disposition and resistance to public health mitigation strategies during COVID-19. *Polit Res Q*. 2023;77(1):239–254. https://doi.org/10.1177/10659129231204234

31. Carpiano RM, Callaghan T, DiResta R, et al. Confronting the evolution and expansion of anti-vaccine activism in the USA in the COVID-19 era. *Lancet*. 2023;401(10380):967–970. https://doi.org/10.1016/S0140-6736(23)00136-8

32. Sylvester S, Motta M, Trujillo KL, Callaghan T. Vaccinating across the aisle: using co-partisan source cues to encourage COVID-19 vaccine uptake in the ideological right. *J Behav Med*. 2023;46(1-2):311–323. https://doi.org/10.1007/s10865-022-00323-4

33. Ayub S, Anugwom GO, Basiru T, et al. Bridging science and spirituality: the intersection of religion and public health in the COVID-19 pandemic. *Front Psychiatry*. 2023;14:1183234. https://doi.org/10.3389/fpsyt.2023.1183234

Health Care Stereotype Threat During the COVID-19 Pandemic Among Sexual and Gender Minority Individuals

Wendy D. Manning, PhD, Claire Kamp Dush, PhD, and Kristen Gustafson, MA

See also Turpin, p. 265.

Objectives. To determine the levels and differentials in health care stereotype threat experienced during the COVID-19 pandemic by individuals with sexual or gender minority identities.

Methods. The National Couples' Health and Time Use Study is a national cross-sectional US population–based sample of partnered individuals interviewed during the pandemic between September 2020 and April 2021 with oversamples of sexual and gender minority individuals. The analytic sample consisted of 3614 individuals (n = 2043 heterosexual and n = 1571 sexual minority individuals along with 3489 cisgender and 125 noncisgender people).

Results. Individuals with sexual minority identities experienced significantly more health care stereotype threat than heterosexual people. Cisgender women and those with another gender identity experienced significantly more health care stereotype threat than cisgender men. These results persisted after the inclusion of indicators of health conditions, insurance, COVID-19 experience, and sociodemographic factors.

Conclusions. Gender and sexual minority–identifying people reported high levels of worries about health discrimination. Our work suggests that providing positive health care experiences may reduce these worries and offer a potential antidote to sexual and gender minority health disparities that are driven by structural and interpersonal discrimination. These findings support calls for the further education and transformation of health care provision and systems. (*Am J Public Health*. 2025;115(3):425–433. https://doi.org/10.2105/AJPH.2024.307926)

AJPH March 2025, Vol. 115, No. 3

The disparities in the health and well-being of sexual and gender–diverse people that existed before the COVID-19 pandemic are well described in a large body of research ranging from cardiac health to mental illness to substance use.[1–4] These health differentials continued into the COVID-19 pandemic.[5–11] Before the pandemic, it was clear that an important barrier to receiving health care—and an underlying reason for a substantial share of sexual and gender minority health disparities—was anticipating or experiencing discrimination in the health care setting.[12–20] Our study builds on this work and examined whether health care stereotype threat reported during the pandemic was greater for sexual and gender–diverse people at the bivariate level and after adjusting for health conditions and insurance as well as sociodemographic indicators.

According to evidence from before the onset of the COVID-19 pandemic, sexual and gender minority individuals faced discrimination on a regular basis with nearly 4 in 10 (36%) reporting discrimination in the last year.[12] Discrimination is characterized as a form of stigma and unfair treatment that impacts health both directly and via heightened stress and behaviors.[18,21,22] Specifically, health care discrimination is consequential as it has the potential to make individuals reluctant to seek care, delay appointments, and avoid preventive health care, and, as a result, leads to postponed diagnoses and treatments.[20] Experiences with discrimination influence the lives of lesbian, gay, bisexual, and transgender (LGBT)–identifying people as two thirds (68.5%) reported that it impacted their psychological well-being, and two fifths (44%) their physical well-being.[23] Furthermore, discrimination contributed to heightened levels of suicidal intentions among sexual minority young adults[16] and alcohol use among sexual minority adults.[24]

Research specifically on discrimination in the health care setting is more limited. A handful of studies indicate that sexual and gender–diverse individuals have experienced discrimination and unfair treatment specifically in health care settings. A large national survey of LGBT adults with HIV indicated 56% reported some form of health care discrimination including harsh or abusive language, refusals to touch, and blaming for their health status.[25] Similarly, in the 2015–2017 California Health Interview Survey, gay, lesbian, and bisexual adults more often reported receiving unfair health care treatment than heterosexual adults, and in another study of 489 lesbian, gay, bisexual, transgender, and queer (LGBTQ) adults, 16% of LGBTQ individuals reported health care discrimination.[26,27] The prevalence of health care discrimination was highest in middle age among lesbian, gay, and bisexual (LGB) adults in the 2012–2013 National Epidemiologic Survey of Alcohol and Related Conditions III. The peak age of health care discrimination experience (23%) was age 55 for LGB adults, likely tied in to growing demands for health care as individuals age.[28]

A related body of work focused on stereotype threat and LGB health and is based on worries about being negatively judged because of a stereotype. Health care stereotype threat is defined as "the threat of being personally reduced to group stereotypes that commonly operate within the health-care domain."[29–32(p191)] Individuals who report health care stereotype threat or in other words anticipate discrimination are likely avoiding important health care visits. Stereotype threat is based on individual reports of subjective appraisals (defined as worries) related to their treatment in the health care realm. The effects of this threat on health outcomes depended on the strength of the identity in experiment-based work on race.[33] This framework aligns with health care discrimination research, and we focused on health care stereotype threat. Empirical evidence based on data collected before the pandemic indicates that substantial shares of LGBTQ individuals postponed or avoided health care because of discrimination or anticipated discrimination.[12,27,34–36] Analyses of LGB adults show that health care stereotype threat is linked to more frequent poor physical health days and psychological distress.[30] There are few studies focusing on health care stereotype threat during the COVID-19 pandemic.

METHODS

The National Couples' Health and Time Study is a nationally representative sample of 3642 partnered respondents with oversamples of racial, ethnic, and sexual minority people. Respondents' ages ranged from 20 to 60 years, and they were individuals who were married or cohabiting at the time of data collection. The respondents were part of the Gallup Panel, and data were collected online from September 2020 to April 2021. An asset of the Gallup Panel was that it allowed an oversample of sexual minority respondents as they were identified as part of panel membership. These data were especially well suited for these analyses because of the breadth of questions, timing of data collection, and the large, population-based sample of sexual and gender minority people. Given the oversampling, it was important that Gallup generated sample weights based on national estimates, and person-level weights were applied to all analyses. These data are publicly available for download at the Inter-university Consortium for Political and Social Research (https://www.icpsr.umich.edu/web/DSDR/studies/38417).[37]

The analytic sample was limited to those without missing responses on the health care stereotype threat measures (n = 3632). The final sample was restricted to those who responded to questions on COVID-19, identity centrality, and having a health condition (n = 3618). The final sample excluded 4 additional respondents who did not respond to questions about gender or education (n = 3614). More details about the study are provided in this paper.[38]

Measures

Health care stereotype threat draws on 3 items used in the Generations Study.[33,39] Respondents were asked when seeking health care to indicate on a 5-point scale how much they agreed or disagreed with 3 statements: "I worry about being negatively judged"; "I worry that diagnoses of me/my health may be negatively affected because of who I am"; and "I worry that I might confirm negative stereotypes about people like me." Responses ranged from 1 = "Strongly Disagree" to 5 = "Strongly Agree," and items were averaged. The Cronbach α was 0.84.

Respondents were asked to "select all that apply" when asked about 11 sexual identities including "heterosexual or straight," "gay or lesbian," "bisexual," "same-gender loving," "queer," "pansexual," "omnisexual," "asexual," "don't know," "questioning," and "something else." We coded respondents into 4 mutually exclusive sexual identity categories. Respondents who reported being only heterosexual and no other sexual identities were coded as heterosexual; respondents who reported a gay or lesbian identity along with any other identity were coded as gay or lesbian; respondents who reported a bisexual identity and another identity except gay or lesbian were coded as bisexual, and those who did not report exclusively heterosexual, gay or lesbian, or bisexual are coded as "another." Among the most common sexual identities included in the "another" group were exclusively pansexual (n = 62) and exclusively queer (n = 49). We acknowledge there are many ways to code sexual identities, and we have tested differing strategies and obtained similar results.

Gender identity was measured based on respondents' answers to 2 questions: gender identity and sex assigned at birth. Gender identity was asked as "Which of the following best describes your gender?" Responses were 1 = "Man"; 2 = "Woman"; 3 = "Trans man"; 4 = "Trans woman"; 5 = "Do not identify as any of the above." Sexual identity at birth was asked as "What sex appears on your birth certificate? 1 = "Male"; 2 = "Female"; 3 = "Don't know/does not apply." For analysis, we categorized individuals as noncisgender when their sex at birth did not match their gender identity response of "Man" or "Woman" as well as individuals who reported "Trans woman, "Trans man," or "Do not identify as any of the above." For example, our coding allowed someone who identified as a man but was assigned female at birth to be considered noncisgender. The three mutually exclusive categories were cisgender man, cisgender woman, and transgender or another gender identity. The sample did not have sufficient sample sizes to distinguish the noncisgender identities.

Centrality of sexual identity was measured by respondents reporting how much they agreed or disagreed with the statement, "My sexual orientation/identity is a central part of my identity." Responses ranged from 1 = "Strongly Disagree" to 5 = "Strongly Agree."

Access to health insurance was measured by respondents' reports of whether they had some form of health insurance. This variable was coded as 0 indicating that the respondent reported "I currently do not have health insurance" and 1 indicating the respondent reported that they had insurance including through their current or former employer or union, purchased through healthcare.gov or a health insurance marketplace, or Medicaid.

Current health conditions were measured by respondents' reports of currently having 1 of 22 health conditions: arthritis, asthma, blood clots, cancer, chronic obstructive pulmonary disease, Crohn's, diabetes, emphysema, heart attack, heart condition, high blood sugar, high cholesterol, HIV, hypertension, kidney disease, liver disease, osteoporosis, prediabetes, sleep disorder, stroke, thyroid problems, and ulcer. The variable was coded as 1 if respondents indicated they currently had any of the conditions and 0 otherwise.

Experience with COVID-19 was measured by "Have you ever been ill, or suspected you may be ill, with coronavirus (COVID-19)?" Responses ranged from 1 = "Yes, I have had coronavirus or suspected I had coronavirus in the past"; 2 = "Yes, I currently have or suspect I have coronavirus"; and 3 = "No, I have not had or suspected I had coronavirus." This variable was coded as 0 = "Never Had/Suspected COVID-19" and 1 = "Had or Suspected COVID-19."

The models included age as a continuous variable ranging from 20 to 60 years. Race/ethnicity was coded into a mutually exclusive 6-category variable (non-Hispanic White, non-Hispanic Black, non-Hispanic Asian, Hispanic/Latinx, non-Hispanic multiracial, and another). Education was coded into 3 categories (high school or less, some college, college degree) and marital status distinguished respondents who were married and cohabiting. To account for the timing of the interview, month of interview was included as a series of dummy variables ranging from September to April.

Statistical Analysis

The analyses were primarily descriptive. The distribution of the sample across the independent variables is presented in Table 1. We provided the levels of health care stereotype threat for respondents according to their sexual and gender identity and compared differences using bivariate ordinary least squares models. These findings are presented in Figure 1 with heterosexual respondents as the reference group for sexual identity and cisgender women as the reference group for gender identity. Table 2 presents the multivariable ordinary least square regression model results. We selected this method given the distribution of responses based on the scale but obtained similar results when relying on an ordered logistic regression model. We conducted outlier analysis and used variance inflation factor estimates to check for multicollinearity. Data collection included oversamples of sexual minority individuals to ensure the analyses were representative; sample weights were applied to all analyses. We conducted statistical analyses with Stata version 16.1 (StataCorp LP, College Station, TX).

TABLE 1— Characteristics of Sample of Married and Cohabiting Individuals: United States, National Couples' Health and Time Use Study, September 2020–April 2021

	Unweighted No. (Weighted %) or Mean (Range)	95% CI
Dependent variable		
Health discrimination	2.2 (1–5)	2.1, 2.2
Independent variables		
Sexual identity		
Heterosexual or straight	2043 (96.8)	96.5, 97.1
Gay or lesbian	798 (1.2)	1.0, 0.1
Bisexual	535 (1.4)	1.2, 1.6
Another	238 (0.7)	0.6, 0.9
Gender		
Cisgender man	1750 (48.4)	46.0, 50.8
Cisgender woman	1704 (50.6)	48.2, 53.0
Transgender or another	160 (1.0)	0.6, 1.4
Age, y	43.2 (20–60)	42.7, 43.7
Race/ethnicity		
Non-Hispanic White	2137 (56.2)	53.8, 58.5
Non-Hispanic Black	310 (7.4)	6.5, 8.5
Non-Hispanic Asian	200 (6.7)	5.6, 7.8
Hispanic	572 (21.6)	19.6, 23.7
Non-Hispanic multiracial	198 (3.4)	2.8, 4.1
Another	197 (4.8)	4.0, 5.8
Education		
High school or less	635 (31.2)	29.0, 33.5
Some college	705 (22.3)	20.3, 24.4
College degree	2274 (46.5)	44.2, 48.9
Marital status		
Married	2662 (80.8)	78.8, 82.6
Cohabiting	952 (19.2)	17.4, 21.2
Sexual identity centrality	3.2 (1–5)	3.1, 3.2
Health indicators		
Reported health condition		
No current health condition	1864 (57.9)	55.6, 60.3
Currently have health condition	1750 (42.1)	39.7, 44.4
Health insurance		
No health insurance	217 (7.2)	6.0, 8.6
Have health insurance	3397 (92.8)	91.4, 94.0
COVID-19		
Never had or suspected COVID-19	2874 (78.9)	76.9, 80.8
Had or suspected COVID-19	740 (21.1)	19.2, 23.1
Month of survey		
September	1224 (21.7)	19.7, 23.7
October	178 (3.8)	2.9, 4.8
November	363 (13.7)	12.1, 15.5

Continued

RESULTS

The weighted mean level of health discrimination among this sample of partnered adults aged 20 to 60 years was 2.18, slightly below the midpoint (Table 1). Based on weighted estimates, the sample included 3.0% sexual minority participants and 0.3% transgender or noncisgender participants. About half (56.15%) of the sample identified as non-Hispanic White, one fifth (21.61%) as Hispanic, and 7.43% as non-Hispanic Black. The mean age of the sample was 43 years. Nearly half of the sample had a college degree, and the majority were married. About two fifths reported a current health condition, the vast majority had health insurance, and about one fifth had or suspected they had COVID-19 by the time of interview. Most were interviewed in the month of September.

The mean levels of health care stereotype threat at the bivariate level are shown in Figure 1 based on sexual and gender identities. Health care stereotype threat was higher for gay or lesbian respondents in partnerships than for than heterosexual respondents living with a partner or spouse (Figure 1). Respondents who identified as bisexual or "another" sexual identity reported higher levels of health care stereotype threat than gay or lesbian respondents. The next panel of Figure 1 showed that average levels of health care stereotype threat were higher for cisgender women than men, and respondents who were not cisgender had higher levels of health care stereotype threat than cisgender women.

Table 2 presents the parameter estimates from the multivariable ordinary least squares regression models. Consistent with the bivariate results, gay- or lesbian-identifying respondents reported

TABLE 1— Continued

	Unweighted No. (Weighted %) or Mean (Range)	95% CI
December	348 (7.0)	5.9, 8.3
January	765 (29.3)	27.1, 31.6
February	178 (3.6)	0.3, 4.7
March	446 (17.5)	15.8, 19.4
April	112 (3.5)	2.8, 4.4

Note. CI = confidence interval. The full sample (n = 3614) is included in means and CIs for continuous indicators.

higher levels of health care stereotype threat than heterosexual respondents. Bisexual-identifying respondents indicated higher levels of health care stereotype than their heterosexual counterparts. Individuals who reported "another" sexual identity (not heterosexual, bisexual, or gay or lesbian) had greater levels of health care stereotype threat. In this model, respondents identifying as bisexual or another sexual identity shared similar levels of health care stereotype threat as gay or lesbian respondents (*P* = .57 and *P* = .83, respectively; results not shown). Cisgender men experienced lower levels of health care stereotype threat than cisgender women, and respondents who were transgender or noncisgender reported higher levels of health care stereotype threat than cisgender men.

In addition, levels of health care stereotype threat were higher among non-Hispanic Black respondents compared with any other racial or ethnic group. Cohabiting individuals indicated higher levels of health care stereotype threat. Individuals with a health condition reported more health care stereotype threat, but having health insurance was not associated with health care stereotype threat. Recent COVID-19 experience was associated with lower levels of health care stereotype threat, perhaps because most individuals with COVID-19 did not need to seek medical care or accessed telemedicine. Sexual identity centrality was not associated with levels of health care stereotype threat. Higher reports of health care stereotype threat were reported in September 2020 and March 2021 (results not shown). None of these factors appeared to account for the disparities according to gender and sexual identity in health care stereotype threat. There did not appear to be issues related to multicollinearity

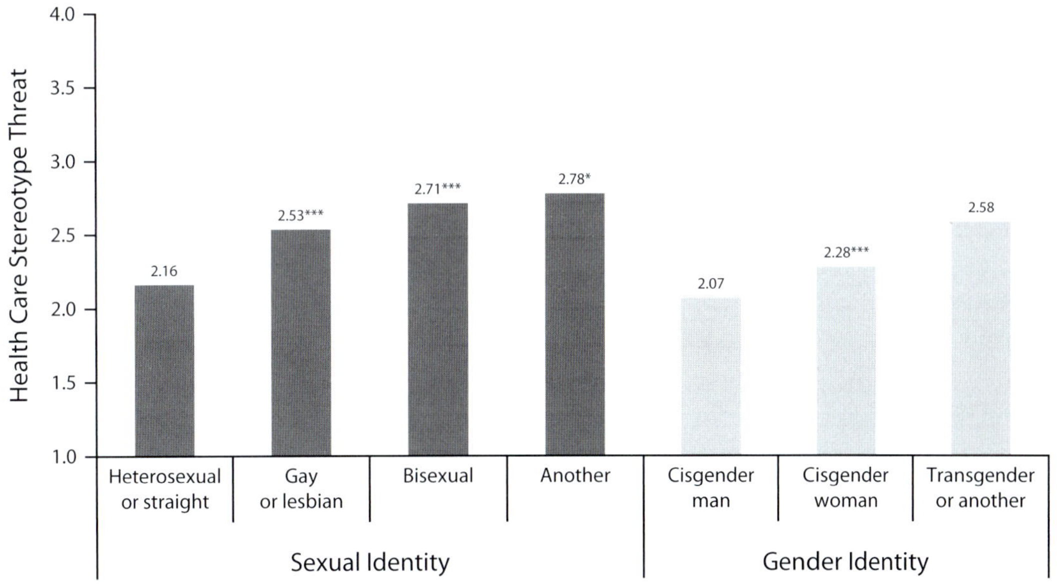

FIGURE 1— Health Care Stereotype Threat According to Sexual and Gender Identities: United States, National Couples' Health and Time Study, September 2020–April 2021

Note. Weighted mean levels of health care stereotype threat and significance testing using ordinary least squares models. Reference groups were heterosexual or straight (sexual identity) and cisgender man (gender identity).
$^{*}P \le .05$; $^{**}P \le .01$; $^{***}P \le .001$.

TABLE 2— Ordinary Least Squares Regression Model Predicting Health Care Stereotype Threat: United States, National Couples' Health and Time Use Study, September 2020–April 2021

	b (95% CI)
Sexual identity	
Heterosexual or straight (Ref)	0
Gay or lesbian	0.30 (0.14, 0.46)
Bisexual	0.35 (0.15, 0.56)
Another	0.34 (0.00, 0.67)
Gender identity	
Cisgender man (Ref)	0
Cisgender woman	0.20 (0.11, 0.30)
Transgender or another	0.38 (0.01, 0.82)
Age	−0.01 (−0.01, 0.08)
Race/ethnicity	
Non-Hispanic Black (Ref)	0
Non-Hispanic White	−0.58 (−0.73, −0.42)
Non-Hispanic Asian	−0.22 (−0.45, 0.02)
Hispanic	−0.51 (−0.69, −0.33)
Non-Hispanic multiracial	−0.52 (−0.75, −0.28)
Another	−0.46 (−0.69, −0.24)
Education	
High school or less (Ref)	0
Some college	0.09 (−0.04, 0.23)
College degree	0.09 (−0.04, 0.22)
Marital status	
Cohabiting (Ref)	0
Married	−0.26 (−0.39, −0.13)
Sexual identity centrality	0.03 (−0.01, 0.07)
Health indicators	
Reported health condition	
No current health condition (Ref)	0
Current health condition	0.16 (0.06, 0.26)
Health insurance	
No health insurance (Ref)	0
Have health insurance	−0.14 (−0.34, 0.06)
COVID-19	
Never had or suspected COVID-19 (Ref)	0
Had or suspected COVID-19	−0.12 (−0.23, −0.01)
Model statistics	F (25, 3589) = 9.37***
R^2	0.0863

Note. CI = confidence interval. Month of interview is included in the model, coefficients not reported.
***$P \le .001$

as the highest variance inflation factor was 2.29 and most were below 1.5, and our outlier analysis of residuals indicated outliers were not driving the findings for those with marginalized identities.

DISCUSSION

During the COVID-19 pandemic, there was likely a growing demand for health care, but little is known about how individuals who do not identify as cisgender or heterosexual were treated in health care settings. One reason why individuals with sexual minority identities may have disproportionately experienced the effects of the pandemic is because of their experiences with discrimination and stigma in health care settings.[8] We found that perceptions of health care stereotype threat during the pandemic were higher among respondents with marginalized identities. The basis to these concerns was cultural factors (stigma, negative stereotypes, implicit bias) that are systems of beliefs and norms that mark some individuals as inferior to others leading to prejudice and negative stereotypes. As Williams et al.[20] argued, these cultural indicators as well as structural factors and individual discrimination form the foundation of sexism, racism, and cis-heterosexism at the institutional, community, and societal levels. Marginalized individuals are forced to navigate cultural- and structural-based stigma and discrimination in their everyday lives and, as a result, form negative perceptions about how they will be treated or viewed. Furthermore, their perceptions may be shaped by not only their own experiences but also by those of their friends or family in health care settings. These perceptions of possibly negative encounters are especially harmful in the health care realm when individuals may be the most physically and psychologically vulnerable.

The gender and sexual identity differentials persisted with the inclusion of sociodemographic indicators as well as health-related measures including health conditions and health insurance. We found that individuals identifying as bisexual, gay or lesbian, or "another" shared similar levels of health care stereotype threat. Furthermore, individuals who faced the greatest need for health care, those with a health condition, reported the highest levels of health care stereotype threat. In addition, our findings indicated that respondents who identified as Black suffered from more health care stereotype threat than those of any other race or ethnicity, and these perceptions of anticipated discrimination could drive individuals away from receiving the care they require. These results are consistent with previous studies and provide a pandemic lens on health care stereotype threat. These anticipated concerns about discrimination in health care settings may be responsible for many of the observed health disparities experienced by individuals based on their sexual, gender, and racial/ethnic identification.

These worries about treatment in health care settings may have immediate implications in terms of receiving inadequate health care and ramifications for long-term health and well-being such as decisions to avoid or delay health care visits that may result in late diagnoses and treatments. The implications extend beyond individual health because persons who experience health care stereotype threat may also avoid accessing health care for their children and other family members. Worries about treatment in health care settings may also result in increases in stress and influence many domains of life outside of the health realm, such as stress in the workplace or school or adopting negative coping strategies.

Limitations

Although this study provided new insights into health care stereotype threat, there were a few limitations. First, the data were cross-sectional and collected during the early phase of the COVID-19 pandemic. The lack of prepandemic data means we cannot identify whether these experiences with health care discrimination were elevated during the pandemic. It is possible that individuals with sexual minority identities may have felt more health care discrimination because of greater need for services and potentially reaching out to medical providers with whom they had not interacted during previous appointments. However, individuals with sexual minority identities may have felt less intimidated during the pandemic because of access to telemedicine or the use of masks. We also lack longitudinal data that could assess changes in perceptions of discrimination over the course of the pandemic.

Second, the data were limited to individuals in couples, and further analysis of single individuals is warranted. Those who are in couples may benefit from partner support to buffer against the negative effects of worries about negative treatment that may not be available to single adults, or, alternatively, being in a couple may not be protective because both members experience worries about how they and their spouse or partner will be treated.

Third, this study did not consider intersectional identities, and further attention to individuals who face multiple sources of discrimination or stigma is critical. Note that our health care stereotype threat measure did not specify the particular identity that led to worries about discrimination. It is important to move beyond identifying differentials and specifying the sources of cultural and structural stigma that create discrimination and stigma.

Finally, participants in this study were interviewed during the COVID-19 pandemic, but their perceptions of health care stereotype threat could have been based on experiences that occurred before the pandemic because there was no time referent in the items. However, this measure is based on respondent's own subjective assessments of their worries at the time of interview.

Conclusions

One way to limit health disparities of sexual and gender–diverse populations is to provide health care that is free of threats of discrimination and stigma. Despite the widespread awareness and policies promoting equitable health care, we found elevated perceptions of discrimination in the health care setting among sexual and gender–diverse individuals that are likely responsible for health and well-being disparities. Our work is part of a growing body of research paying attention to the mechanisms driving health disparities.[40] Rather than focus on the marginalized identities of individuals, more attention needs to be focused on determining the ways that sexism, cis-heterosexism, and racism are negatively influencing health and well-being. It is important to acknowledge that these perceptions not only could influence their own well-being but may spill over to the health of their children, spouses or partners, parents, friends, and community members.

This research contributes to calls for greater cultural competence and skill-building in medical education and training for not only physicians but also medical staff, assistants, and receptionists. All sources of contact with the medical system are opportunities to ensure that individuals are treated fairly and with respect. In addition, it is important that health care policies and legislation prohibit health care discrimination based on marginalized identities. Certainly, discrimination and stigma experienced in other settings (e.g., school and work) may extend to concerns about the health care setting, and similarly anticipated discrimination in the health care setting may shape concerns about treatment in other institutional contexts. The ongoing debates regarding sexual and gender–diverse individuals' rights and rolling back of supportive policies create additional burdens and challenges that prevent individuals from receiving health care. These issues not only are important during the public health care crisis but also merit further investigation as we move through the COVID-19 pandemic. AJPH

ABOUT THE AUTHORS

Wendy D. Manning and Kristen E. Gustafson are with the Department of Sociology and Center for Family and Demographic Research at Bowling Green State University. Claire Kamp Dush is with the Department of Sociology and Minnesota Population Center at the University of Minnesota.

CORRESPONDENCE

Correspondence should be sent to Wendy D. Manning, 233 Williams Hall, Bowling Green State University, Bowling Green, OH 43403 (e-mail: wmannin@bgsu.edu). Reprints can be ordered at https://www.ajph.org by clicking the "Reprints" link.

PUBLICATION INFORMATION

Full Citation: Manning WD, Dush CK, Gustafson K. Health care stereotype threat during the COVID-19 pandemic among sexual and gender minority individuals. *Am J Public Health*. 2025;115(3):425–433.

Acceptance Date: November 5, 2024.

DOI: https://doi.org/10.2105/AJPH.2024.307926

ORCID iDs:

Wendy D. Manning https://orcid.org/0000-0002-8063-7380

Claire Kamp Dush https://orcid.org/0000-0003-4307-6825

Kristen Gustafson https://orcid.org/0000-0003-0336-235X

CONTRIBUTORS

W. D. Manning led and conceptualized the study, developed the approach, interpreted the results, and wrote the article. C. K. Dush contributed to the development and writing as well as edited the article. K. E. Gustafson analyzed the data, assisted with the interpretation of the findings, and assisted with the writing and references.

ACKNOWLEDGMENTS

The authors acknowledge support from Eunice Kennedy Shriver National Institute of Child Health and Human Development R01HD094081. Further infrastructure support was provided from the Eunice Kennedy Shriver National Institute of Child Health and Human Development to the Center for Family and Demographic Research at Bowling Green State University (P2CHD050959), Minnesota Population Center at University of Minnesota (P2CHD041023), and the Institute for Population Research at the Ohio State University (P2CHD058484).

Note. The content is solely the responsibility of the authors and does not necessarily represent the official views of the Eunice Kennedy Shriver National Institute of Child Health and Human Development or the National Institutes of Health.

CONFLICTS OF INTEREST

The authors have no conflicts of interest to declare.

HUMAN PARTICIPANT PROTECTION

The project received institutional review board approval from Bowling Green State University. The procedures to collect the data along with informed consent were approved by the Ohio State University institutional review board and are in accordance with the Declaration of Helsinki as revised in 2013.

REFERENCES

1. Heslin KC, Hall JE. Sexual orientation disparities in risk factors for adverse COVID-19–related outcomes, by race/ethnicity—Behavioral Risk Factor Surveillance System, United States, 2017–2019. *MMWR Morb Mortal Wkly Rep.* 2021;70:149–154. http://dx.doi.org/10.15585/mmwr.mm7005a1
2. Gonzales G, Przedworski J, Henning-Smith C. Comparison of health and health risk factors between lesbian, gay, and bisexual adults and heterosexual adults in the United States. *JAMA Intern Med.* 2016;176(9):1344–1351. https://doi.org/10.1001/jamainternmed.2016.3432
3. Streed CG, McCarthy E, Haas JS. Association between gender minority status and self-reported physical and mental health in the United States. *JAMA Intern Med.* 2017;177(8):1210–1212. https://doi.org/10.1001/jamainternmed.2017.1460
4. Lynch KE, Shipherd JC, Gatsby E, et al. Sexual orientation-related disparities in health conditions that elevate COVID-19 severity. *Ann Epidemiol.* 2022;66:5–12. https://doi.org/10.1016/j.annepidem.2021.11.006
5. File T, Marlay M. Regardless of household type, LGBT adults struggled more with mental health than non-LGBT adults. US Census Bureau. June 16, 2022. Available at: https://www.census.gov/library/stories/2022/06/lgbt-adults-report-anxiety-depression-during-pandemic.html. Accessed July 6, 2022.
6. Fish JN, Salerno J, Williams ND, et al. Sexual minority disparities in health and well-being as a consequence of the COVID-19 pandemic differ by sexual identity. *LGBT Health.* 2021;8(4):263–272. https://doi.org/10.1089/lgbt.2020.0489
7. Kamp Dush C, Manning WD, Berrigan MN, et al. Stress and mental health: a focus on COVID-19 and racial trauma stress. *RSF.* 2022;8(8):104–134. https://doi.org/10.7758/RSF.2022.8.8.06
8. Manning WD, Dush CK. COVID-19 stress and sexual identities. *Socius.* 2022;8:1–11. https://doi.org/10.1177/23780231221105376
9. Chima C, Shalaby R, Lawal M, et al. COVID-19 pandemic: influence of gender identity on stress, anxiety, and depression levels in Canada. *Trauma Care.* 2022;2(1):11–22. https://doi.org/10.3390/traumacare2010002
10. Heslin KC, Hall JE. Sexual orientation disparities in risk factors for adverse COVID-19–related outcomes, by race/ethnicity—Behavioral Risk Factor Surveillance System, United States, 2017–2019. *MMWR Morb Mortal Wkly Rep.* 2021;70(5):149–154. https://doi.org/10.15585/mmwr.mm7005a1
11. Salerno JP, Devadas J, Pease M, et al. Sexual and gender minority stress amid the COVID-19 pandemic: implications for LGBTQ young persons' mental health and well-being. *Public Health Rep.* 2020;135(6):721–727. https://doi.org/10.1177/0033354920954511
12. Gruberg S, Halpin J, Mahowald L. The state of the LGBTQ community in 2020. Center for American Progress. October 6, 2020. Available at: https://www.americanprogress.org/article/state-lgbtq-community-2020. Accessed July 6, 2022.
13. Fish JN, Baams L. Trends in alcohol-related disparities between heterosexual and sexual minority youth from 2007 to 2015: findings from the Youth Risk Behavior Survey. *LGBT Health.* 2018;5(6):359–367. https://doi.org/10.1089/lgbt.2017.0212
14. Grant JM, Mottet ML, Tanis J, et al. National Transgender Discrimination Survey Report on health and healthcare. National Center for Transgender Equality and the National Gay and Lesbian Task Force. October 2010. Available at: https://cancer-network.org/wp-content/uploads/2017/02/National_Transgender_Discrimination_Survey_Report_on_health_and_health_care.pdf. Accessed December 6, 2024.
15. Hatzenbuehler ML, Jun HJ, Corliss HL, et al. Structural stigma and cigarette smoking in a prospective cohort study of sexual minority and heterosexual youth. *Ann Behav Med.* 2014;47(1):48–56. https://doi.org/10.1007/s12160-013-9548-9
16. Layland EK, Exten C, Mallory AB, et al. Suicide attempt rates and associations with discrimination are greatest in early adulthood for sexual minority adults across diverse racial and ethnic groups. *LGBT Health.* 2020;7(8):439–447. https://doi.org/10.1089/lgbt.2020.0142
17. McCabe SE, Bostwick WB, Hughes TL, et al. The relationship between discrimination and substance use disorders among lesbian, gay, and bisexual adults in the United States. *Am J Public*

Health. 2010;100(10):1946–1952. https://doi.org/10.2105/AJPH.2009.163147

18. Pascoe EA, Richman SL. Perceived discrimination and health: a meta-analytic review. *Psychol Bull*. 2009;135(4):531–554. https://doi.org/10.1037/a0016059
19. Qeaden F, Azagba S, Barbeau WA, et al. Associations between discrimination and substance use among college students in the United States from 2015 to 2019. *Addict Behav*. 2022;125:107164. https://doi.org/10.1016/j.addbeh.2021.107164
20. Williams DR, Lawrence JA, Davis BA, et al. Understanding how discrimination can affect health. *Health Serv Res*. 2019;54(suppl 2):1374–1388. https://doi.org/10.1111/1475-6773.13222
21. Meyer IH. Prejudice, social stress, and mental health in lesbian, gay, and bisexual populations: conceptual issues and research evidence. *Psychol Bull*. 2003;129(5):674–697. https://doi.org/10.1037/0033-2909.129.5.674
22. Williams DR, Yu Y, Jackson JS, et al. Racial differences in physical and mental health: socio-economic status, stress, and discrimination. *J Health Psychol*. 1997;2(3):335–351. https://doi.org/10.1177/135910539700200305
23. Singh S, Durso LE. Widespread discrimination continues to shape LGBT people's lives in both subtle and significant ways. Center for American Progress. May 2, 2017. Available at: https://www.americanprogress.org/article/widespread-discrimination-continues-shape-lgbt-peoples-lives-subtle-significant-ways. Accessed July 6, 2022.
24. Fish JN, Exten C. Sexual orientation differences in alcohol use disorder across the adult life course. *Am J Prev Med*. 2020;59(3):428–436. https://doi.org/10.1016/j.amepre.2020.04.012
25. When healthcare isn't caring. Lamba Legal. 2010. Available at: https://www.lambdalegal.org/health-care-report. Accessed July 6, 2022.
26. Babey SH, Wolstein J, Herman JL, et al. Gaps in healthcare access and health insurance among LGBT populations in California. UCLA School of Law Williams Institute. February 2022. Available at: https://williamsinstitute.law.ucla.edu/publications/gaps-health-care-lgbt-ca. Accessed July 6, 2022.
27. Casey LS, Reisner SL, Findling MG, et al. Discrimination in the United States: experiences of lesbian, gay, bisexual, transgender, and queer Americans. *Health Serv Res*. 2019;54(suppl 2):1454–1466. https://doi.org/10.1111/1475-6773.13229
28. Rice CE, Fish JN, Russell ST, et al. Sexual minority related discrimination across the life course: findings from a national sample of adults in the United States. *J Homosex*. 2021;68(2):252–268. https://doi.org/10.1080/00918369.2019.1648083
29. Fingerhut AW, Abdou CM. The role of healthcare stereotype threat and social identity threat in LGB health disparities. *J Soc Issues*. 2017;73(3):493–507. https://doi.org/10.1111/josi.12228
30. Fingerhut AW, Martos AJ, Choi SK, et al. Healthcare stereotype threat and health outcomes among LGB individuals. *Ann Behav Med*. 2022;56(6):562–572. https://doi.org/10.1093/abm/kaab060
31. Saunders RK, Carr DC, Burdette AM. Health care stereotype threat and sexual and gender minority well-being. *J Health Soc Behav*. 2024;65(1):20–37. https://doi.org/10.1177/00221465231205549
32. Abdou CM, Fingerhut AW, Jackson JS, et al. Healthcare stereotype threat in older adults in the Health and Retirement Study. *Am J Prev Med*. 2016;50(2):191–198. https://doi.org/10.1016/j.amepre.2015.07.034
33. Abdou CM, Fingerhut AW. Stereotype threat among Black and White women in healthcare settings. *Cultur Divers Ethnic Minor Psychol*. 2014;20(3):316–323. https://doi.org/10.1037/a0036946
34. Ayhan CHB, Bilgin H, Uluman OT, et al. A systematic review of the discrimination against sexual and gender in healthcare settings. *Int J Health Serv*. 2019;50(1):44–61. https://doi.org/10.1177/0020731419885093
35. Glick JL, Theall KP, Andrinopoulos KM, et al. The role of discrimination in care postponement among trans-feminine individuals in the US National Transgender Discrimination Survey. *LGBT Health*. 2018;5(3):171–179. https://doi.org/10.1089/lgbt.2017.0093
36. Mirza SA, Rooney C. Discrimination prevents LGBTQ people from accessing healthcare. Center for American Progress. January 18, 2018. Available at: https://www.americanprogress.org/article/discrimination-prevents-lgbtq-people-accessing-health-care. Accessed July 6, 2022.
37. Dush CK, Manning WD. National Couples' Health and Time Study (NCHAT), United States, 2020–2021. Ann Arbor, MI: Inter-university Consortium for Political and Social Research; 2022. https://doi.org/10.3886/ICPSR38417.v1
38. Kamp Dush CM, Manning WD, Berrigan MN, et al. National Couples' Health and Time Study: sample, design, and weighting. *Popul Res Policy Rev*. 2023;42(4):62. https://doi.org/10.1007/s11113-023-09799-7
39. Meyer IH, Frost DM, Hammack PL, et al. Generations Study baseline questionnaire and measure sources. Generations Study. 2016. Available at: https://static1.squarespace.com/static/54f4cc0be4b0014ec19fcbab/t/5b845e68c2241b8b623239f3/1535401577846/Generations+Study+Baseline+Questionnaire+and+Measure+Sources_WEB.pdf. Accessed July 6, 2022.
40. Adams LM, Miller AB. Mechanisms of mental health disparities among minoritized groups: how well are the top journals in clinical psychology representing this work? *Clin Psychol Sci*. 2022;10(3):387–416. https://doi.org/10.1177/21677026211026979

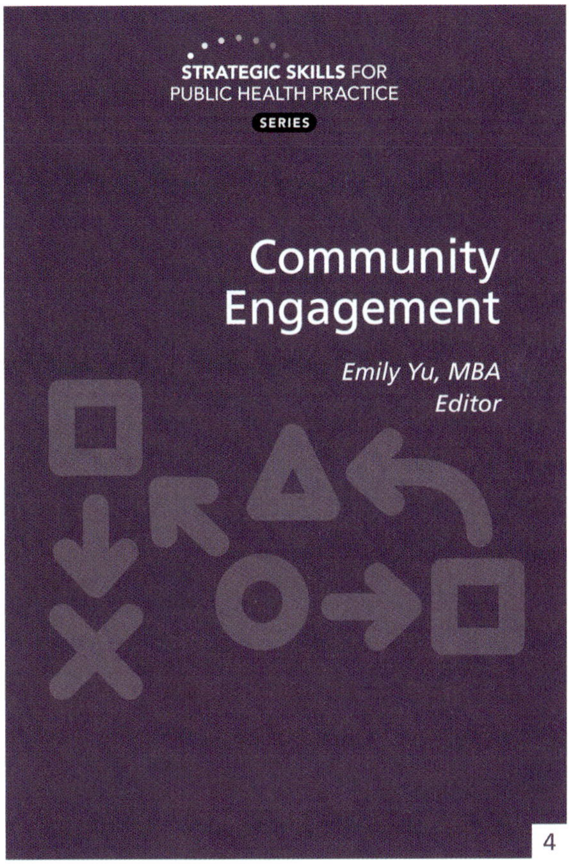

978-087553-3308, 108 PP, DIGITAL & SOFTCOVER

Community Engagement

Edited by Emily Yu, MBA

Community Engagement is the first book to be published from our new *Strategic Skills for Public Health Practice* series. This book brings the concept of community engagement to life through first-person stories, real-world examples and valuable insights from leaders across sectors. Curated specifically for public health practitioners and those interested in supporting community health, the book's chapters, guidance, and perspectives from the field will enhance readers' understanding of community-centered design and provide the tools to support organizational practices that drive better health for all.

APHABOOKSTORE.ORG

APHA PRESS

AN IMPRINT OF AMERICAN PUBLIC HEALTH ASSOCIATION

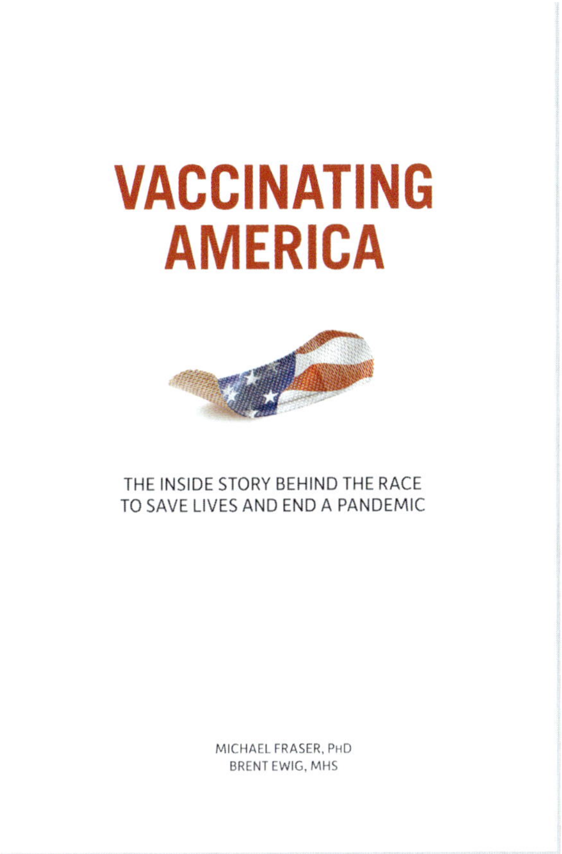

Vaccinating America: The Inside Story Behind the Race to Save Lives, and End a Pandemic

Edited by: Michael Fraser, PhD, Brent Ewig, MHS

2023, 250 PP, SFTCVR, ISBN 978-0-87553-332-2

Vaccinating America spotlights the public servants and heroes who planned and executed this unprecedented program to combat COVID-19 amidst fierce partisan divides, bureaucratic infighting and overwhelming logistical challenges, and doesn't hold back on pointing out those who hindered progress.

APHABOOKSTORE.ORG

APHA PRESS

AN IMPRINT OF AMERICAN PUBLIC HEALTH ASSOCIATION

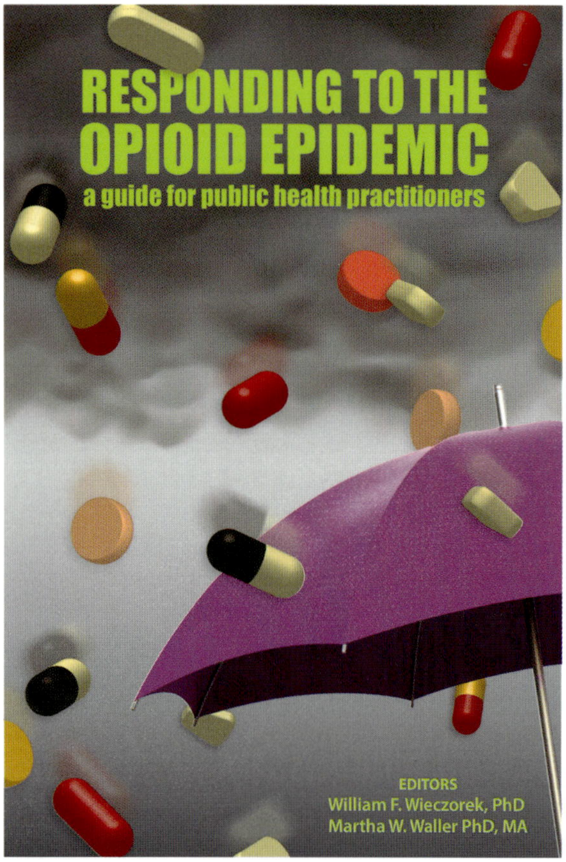

ISBN 978-0-87553-344-5, 400 PP., 2024,
SOFTBOUND/PRINT-ON-DEMAND

Responding to the Opioid Epidemic: A Guide for Public Health Practitioners

Edited by: William F. Wieczorek, PhD and Martha W. Waller PhD, MA

It's impossible to completely prevent the substance misuse defining the opioid epidemic, and it's impossible to treat the problem away. This reality requires a continuum of care (COC) approach, which includes promotion, prevention, case-finding, treatment, and recovery. This book presents research-informed interventions aligned with the COC approach to guide how communities, first responders, lay persons, medical providers, policymakers, treatment providers, and others can respond to the opioid epidemic at an individual, community, state, and national level.

APHABOOKSTORE.ORG

APHA PRESS

AN IMPRINT OF AMERICAN PUBLIC HEALTH ASSOCIATION